T0195199

Advances in Female Pelvic Medicine and Reconstructive Surgery

Editors

HEIDI WENDELL BROWN
REBECCA GLENN ROGERS

OBSTETRICS AND GYNECOLOGY CLINICS OF NORTH AMERICA

www.obgyn.theclinics.com

Consulting Editor
WILLIAM F. RAYBURN

September 2021 • Volume 48 • Number 3

ELSEVIER

1600 John F. Kennedy Boulevard • Suite 1800 • Philadelphia, Pennsylvania, 19103-2899

http://www.theclinics.com

OBSTETRICS AND GYNECOLOGY CLINICS OF NORTH AMERICA Volume 48, Number 3
September 2021 ISSN 0889-8545, ISBN-13: 978-0-323-79709-2

Editor: Kerry Holland
Developmental Editor: Hannah Almira Lopez

© **2021 Elsevier Inc. All rights reserved.**

This periodical and the individual contributions contained in it are protected under copyright by Elsevier, and the following terms and conditions apply to their use:

Photocopying
Single photocopies of single articles may be made for personal use as allowed by national copyright laws. Permission of the Publisher and payment of a fee is required for all other photocopying, including multiple or systematic copying, copying for advertising or promotional purposes, resale, and all forms of document delivery. Special rates are available for educational institutions that wish to make photocopies for non-profit educational classroom use. For information on how to seek permission visit www.elsevier.com/permissions or call: (+44) 1865 843830 (UK)/(+1) 215 239 3804 (USA).

Derivative Works
Subscribers may reproduce tables of contents or prepare lists of articles including abstracts for internal circulation within their institutions. Permission of the Publisher is required for resale or distribution outside the institution. Permission of the Publisher is required for all other derivative works, including compilations and translations (please consult www.elsevier.com/permissions).

Electronic Storage or Usage
Permission of the Publisher is required to store or use electronically any material contained in this periodical, including any article or part of an article (please consult www.elsevier.com/permissions). Except as outlined above, no part of this publication may be reproduced, stored in a retrieval system or transmitted in any form or by any means, electronic, mechanical, photocopying, recording or otherwise, without prior written permission of the Publisher.

Notice
No responsibility is assumed by the Publisher for any injury and/or damage to persons or property as a matter of products liability, negligence or otherwise, or from any use or operation of any methods, products, instructions or ideas contained in the material herein. Because of rapid advances in the medical sciences, in particular, independent verification of diagnoses and drug dosages should be made.

Although all advertising material is expected to conform to ethical (medical) standards, inclusion in this publication does not constitute a guarantee or endorsement of the quality or value of such product or of the claims made of it by its manufacturer.

Obstetrics and Gynecology Clinics (ISSN 0889-8545) is published quarterly by Elsevier Inc., 360 Park Avenue South, New York, NY 10010-1710. Months of issue are March, June, September, and December. Periodicals postage paid at New York, NY, and additional mailing offices. Subscription price per year is $335.00 (US individuals), $944.00 (US institutions), $100.00 (US students), $404.00 (Canadian individuals), $991.00 (Canadian institutions), $100.00 (Canadian students), $459.00 (international individuals), $991.00 (international institutions), and $225.00 (international students). To receive student/resident rate, orders must be accompanied by name of affiliated institution, date of term, and the signature of program/residency coordinator on institution letterhead. Orders will be billed at individual rate until proof of status is received. Foreign air speed delivery is included in all *Clinics* subscription prices. All prices are subject to change without notice. POSTMASTER: Send address changes to *Obstetrics and Gynecology Clinics*, Elsevier Health Sciences Division, Subscription Customer Service, 3251 Riverport Lane, Maryland Heights, MO 63043. **Customer Service: Telephone: 1-800-654-2452 (U.S. and Canada); 314-447-8871 (outside U.S. and Canada). Fax: 314-447-8029. E-mail: journalscustomerservice-usa@elsevier.com (for print support); journalsonlinesupport-usa@elsevier. com (for online support).**

Reprints. For copies of 100 or more of articles in this publication, please contact the Commercial Reprints Department, Elsevier Inc., 360 Park Avenue South, New York, New York 10010-1710. Tel.: 212-633-3874; Fax: 212-633-3820; E-mail: reprints@elsevier.com.

Obstetrics and Gynecology Clinics of North America is also published in Spanish by McGraw-Hill Interamericana Editores S.A., P.O. Box 5-237, 06500, Mexico; in Portuguese by Reichmann and Affonso Editores, Rio de Janeiro, Brazil; and in Greek by Paschalidis Medical Publications, Athens, Greece.

Obstetrics and Gynecology Clinics of North America is covered in MEDLINE/PubMed (Index Medicus), Excerpta Medica, Current Concepts/Clinical Medicine, Science Citation Index, BIOSIS, CINAHL, and ISI/BIOMED.

Printed in the United States of America.

Contributors

CONSULTING EDITOR

WILLIAM F. RAYBURN, MD, MBA
Adjunct Professor, Department of Obstetrics and Gynecology, College of Graduate Studies, Medical University of South Carolina, Charleston, South Carolina; Associate Dean, Continuing Medical Education and Professional Development, Distinguished Professor and Emeritus Chair, Department of Obstetrics and Gynecology, University of New Mexico School of Medicine, Albuquerque, New Mexico, USA

EDITORS

HEIDI WENDELL BROWN, MD, MAS
Assistant Professor, Department of Obstetrics and Gynecology, University of Wisconsin-Madison School of Medicine and Public Health, Madison, Wisconsin, USA

REBECCA GLENN ROGERS, MD
Professor, Department of Obstetrics and Gynecology, Albany Medical College, Albany, New York, USA

AUTHORS

DANIELLE D. ANTOSH, MD
Department of Obstetrics and Gynecology, Houston Methodist Hospital, Houston, Texas, USA

LAUREN CALDWELL, MD
Fellow, Female Pelvic Medicine and Reconstructive Surgery, Department of Women's Health, The University of Texas at Austin, Dell Medical School, Austin, Texas, USA

ERIN C. CROSBY, MD
Associate Professor, Department of Obstetrics and Gynecology, Division of Urogynecology and Pelvic Reconstructive Surgery, Albany Medical College, Albany, New York, USA

CARLY CROWDER, MD
Department of Obstetrics and Gynecology, University of California, Irvine, Orange, California, USA

ALEXIS ANNE DIETER, MD
Associate Professor, Department of Obstetrics and Gynecology, MedStar Washington Hospital Center, Georgetown University School of Medicine, Washington, DC, USA

ALEX DIGESU, MD, PhD
Consultant Urogynaecologist, Department of Obstetrics and Gynaecology, St Marys Hospital, Imperial College Healthcare NHS Trust, London, United Kingdom

TOLA B. FASHOKUN, MD
Female Pelvic Medicine and Reconstructive Surgery Faculty, Institute of Female Pelvic Medicine, Sinai Hospital of Baltimore, Baltimore, Maryland, USA

CARA L. GRIMES, MD, MAS
Associate Professor, Obstetrics and Gynecology and Urology, New York Medical College, Hawthorne, New York, USA

CHRISTINE A. HEISLER, MD, MS
Assistant Professor, Departments of Obstetrics and Gynecology, and Urology, University of Wisconsin-Madison School of Medicine and Public Health, Madison, Wisconsin, USA

LISA C. HICKMAN, MD
Urogynecologist, Division of Female Pelvic Medicine and Reconstructive Surgery, Department of Obstetrics and Gynecology, The Ohio State University Wexner Medical Center, Columbus, Ohio, USA

KATHERINE E. HUSK, MD
Assistant Professor, Department of Obstetrics and Gynecology, Division of Urogynecology and Pelvic Reconstructive Surgery, Albany Medical College, Albany, New York, USA

PETER C. JEPPSON, MD
Division of Female Pelvic Medicine and Reconstructive Surgery, Department of Obstetrics and Gynecology, Albuquerque, New Mexico, USA

GEORGE A. KUCHEL, MD
Professor, UConn Center on Aging, University of Connecticut, Farmington, Connecticut, USA

ANNETTA M. MADSEN, MD
Division of Female Pelvic Medicine and Reconstructive Surgery, Department of Obstetrics and Gynecology, Mayo Clinic, Rochester, Minnesota USA

SARAH E. McACHRAN, MD, FACS
Associate Professor, Department of Urology, University of Wisconsin-Madison School of Medicine and Public Health, Madison, Wisconsin, USA

NADIA N. MEGAHED, MD
Department of Obstetrics and Gynecology, Houston Methodist Hospital, Houston, Texas, USA

ISUZU MEYER, MD, MSPH
Assistant Professor, Division of Urogynecology and Pelvic Reconstructive Surgery, Department of Obstetrics and Gynecology, The University of Alabama at Birmingham, Birmingham, Alabama, USA

CATHERINE CHANDLER MOODY, MD
Obstetrics and Gynecology Resident, PGY3, Department of Obstetrics and Gynecology, Sinai Hospital of Baltimore, Baltimore, Maryland, USA

KAREN NOBLETT, MD, MBA
Professor, Department of Obstetrics and Gynecology, University of California, Irvine, Orange, California, USA

CANDACE PARKER-AUTRY, MD
Assistant Professor, Department of Urology, Wake Forest School of Medicine, Winston-Salem, North Carolina, USA

USHMA J. PATEL, MD
Department of Obstetrics and Gynecology, University of Wisconsin-Madison School of Medicine and Public Health, Madison, Wisconsin, USA

JULIE PECK, MB BS, BAO
St Francis Hospital Trinity Health, Hartford, Connecticut, USA

TRANG X. PHAM, MD
Clinical Fellow, Female Pelvic Medicine and Reconstructive Surgery, Department of Obstetrics and Gynecology, University of Oklahoma Health Sciences, Oklahoma City, Oklahoma, USA

KATIE PROPST, MD
Urogynecologist, Urogynecology and Reconstructive Pelvic Surgery, OB/Gyn and Women's Health Institute, Cleveland Clinic, Cleveland, Ohio, USA

LIESCHEN H. QUIROZ, MD
Professor, Female Pelvic Medicine and Reconstructive Surgery, Department of Obstetrics and Gynecology, University of Oklahoma Health Sciences, Oklahoma City, Oklahoma, USA

HOLLY E. RICHTER, PhD, MD
Professor, Division of Urogynecology and Pelvic Reconstructive Surgery, Department of Obstetrics and Gynecology, The University of Alabama at Birmingham, Birmingham, Alabama, USA

TASHA SERNA-GALLEGOS, MD
Division of Female Pelvic Medicine and Reconstructive Surgery, Department of Obstetrics and Gynecology, Albuquerque, New Mexico, USA

EMILY C. SERRELL, MD
Resident, Department of Urology, University of Wisconsin-Madison School of Medicine and Public Health, Madison, Wisconsin, USA

JONATHAN P. SHEPHERD, MD, MSc
St Francis Hospital Trinity Health, Hartford, Connecticut, USA

STEVEN EDWARD SWIFT, MD
Consultant Urogynaecologist, Department of Obstetrics and Gynecology, Medical University of South Carolina, Charleston, South Carolina, USA

VISHA TAILOR, MBBS, BSc
Urogynaecology Sub-speciality Trainee, Department of Obstetrics and Gynaecology, St Mary's Hospital, Imperial College Healthcare NHS Trust, London, United Kingdom

MIRIAM C. TOAFF, MD, MS
PGY-3, Obstetrics and Gynecology, New York Medical College, Hawthorne, New York, USA

AMANDA B. WHITE, MD
Associate Professor, Female Pelvic Medicine and Reconstructive Surgery, Department of Women's Health, The University of Texas at Austin, Dell Medical School, Austin, Texas, USA

Contents

This article discusses a few of the most prominent controversies currently confronting providers and patients when planning for surgical repair of pelvic organ prolapse including preoperative counseling and patient preparedness, preoperative urodynamics and concomitant anti-incontinence procedures, uterine preservation, total versus supracervical hysterectomy at the time of sacrocolpopexy, same-day discharge, and use of telemedicine for routine postoperative care. These current controversies reflect some of the larger questions and themes confronting the field at this time, and this discussion serves to highlight opportunities for further research and stimulate the constructive debate that moves the field forward.

Synthetic midurethral slings offer optimal cure rates for the minimally invasive treatment of stress urinary incontinence in women. Performed via a retropubic or transobturator technique, midurethral sling approaches demonstrate comparable efficacy, with unique adverse event profiles. Single incision slings were introduced to minimize the complication of groin pain with full-length transobturator slings and enhance operative recovery. The earliest therapies for stress urinary incontinence including urethral bulking, retropubic colposuspension, and autologous sling offer alternative methods of surgical management without using synthetic mesh. These methods boast satisfactory efficacy with low rates of complications, and may be ideal for appropriately selected patients.

Fecal incontinence is a highly prevalent and debilitating condition that negatively impacts quality of life. The etiology is often multifactorial and treatment can be hindered by lack of understanding of its mechanisms and available treatment options. This article reviews the evidence-based update for the management of fecal incontinence.

Surgical management is based on the size and location of injury and should be performed by an experienced surgeon with thorough knowledge of pelvic anatomy, surgical technique, and postoperative management.

Tasha Serna-Gallegos and Peter C. Jeppson

Female pelvic fistulae are a pathologic connection between the urinary or gastrointestinal tract and the genital tract. Although this condition has been present for millennia, successful surgical treatments have only been described for the past few hundred years. In developed nations, the most common cause of genitourinary fistulae is benign gynecologic surgery, but worldwide it is obstetric trauma. Fistulae management is rooted in surgical intervention with the highest probability of success associated with the first repair.

Annetta M. Madsen, Lisa C. Hickman, and Katie Propst

Often considered a condition of aging women, pelvic floor disorders may initially present in pregnancy and postpartum, having a negative impact on quality of life during this important time in a woman's life. This review outlines the clinical approach to implementing pelvic health into obstetric care through education and promotion of pelvic health in pregnancy, screening for pelvic floor disorders routinely, and providing support through resources, treatment, and referrals if pelvic floor disorders develop during pregnancy and postpartum.

Catherine Chandler Moody and Tola B. Fashokun

This article provides an overview of 2 conditions that defy straightforward characterization and treatment: interstitial cystitis/painful bladder syndrome often coexists with high tone pelvic floor dysfunction. These conditions are common in gynecologic patients who present with chronic pelvic pain and are often misdiagnosed due to their syndromic nature and amorphous definitions. Clinicians should maintain a high level of suspicion for these processes in patients with chronic pelvic pain or recurrent urinary tract infection symptoms. Optimal treatment uses a multimodal approach to alleviate symptoms.

Emily C. Serrell and Sarah E. McAchran

Urethral and periurethral masses in women include both benign and malignant entities that can be difficult to clinically differentiate. Primary urethral carcinoma is rare and the optimal treatment modality may vary depending on the stage at presentation. Because cancer-free survival is poor, clinicians should have a high index of suspicion when evaluating a urethral mass. Some benign-appearing urethral masses may be safely observed.

and mobility disability. The geriatric incontinence syndrome may represent a poorly characterized phenotype of UI among older women, which in many ways reflects unhealthy aging. In this article, we explore the evidence behind these concepts together with potential impact on the diagnosis and management of UI in this group.

Sacral neuromodulation (SNM) has been available in the United States for more than 20 years and is a guideline-recommended therapy by both the American Urological Association and the American Society of Colon and Rectal Surgeons, with proven long-term success for urinary urgency incontinence, urinary urgency frequency, nonobstructive urinary retention, and fecal incontinence. Initially the therapy involved a more invasive surgical approach that included a large cut down over the sacrum. This article reviews recent advancements in SNM therapy including updates in best practices for implant technique, technological innovations, and the new clinical literature relevant to contemporary practice.

Advances in Female Pelvic Medicine and Reconstructive Surgery

OBSTETRICS AND GYNECOLOGY CLINICS

SERIES OF RELATED INTEREST

Clinics in Perinatology
www.perinatology.theclinics.com
Pediatric Clinics of North America
https://www.pediatrics.theclinics.com

THE CLINICS ARE AVAILABLE ONLINE!
Access your subscription at:
www.theclinics.com

Foreword

Aiding the Increasing Numbers of Women with Pelvic Floor Disorders

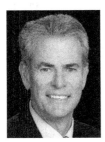

William F. Rayburn, MD, MBA
Consulting Editor

This issue of the *Obstetrics and Gynecology Clinics of North America*, edited by Heidi Brown, MD and Rebecca Rogers, MD, is an update on advances in the field of urogynecology, or female pelvic medicine and reconstructive surgery (FPMRS). The readers have become aware of the expansion in knowledge since the *Obstetrics and Gynecology Clinics of North America* issue was published in 2016 before the field became a recognized subspecialty. Newer surgical and nonsurgical treatments are presented about conditions that affect the pelvic floor, including the supporting muscles and connective tissues. Common problems, such as urinary and fecal incontinence or leakage, pelvic organ prolapse, urinary tract infections, and urinary tract injury, are well covered by the distinguished authors.

Some form of pelvic floor disorders (PFDs) affects more than 30 million women in the United States, with elderly women being at increased risk. With the aging population, the prevalence of symptomatic PFDs has been projected to be about 44 million by 2050, which is predicted to result in a significant increase in surgical procedures performed for these conditions. These projections may underestimate the prevalence, as they are founded on population projections based on the 200 US Census.

While the ideal ratio of patients with PFD per FPMRS subspecialist is unknown, the current ratio is high and may pose further concern about access to care for affected women. It is expected that more obstetrician-gynecologists (ob-gyns) who are comfortable managing the complexities of PFDs will be necessary to care for the greater number of affected women. Most FPMRS subspecialists are geographically concentrated in urban areas, and many women live more remotely. This geographic maldistribution will likely persist, and patients with PFDs will continue to seek

https://doi.org/10.1016/j.ogc.2021.05.013
0889-8545/21/© 2021 Published by Elsevier Inc.
obgyn.theclinics.com

evaluation and treatment from ob-gyns, thus affirming the need to optimize education for all ob-gyns residents.

The American Board of Medical Specialties approved FPMRS as a certified subspecialty in 2011. Today, most departments of obstetrics and gynecology at US medical schools have FPMRS divisions, with approximately 50 departments having a fellowship program. Therefore, residents are exposed to more about this subspecialty as they rotate on their assigned subspecialty blocks. Each FPMRS division and any fellowship training program define their scope of practice, set standards of care and practice guidelines, provide care in complex cases, serve as trusted referral sources, and advocate for evidence-based care. A probable concern would be a decreased comfort level among ob-gyns, both in academic medicine and in the community, in providing advanced reconstructive surgery to patients with PFDs.

The preface introduces the reader as to where we are in 2021. The issue focuses on improved diagnostic and management skills with potentially less morbidity during the past decade. Topics of active current interest include advances in telemedicine in urogynecology, transvaginal grafts, PFDs in pregnancy and the postpartum period, and neuromodulation. Updates are provided about urinary tract concerns: recurrent infections, injury during gynecologic surgery, painful bladder syndrome, and urethral masses.

I appreciate the efforts of Dr Brown and Dr Rogers and their team of experienced authors for their timely, thoughtful, and comprehensive recommendations about the many topics mentioned above. Regardless of whether the patient's care is provided by an ob-gyn alone or in conjunction with an FPMRS subspecialist, it is important to clearly identify measures to monitor for the initial evaluation and follow-up care. Sufficient and timely communication of information during any referral or handoff is critical for more optimal care and safety.

William F. Rayburn, MD, MBA
Department of Obstetrics and Gynecology
University of New Mexico School of Medicine
MSC 10 5580, 1 University of New Mexico
Albuquerque, NM 87131-0001, USA

E-mail address:
wrayburnmd@gmail.com

Preface

Female Pelvic Medicine and Reconstructive Surgery: Where Are We in 2021?

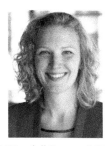 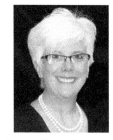

Heidi Wendell Brown, MD, MAS   Rebecca Glenn Rogers, MD
Editors

The field of urogynecology, or female pelvic medicine and reconstructive surgery (FPMRS), has expanded tremendously in the last decade. While the American Urogynecologic Society was founded in 1979, it was more than 30 years later, in 2012, that FPMRS was first officially recognized as a subspecialty by the Accreditation Council for Graduate Medical Education (ACGME). Following a 3-year fellowship, FPMRS-trained subspecialists in OB/GYN complete both written and oral board examinations through the American Board of Obstetrics and Gynecology. FPMRS subspecialists in urology complete a 2- or 3-year fellowship and then a written board examination through the American Board of Urology.

Our growing workforce of fellowship-trained subspecialists brings expertise in the diagnosis and treatment of not just pelvic organ prolapse and urinary incontinence but also a myriad other pelvic floor disorders. In this issue, we have asked leaders in the field to provide a snapshot of the state of the science with Dr Deiter's article regarding surgery for prolapse and Dr Caldwell's article on surgery for incontinence. We have included FPMRS debates about uterine preservation versus hysterectomy and the role of mesh augmentation in our surgeries by Dr Tailor. We present current information about treatment for accidental bowel leakage from Dr Meyer and defecatory dysfunction from Dr Crosby. These disorders are common and often overlooked in summaries of urogynecologic care. Dr Grimes provides a timely FPMRS telehealth overview in light of the changes that have occurred during the global COVID-19 pandemic.

We asked our authors to highlight advances in FPMRS conditions often treated without surgery. Dr Shepherd updates us on urinary tract infections in 2021, and Dr Madsen tackles recognition and management of pelvic floor disorders in pregnant

https://doi.org/10.1016/j.ogc.2021.05.012
0889-8545/21/© 2021 Elsevier Inc. All rights reserved.

and postpartum women. Dr Fashokun describes our current understanding of painful bladder syndrome and its intersection with pelvic floor dysfunction, and Dr Antosh addresses sexual function following pelvic floor surgery.

Our authors provide updates in surgical management of FPMRS conditions. Dr Noblett describes recent advances in neuromodulation, including rechargeable and MRI-compatible implants. Dr Heisler describes approaches to detection and management of urinary tract injury in gynecologic surgery, while Dr Jeppson provides an overview of female pelvic fistulae. For those interested in FPMRS images, urologist Dr McAchran provides many photos of urethral masses, and Dr Quiroz updates us on radiologic diagnostic approaches in FPMRS.

The progress made in the decade since FPMRS was first recognized by ACGME is remarkable. We hope that you enjoy reading these articles highlighting this progress as much as we enjoyed working with our expert authors to bring them to you.

Heidi Wendell Brown, MD, MAS
Department of Obstetrics and Gynecology
University of Wisconsin School of Medicine
and Public Health
202 South Park Street, 2-East
Madison, WI 53715, USA

Rebecca Glenn Rogers, MD
Department of Obstetrics and Gynecology
Albany Medical College
391 Myrtle Avenue, Suite 200
Albany, NY 12208, USA

E-mail addresses:
hwbrown2@wisc.edu (H.W. Brown)
rogersr2@amc.edu (R.G. Rogers)

Pelvic Organ Prolapse
Controversies in Surgical Treatment

Alexis Anne Dieter, MD

KEYWORDS

- Urogynecology • Pelvic organ prolapse • Reconstructive surgery • Prolapse repair

KEY POINTS

- This article reviews some of the current controversies confronting providers and patients when determining what is the best perioperative plan for women choosing to undergo surgery to treat pelvic organ prolapse.
- These controversies include preoperative counseling and patient preparedness, preoperative urodynamics and concomitant anti-incontinence procedures, uterine preservation, total versus supracervical hysterectomy at the time of sacrocolpopexy, same day discharge, and use of telemedicine for routine postoperative care.

INTRODUCTION

Patients often ask, "what is the best surgery to fix my problem?" This is a seemingly simple question that involves a clear understanding of what the actual "problem" is and what perceived risks the patient is willing to take on in return for the potential benefits to achieve their desired goals. In a field where most surgical procedures are elective, patients have high expectations for postoperative outcomes and providers aim to meet them. In striving to meet those expectations and examining the relationship between patient goals and provider perspectives, it has become apparent that often what a provider considers a success or complication may not be the case for the patient and vice versa. This lack of understanding is the root of some of the "controversies" (or debates) regarding pelvic organ prolapse surgery that currently demand attention and research. Other current controversies exist because of a lack of sufficient data to give a clear picture regarding the balance of outcomes and risks with different approaches to surgery and perioperative care. This article discusses a few of the most prominent controversies currently confronting providers and patients when planning for surgical repair of pelvic organ prolapse (POP).

Department of Obstetrics and Gynecology, MedStar Washington Hospital Center, Georgetown University School of Medicine, 106 Irving Street, Northwest, Suite 405 South, Washington, DC 20010, USA
E-mail address: alexis.a.dieter@medstar.net

Obstet Gynecol Clin N Am 48 (2021) 437–448
https://doi.org/10.1016/j.ogc.2021.05.001
0889-8545/21/© 2021 Elsevier Inc. All rights reserved.

obgyn.theclinics.com

PREOPERATIVE COUNSELING, DECISION-MAKING, AND PATIENT PREPAREDNESS

In most practices the process of deciding on a surgery and obtaining preoperative informed consent from the patient involves an informal discussion between the provider and patient reviewing options for management, the potential risks and the expected outcomes, and ultimately electing on and finalizing the plan for surgery. The specific details and the exact processes included in these discussions can vary significantly from one provider or practice to another with providers infrequently or at most informally assessing patient literacy or understanding.[1] As clinicians have become more aware of health literacy (HL), knowledge of patients' understanding of these discussions and the influence of their understanding on recovery and success following surgery has become of more interest and value.

In 2018 a cross-sectional study assessing HL in a urogynecology clinic population (mean age 61 years; 85% white race; 54% college education) Sripad and colleagues[2] found 95% of patients demonstrated adequate HL. Anger and colleagues[3] also demonstrated high HL in a urogynecologic population; but, when Anger and coauthors[3] assessed understanding of pelvic floor disorders, they found that, despite high HL, patients had a poor understanding of their pelvic floor disorders with their comprehension worsening with older age.

For prolapse surgery specifically, there has been significant focus on patient preparedness and the process of informed consent as it relates to outcomes. In a 2017 study Hallock and colleagues[4] examined a population with similar demographics as Sripad's (mean age 58 years, 87% white, 51% with at least some college education) and they found that high satisfaction with the decision for surgery correlated with increasing knowledge of the plan for surgery (regardless of HL, age, race, education level, or anxiety score). A particularly significant study was performed by Kenton and colleagues[5] who examined a group of women undergoing reconstructive pelvic surgery, and found that increased patient-reported preparedness for reconstructive prolapse surgery was associated with improved patient-perceived surgical outcomes including satisfaction, symptom improvement, and quality of life after surgery. These findings highlight the importance of patient understanding and the need for interventions focused on increasing comprehension surrounding the specific pelvic floor disorders affecting women and their preparedness for surgery to optimize care and postoperative outcomes for patients.

In this regard, researchers have made efforts to assess strategies aiming to increase patient preparedness for surgery. A few of the strategies that have been studied include the following:

- Peer support: Madsen and colleagues[6] performed a multicenter study to compare peer support (via group or one-on-one) and usual care in women undergoing pelvic reconstructive surgery. They found that the proportion of women feeling prepared (as measured by the preoperative preparedness questionnaire) was equal between the groups (66% peer support vs 63% usual care; $P = .9$) but a greater proportion of those randomized to peer support reported improved preparedness from baseline (71% peer support vs 44% usual care; $P = .001$).
- Preoperative patient telephone call: Halder and colleagues[7] performed a randomized trial to assess how the addition of a semiscripted checklist-driven preoperative provider-initiated telephone call to the usual preoperative care affected patient preparedness as assessed via the patient preparedness questionnaire in patients undergoing POP and/or stress urinary incontinence (SUI) surgery. They found that the addition of a preoperative telephone call resulted in a higher

proportion of patients feeling prepared for surgery but was not correlated with patient-reported outcomes in the 4 to 8 weeks postoperatively.

- Preoperative patient education video: Greene and colleagues[8] found that the addition of a preoperative patient education video at the preoperative visit before prolapse sacrocolpopexy surgery did not increase patient preparedness for surgery, with most patients in both groups feeling prepared for surgery. The authors found that greater preparedness correlated with patient perception of time spent with the patient, but not the actual time spent.
- Preoperative risk calculator to assist in patient counseling: Miranne and colleagues[9] studied patient satisfaction with the decision for concomitant sling at time of prolapse repair randomizing patients to either standard preoperative counseling or preoperative counseling with the use of a validated online risk calculator for de novo SUI after prolapse surgery. They found that at 3 months postoperatively there was no difference between groups in patient-reported satisfaction with regards to concomitant midurethral sling placement during POP surgery (**Box 1**).

These findings highlight the difficulty in defining and in measuring patient-perceived preparedness, and the challenge of improving communication surrounding the decision for surgery and a comprehension of surgical risks and outcomes. It is promising that these studies found high preparedness and satisfaction among participants overall, indicating that patients overall feel well-prepared for undergoing pelvic organ prolapse surgery. More research is needed to clearly delineate the relationships between understanding, preparedness, and outcomes to help inform the development of effective strategies that optimize understanding and preparedness and, as a result, patient outcomes following prolapse surgery.

PREOPERATIVE URODYNAMICS AND CONCOMITANT ANTI-INCONTINENCE SURGERY

Nearly 15 years ago the landmark Colpopexy and Urinary Reduction Efforts (CARE) randomized trial was published, which found that women undergoing abdominal sacrocolpopexy who did not have symptomatic SUI had significantly reduced postoperative stress incontinence symptoms when they had a concomitant Burch colposuspension at the time of their prolapse repair.[11,12] Visco and colleagues[13] then found that those patients with urodynamic stress incontinence during prolapse reduction testing were at the highest risk of de novo SUI postoperatively. These findings were repeated in the outcomes following vaginal prolapse repair and midurethral sling (OPUS) randomized trial, which compared midurethral sling versus no sling at time of vaginal reconstructive prolapse repair in women with prolapse who did not have incontinence symptoms.[14] Wei and colleagues[14] similarly found that women who demonstrated preoperative SUI with reduction (either via urodynamics or via in

---

Box 1
Tools for clinicians and researchers in assessing preoperative preparedness and satisfaction with decision for surgery

- Satisfaction with decision scale for pelvic floor disorders[10]
- Decision regret scale-pelvic floor disorders[10]
- Preoperative preparedness questionnaire (patient preparedness questionnaire)[5]

office stress testing) were at a higher risk of postoperative SUI when compared with women who did not demonstrate stress incontinence with reduction. These data have led some practitioners to argue for the routine use of preoperative urodynamics to evaluate for occult SUI in women undergoing prolapse repair surgery to identify high-risk patients who would most benefit from a concomitant anti-incontinence procedure, and, conversely, these data have led other providers to argue against routine urodynamics assessment before POP surgery.

Urodynamic testing offers the additional benefits of providing a complete evaluation of bladder function and emptying mechanisms but does add cost and uses additional provider resources, patient time, and potentially delays surgery because of the need to coordinate additional visits to obtain and review results before finalizing a plan for surgery. The OPUS trial showed that while concomitant midurethral sling lowered rates of postoperative SUI, concomitant sling had a higher rate of urinary tract infection and bladder perforation and only a minority of women who did not have concomitant anti-incontinence procedure at the time of prolapse repair went on to have a subsequent anti-incontinence surgery.[14] A 2014 systematic review and meta-analysis found that concomitant sling reduced postoperative SUI, but women with concomitant midurethral sling had higher rates of short-term voiding difficulty and adverse events.[15] These data have led some providers to forego preoperative urodynamics and concomitant sling at the time of prolapse repair and instead opt for a staged approach to perform anti-incontinence surgery only if bothersome SUI develops postoperatively.

To assist practitioners and patients in making an informed and more personalized decision regarding a staged versus concomitant sling, Jelovsek and colleagues[16,17] have produced and validated a risk calculator to predict likelihood of developing postoperative de novo SUI. This risk calculator can provide an individualized estimate of the risk of postoperative SUI with or without concomitant midurethral sling at the time of a prolapse repair surgery. However, when assessing the effect of adding the use of a risk calculator to preoperative counseling, Miranne and colleagues[9] found similar rates of postoperative satisfaction with the decision regarding concomitant sling whether or not the risk calculator was used. The utility of these types of risk calculators and how best to incorporate them into clinical practice needs further assessment and research to determine what is the most effective use for such information (**Box 2**).

A Cochrane systematic review published in 2018 summarized the current evidence nicely in concluding that in women with POP and symptomatic or occult SUI "a concurrent MUS probably reduces postoperative SUI and should be discussed in counseling."[18] At this time there is no clear "best" answer and the debate about the utility and benefit of routine, selective, or no preoperative urodynamics in patients

---

Box 2
Risk calculator for SUI after POP surgery

https://riskcalc.org/FemalePelvicMedicineandReconstructiveSurgery/

Data needed for the model:
- Age
- Body mass index
- Vaginal births
- Diabetes
- Urinary leakage with urgency
- $\pm$ Preoperative stress test result (ok if not available)

planning surgical repair of their prolapse continues. The lack of a consensus highlights the importance of a clear discussion with the patient, providing her with a review of the options available and the various utility of each decision. This discussion and the balance of provider perceptions with patient perceptions of various risks and potential complications provides an additional opportunity for providers to assess their patient's values, comprehension, and preparedness in making an informed decision regarding their care.

UTERINE PRESERVATION AT THE TIME OF PROLAPSE REPAIR

In the United States, hysterectomy has commonly been performed when repairing uterovaginal prolapse; however, recent data have called into question the theory that concomitant hysterectomy is the preferred or even the optimal surgery. It is known that prior hysterectomy is a risk factor for pelvic organ prolapse and this begs the question: should the uterus be removed at the time of pelvic organ prolapse repair?

In an enlightening 2013 study performed by Korbly and colleagues,[19] the research team interviewed women with prolapse symptoms who were being evaluated for initial urogynecologic evaluation to assess views on uterine preservation at the time of prolapse repair. The authors found that when asked about various options in prolapse repair, a higher proportion of women preferred an option that included uterine preservation compared with hysterectomy.[19]

Women may desire uterine preservation for a variety reasons including a feeling of femininity, attachment to their womb, a belief that it will preserve sexual function, a wish to minimize surgery, and others. To examine the evidence and help inform provider and patients regarding the outcomes of uterine-preserving prolapse repair, the Society for Gynecologic Surgeons Systematic Review Group performed a systematic review and meta-analysis in 2018, which examined uterine preservation as compared with hysterectomy in pelvic organ prolapse surgery.[20] In this systematic review, Meriwether and colleagues[20] included 96 papers representing 94 original studies, 57 of which were comparative investigations. After reviewing these data, the authors concluded that, when compared with prolapse repair with concomitant hysterectomy, uterine preservation at the time of prolapse repair is associated with lower rates of mesh exposure, faster operative time, and a lower risk of bleeding, and that "the majority of comparative trials on the topic do not show substantive differences in prolapse outcomes or recurrence."[20] This review provided sound evidence to challenge the current paradigm and for keeping the uterus in situ at the time of prolapse repair but had limited data at 3 years or more following repair.

In the following year, Nager and colleagues[21] from the Pelvic Floor Disorders Network published 3-year outcomes of the study of uterine prolapse procedures randomized trial (SUPeR trial) comparing total vaginal hysterectomy with suture uterosacral apical suspension versus transvaginal mesh hysteropexy. Schulten and colleagues[22] published 5-year outcomes of the Sacrospinous Fixation Versus Vaginal Hysterectomy in Treatment of Uterine Prolapse $\geq$ Two (SAVE U) randomized trial comparing sacrospinous hysteropexy versus vaginal hysterectomy and uterosacral ligament suspension.

- SUPeR Trial 3-year outcomes: At 3 years postoperatively, vaginal mesh hysteropexy as compared with vaginal hysterectomy with uterosacral ligament suspension did not result in a significantly lower rate of the composite primary outcome (retreatment of prolapse, prolapse beyond hymen, or prolapse symptoms) with a 36-month adjusted failure incidence of 26% in the mesh hysteropexy cohort compared with 38% with vaginal hysterectomy and uterosacral suspension cohort.[21]

- SAVE U Trial 5-year outcomes: At 5 years postoperatively, there was a significantly higher rate of composite success in the sacrospinous hysteropexy group (87%) as compared with the vaginal hysterectomy and uterosacral ligament suspension group (76%) with no differences in secondary outcomes.[22]

These data provide compelling evidence in support of incorporating uterine-sparing prolapse procedures into practice and discussing uterine preservation in the preoperative discussion between patient and provider when making a plan for pelvic organ prolapse repair surgery.

When considering a uterine-sparing procedure, in 2019 the Food and Drug Administration recalled the product used for mesh transvaginal hysteropexy procedures[23] leaving two evidence-based options for uterine-preserving reconstructive surgery for apical prolapse: sacrohysteropexy or vaginal native tissue hysteropexy.[24]

In comparing outcomes of the various hysteropexy procedures, Meriwether and colleagues[25] published a systematic review examining the evidence supporting the different types of uterine-preserving surgeries for prolapse repair, including sacrohysteropexy via abdominal, laparoscopic, or robotic approach; vaginal mesh hysteropexy; vaginal native-tissue hysteropexy; Manchester procedure; and Le Fort colpocleisis. This study was a planned secondary analysis of the original systematic review examining uterine-sparing versus hysterectomy at time of prolapse repair. In this secondary review, Meriwether and colleagues[20] found there were limited comparative data to enable an informed decision regarding one type of hysteropexy procedure as compared with another, but that the available data indicated few differences in recurrence when comparing one type of hysteropexy procedure to another. Because of the lack of evidence to support one hysteropexy procedure as compared with the other options, surgeon experience and patient preference are best to act as the guides in circumstances where a prolapse repair surgery that preserves the uterus is desired (**Box 3**).

TYPE OF HYSTERECTOMY TO PERFORM AT THE TIME OF MESH SACROCOLPOPEXY

In a woman with a uterus who elects to undergo an abdominal sacrocolpopexy there are several approaches for performing a concomitant hysterectomy: vaginally, laparoscopically, robotically, or abdominally. When performing the hysterectomy via an abdominal approach the surgeon has the option to remove or preserve the cervix. Proponents of supracervical hysterectomies argue that it reduces the risk of infection by avoiding potential vaginal contamination of the mesh graft, and that preserving the cervix leaves a thicker layer of tissue at the vaginal apex reducing the risk of apical vaginal mesh exposure.[26] In contrast, surgeons who support performing a total hysterectomy argue that cervical removal reduces risk of

---

Box 3
Potential benefits of uterine preservation

- Faster recovery
- Less risk of significant bleeding
- Shorter operative time
- Patient preference

prolapse recurrence and reduces risk of cervical cancer/dysplasia, and, in women who are premenopausal, prevents episodic bleeding and avoids the need for intra-abdominal morcellation.[27–29]

- National trends and practice patterns: Using the American College of Surgeons National Surgical Quality Improvement Program database, several studies have recently examined the rate of total versus supracervical hysterectomy at the time of sacrocolpopexy.[30–32] The two studies that sampled thousands of procedures between 2010 and 2017 found that total hysterectomy is more commonly performed at a rate of 53% to 56% of all laparoscopic/robotic hysterectomies during sacrocolpopexy.[31,32] In their study examining the 2014 to 2016 National Surgical Quality Improvement Program database, Slopnick and colleagues[31] reported that in patients undergoing minimally invasive sacrocolpopexy with concomitant hysterectomy, performance of a total hysterectomy was associated with younger age, greater uterine weight, and non-White race with no differences found in postoperative 30-day complications between the two routes. Similarly Winkelman and colleagues[32] found a higher rate of total hysterectomies compared with supracervical at time of colpopexy; but, in contrast to Slopnick's study, they found no significant difference in characteristics between groups and they found a significantly higher rate of blood transfusion and deep surgical site infection associated with total hysterectomy.
- Risk of recurrence: One recent retrospective cohort study showed an increased risk of recurrent anatomic prolapse following supracervical hysterectomies but others have failed to show a difference.[27,28,33] In a 2019 a study performed by Maldonado and colleagues[34] the research team used human cadavers to assess the ability of abdominal sacrocolpopexy with total hysterectomy as compared with supracervical hysterectomy to resist downward traction as a measure of functional anatomic support. The authors found no difference in the ability of the cervices compared with vaginal cuff to resist downward traction of successive weights after sacrocolpopexy indicating that either approach should result in sufficient strength of repair.
- Risk of mesh exposure: As with the risk of recurrence, studies examining the risk of mesh exposure between supracervical hysterectomy compared with total hysterectomy report conflicting results.
  - Vaginal hysterectomy versus supracervical hysterectomy: One study by Nosti and colleagues[28] comparing vaginal hysterectomy versus laparoscopic supracervical hysterectomy at time of laparoscopic sacrocolpopexy found no difference in mesh-related complications (1.6% vs 1.7%) and no difference in intraoperative/postoperative complications with decreased operative time with total vaginal hysterectomy (TVH). However, Tan-Kim and colleagues[35] found the opposite when examining patients undergoing minimally invasive sacrocolpopexy, showing that vaginal hysterectomy was associated with a higher but not statistically significant rate of mesh erosion compared with supracervical hysterectomy (23% total vs 5% supracervical; $P = .109$).
  - Total vaginal/laparoscopic-assisted vaginal versus laparoscopic supracervical hysterectomy: When comparing total vaginal/laparoscopic-assisted vaginal hysterectomy versus laparoscopic supracervical hysterectomy Warner and colleagues[36] found higher mesh exposure with total hysterectomy compared with supracervical hysterectomy (4.9% [9/185] vs 0% [0/92]; $P = .032$) and higher mesh exposure in patients undergoing open cuff laparoscopic suturing

than transvaginal suturing (14.3% [5/35] vs 2.7% [4/150]; relative risk, 5.4; $P = .013$).

○ Robotic total versus robotic supracervical hysterectomy: A study by Crane and colleagues[37] examining mesh exposure in women who underwent robotic sacrocolpopexy with either total versus supracervical hysterectomy found that of the women in the study who had a mesh exposure, all of them had had a robotic total hysterectomy but this was not statistically significant when compared with women who had undergone supracervical hysterectomy ($P = .55$) (**Box 4**).

LENGTH OF STAY

The main goal of vaginal and laparoscopic/robotic minimally invasive procedures is faster recovery and return to normal function. In the last 20 years, enhanced recovery after surgery protocols have become widely adopted and have helped to improve recovery in the immediate postoperative period. One aspect of this expedited recovery is the potential for patients to go home on the day of surgery and same-day discharge has been increasingly used following pelvic organ prolapse surgery including after hysterectomy and sacrocolpopexy procedures performed via minimally invasive routes. Because this is a recent advancement in the field, there are limited data regarding the use of same-day discharge following pelvic organ prolapse surgeries. So far studies have shown similar outcomes in patients discharged home on the day of surgery but larger studies are needed.[38–40] One of the largest studies to date to specifically examine this topic was a recent paper by Berger and colleagues[38] published in 2020 that used data from the Kaiser Permanente managed care organization to compare the 30-day postoperative outcomes in patients discharged home same day (discharged before midnight on postoperative day 0) versus those discharged home on postoperative day 1 after undergoing minimally invasive pelvic reconstructive procedures with and without concomitant hysterectomy. Of the more than 13,000 patients included, approximately 40% (about 5500) were discharged home on the day of surgery. The authors found no differences in 30-day readmission rates or emergency department visits within 30 days for the overall population and when comparing specific prolapse surgeries or concomitant minimally invasive hysterectomy.[38–40] These data provide reassuring evidence that same day discharge after pelvic organ prolapse repair is a safe and feasible option for many women.

Box 4
Factors favoring total hysterectomy (as compared with hysteropexy or supracervical hysterectomy)

- Cervical dysplasia

- Known endometrial hyperplasia, high risk for uterine malignancy, or unevaluated postmenopausal bleeding

- Cervical elongation[a]

- Elongated vaginal length such that shortening total vaginal length is needed to enable either proper placement of mesh graft on the sacrum at time of sacrocolpopexy or for sufficient suspension of the vaginal apex at the time of native tissue repair

[a]Unless Manchester procedure or concomitant trachelectomy will be performed.

IN-PERSON VERSUS VIRTUAL POSTOPERATIVE CARE

Telemedicine has been steadily gaining availability but with the COVID-19 pandemic the accessibility to telemedicine has dramatically risen. Before the pandemic Thompson and colleagues[41] performed a noninferiority randomized trial comparing in-person visits with telephone interviews for postoperative checks at 2, 6, and 12 weeks following pelvic floor surgery. Patient satisfaction was not inferior in the telephone interview cohort as compared with in-person visits with no differences in clinical outcomes or adverse events. As clinicians discover and use new technologies and practices, this area of surgery and postoperative care will continue to change. At this point in time few studies have assessed outcomes or patient/provider satisfaction with postoperative evaluation and follow-up using telemedicine, but those that have been performed reveal promising results, which would support further research and increased flexibility in offering telemedicine for routine postoperative care.[42]

SUMMARY

Female pelvic medicine and reconstructive surgery is a young field and there is still a lot to learn about the "best practices" for pelvic organ prolapse repair surgery. The robust research that has been and continues to be performed is exciting and each study provides new insights that allow providers and patients to come to a clearer understanding of one another and gain a greater comprehension of the various options available at each step in the perioperative pathway. The current controversies discussed here provide an overview of some of the larger questions the field is confronted by at this time, highlight opportunities for further research, and aim to further stimulate the discussion and debate that continues to move the field forward as clinicians strive to improve the lives of the millions of women affected by pelvic organ prolapse, and more specifically those women who elect for a surgical approach to therapy.

CLINICS CARE POINTS

- Patient satisfaction, success, and quality of life is increased with better preparedness for pelvic organ prolapse repair surgery.
- Women planning to undergo pelvic organ prolapse surgery are candidates for preoperative evaluation for occult stress urinary incontinence to provide additional information and guide counseling.
- Preoperative counseling on the management of uterovaginal prolapse should include discussion of uterine-sparing prolapse repair surgeries in patients who are appropriate candidates for uterine preservation.
- Supracervical hysterectomy at the time of mesh sacrocolpopexy for reconstructive repair of uterovaginal prolapse is performed commonly and in appropriate candidates may confer a benefit of decreasing the risk of mesh exposure at the vaginal apex.
- Same-day discharge seems to be a safe option following pelvic organ prolapse surgery including for women undergoing concomitant minimally invasive hysterectomy.
- Telemedicine is a viable option for routine postoperative care in the appropriate patient population and clinical setting.

DISCLOSURE

The author has nothing to disclose.

REFERENCES

1. Abed H, Rogers R, Helitzer D, et al. Informed consent in gynecologic surgery. Am J Obstet Gynecol 2007;197(6):674.e1-5.
2. Sripad AA, Rupp BM, Gage JL, et al. Health literacy in women presenting to a urogynecology practice. Female Pelvic Med Reconstr Surg 2018;24(6):435–9.
3. Anger JT, Lee UJ, Mittal BM, et al. Health literacy and disease understanding among aging women with pelvic floor disorders. Female Pelvic Med Reconstr Surg 2012;18(6):340–3.
4. Hallock JL, Rios R, Handa VL. Patient satisfaction and informed consent for surgery. Am J Obstet Gynecol 2017;217(2):181.e1-7.
5. Kenton K, Pham T, Mueller E, et al. Patient preparedness: an important predictor of surgical outcome. Am J Obstet Gynecol 2007;197(6):654.e1-6.
6. Madsen AM, Rogers RG, Dunivan GC, et al. Perioperative peer support and surgical preparedness in women undergoing reconstructive pelvic surgery. Int Urogynecol J 2020;31(6):1123–32.
7. Halder GE, White AB, Brown HW, et al. A randomized control trial evaluating preoperative telephone calls on surgical preparedness in urogynecology. Int Urogynecol J 2021. [Epub ahead of print].
8. Greene KA, Wyman AM, Scott LA, et al. Evaluation of patient preparedness for surgery: a randomized controlled trial. Am J Obstet Gynecol 2017;217(2):179.e1-7.
9. Miranne JM, Gutman RE, Sokol AI, et al. Effect of a new risk calculator on patient satisfaction with the decision for concomitant midurethral sling during prolapse surgery: a randomized controlled trial. Female Pelvic Med Reconstr Surg 2017;23(1):17–22.
10. Sung VW, Kauffman N, Raker CA, et al. Validation of decision-making outcomes for female pelvic floor disorders. Am J Obstet Gynecol 2008;198(5):575.e1-6.
11. Brubaker L, Cundiff GW, Fine P, et al. Abdominal sacrocolpopexy with Burch colposuspension to reduce urinary stress incontinence. N Engl J Med 2006;354(15):1557–66.
12. Brubaker L, Nygaard I, Richter HE, et al. Two-year outcomes after sacrocolpopexy with and without Burch to prevent stress urinary incontinence. Obstet Gynecol 2008;112(1):49–55.
13. Visco AG, Brubaker L, Nygaard I, et al. The role of preoperative urodynamic testing in stress-continent women undergoing sacrocolpopexy: the Colpopexy and Urinary Reduction Efforts (CARE) randomized surgical trial. Int Urogynecol J Pelvic Floor Dysfunct 2008;19(5):607–14.
14. Wei JT, Nygaard I, Richter HE, et al. A midurethral sling to reduce incontinence after vaginal prolapse repair. N Engl J Med 2012;366(25):2358–67.
15. van der Ploeg JM, van der Steen A, Oude Rengerink K, et al. Prolapse surgery with or without stress incontinence surgery for pelvic organ prolapse: a systematic review and meta-analysis of randomised trials. BJOG 2014;121(5):537–47.
16. Jelovsek JE, Chagin K, Brubaker L, et al. A model for predicting the risk of de novo stress urinary incontinence in women undergoing pelvic organ prolapse surgery. Obstet Gynecol 2014;123(2 Pt 1):279–87.
17. Jelovsek JE, Ploeg JMV, Roovers JP, et al. Validation of a model predicting de novo stress urinary incontinence in women undergoing pelvic organ prolapse surgery. Obstet Gynecol 2019;133(4):683–90.

18. Baessler K, Christmann-Schmid C, Maher C, et al. Surgery for women with pelvic organ prolapse with or without stress urinary incontinence. Cochrane Database Syst Rev 2018;8:CD013108.
19. Korbly NB, Kassis NC, Good MM, et al. Patient preferences for uterine preservation and hysterectomy in women with pelvic organ prolapse. Am J Obstet Gynecol 2013;209(5):470.e1-6.
20. Meriwether KV, Antosh DD, Olivera CK, et al. Uterine preservation vs hysterectomy in pelvic organ prolapse surgery: a systematic review with meta-analysis and clinical practice guidelines. Am J Obstet Gynecol 2018;219(2):129–46.e2.
21. Nager CW, Visco AG, Richter HE, et al. Effect of vaginal mesh hysteropexy vs vaginal hysterectomy with uterosacral ligament suspension on treatment failure in women with uterovaginal prolapse: a randomized clinical trial. JAMA 2019;322(11):1054–65.
22. Schulten SFM, Detollenaere RJ, Stekelenburg J, et al. Sacrospinous hysteropexy versus vaginal hysterectomy with uterosacral ligament suspension in women with uterine prolapse stage 2 or higher: observational follow-up of a multicentre randomised trial. BMJ 2019;366:l5149.
23. Available at: https://www.fda.gov/medical-devices/urogynecologic-surgical-mesh-implants/fdas-activities-urogynecologic-surgical-mesh. Accessed November 28, 2020.
24. Developed by the Joint Writing Group of the American Urogynecologic S, the International Urogynecological Association. Individual contributors are noted in the acknowledgment s. Joint Report on Terminology for Surgical Procedures to Treat Pelvic Organ Prolapse. Female Pelvic Med Reconstr Surg 2020;26(3):173–201.
25. Meriwether KV, Balk EM, Antosh DD, et al. Uterine-preserving surgeries for the repair of pelvic organ prolapse: a systematic review with meta-analysis and clinical practice guidelines. Int Urogynecol J 2019;30(4):505–22.
26. Nygaard IE, McCreery R, Brubaker L, et al. Abdominal sacrocolpopexy: a comprehensive review. Obstet Gynecol 2004;104(4):805–23.
27. Myers EM, Siff L, Osmundsen B, et al. Differences in recurrent prolapse at 1 year after total vs supracervical hysterectomy and robotic sacrocolpopexy. Int Urogynecol J 2015;26(4):585–9.
28. Nosti PA, Carter CM, Sokol AI, et al. Transvaginal versus transabdominal placement of synthetic mesh at time of sacrocolpopexy. Female Pelvic Med Reconstr Surg 2016;22(3):151–5.
29. Vallabh-Patel V, Saiz C, Salamon C, et al. Prevalence of occult malignancy within morcellated specimens removed during laparoscopic sacrocolpopexy. Female Pelvic Med Reconstr Surg 2016;22(4):190–3.
30. Cardenas-Trowers O, Stewart JR, Meriwether KV, et al. Perioperative outcomes of minimally invasive sacrocolpopexy based on route of concurrent hysterectomy: a secondary analysis of the national surgical quality improvement program database. J Minim Invasive Gynecol 2020;27(4):953–8.
31. Slopnick EA, Roberts K, Sheyn DD, et al. Factors influencing selection of concomitant total versus supracervical hysterectomy at the time of sacrocolpopexy and associated perioperative outcomes. Female Pelvic Med Reconstr Surg 2020. https://doi.org/10.1097/SPV.0000000000000950.
32. Winkelman WD, Modest AM, Richardson ML. The surgical approach to abdominal sacrocolpopexy and concurrent hysterectomy: trends for the past decade. Female Pelvic Med Reconstr Surg 2020;27(1):e196–201.

33. Davidson ERW, Thomas TN, Lampert EJ, et al. Route of hysterectomy during minimally invasive sacrocolpopexy does not affect postoperative outcomes. Int Urogynecol J 2019;30(4):649–55.
34. Maldonado PA, Norris KP, Florian-Rodriguez ME, et al. Sacrocolpopexy with concomitant total vs supracervical hysterectomy: functional support comparisons in cadavers. Female Pelvic Med Reconstr Surg 2019;25(3):213–7.
35. Tan-Kim J, Menefee SA, Luber KM, et al. Prevalence and risk factors for mesh erosion after laparoscopic-assisted sacrocolpopexy. Int Urogynecol J 2011; 22(2):205–12.
36. Warner WB, Vora S, Hurtado EA, et al. Effect of operative technique on mesh exposure in laparoscopic sacrocolpopexy. Female Pelvic Med Reconstr Surg 2012;18(2):113–7.
37. Crane AK, Geller EJ, Sullivan S, et al. Short-term mesh exposure after robotic sacrocolpopexy with and without concomitant hysterectomy. South Med J 2014;107(10):603–6.
38. Berger AA, Tan-Kim J, Menefee SA. Comparison of 30-day readmission after same-day compared with next-day discharge in minimally invasive pelvic organ prolapse surgery. Obstet Gynecol 2020;135(6):1327–37.
39. Kisby CK, Polin MR, Visco AG, et al. Same-day discharge after robotic-assisted sacrocolpopexy. Female Pelvic Med Reconstr Surg 2019;25(5):337–41.
40. Romanova AL, Carter-Brooks C, Ruppert KM, et al. 30-Day unanticipated health-care encounters after prolapse surgery: impact of same day discharge. Am J Obstet Gynecol 2020;222(5):482.e1-8.
41. Thompson JC, Cichowski SB, Rogers RG, et al. Outpatient visits versus telephone interviews for postoperative care: a randomized controlled trial. Int Urogynecol J 2019;30(10):1639–46.
42. Grimes CL, Balk EM, Crisp CC, et al. A guide for urogynecologic patient care utilizing telemedicine during the COVID-19 pandemic: review of existing evidence. Int Urogynecol J 2020;31(6):1063–89.

Stress Urinary Incontinence
Slings, Single-Incision Slings, and Nonmesh Approaches

Lauren Caldwell, MD, Amanda B. White, MD*

KEYWORDS

- Sling • Stress urinary incontinence • Urethral bulking • Colposuspension
- Fascial sling

KEY POINTS

- Midurethral sling surgery offers a minimally invasive approach for the treatment of stress urinary incontinence in women.
- Retropubic and transobturator slings demonstrate comparable efficacy, though with unique adverse event profiles.
- Single incision slings may optimize patient experience through decreased pain and faster return to normal activity.
- Surgical treatments of stress urinary incontinence not requiring the use of synthetic mesh include urethral bulking, retropubic colposuspension, and the autologous sling.
- Although synthetic slings have quickly become the standard of care for stress urinary incontinence, nonmesh therapies are well-established and offer favorable cure rates for the complex or mesh-averse patient.

SYNTHETIC MIDURETHRAL SLINGS

Since the introduction of the tension-free vaginal tape (TVT) by Ulmsten and Petros in 1995, the most common surgical treatment for symptomatic stress urinary incontinence has been the midurethral sling. The midurethral sling has largely replaced nonmesh alternatives, including the Burch retropubic urethropexy and the autologous pubovaginal sling, owing to the minimally invasive approach of the midurethral sling. Given comparable efficacy, along with decreased surgical time and recovery, the synthetic midurethral sling is considered the standard of care for the surgical treatment of stress urinary incontinence.[1] With more than 250,000 procedures performed annually in the United States, and a 27% increase in the number of procedures performed in the last decade, the prevalence of sling surgery continues to increase.[2–4]

Female Pelvic Medicine and Reconstructive Surgery, Department of Women's Health, University of Texas at Austin, Dell Medical School, 1301 West 38th Street, Suite 705, Austin, TX 78705, USA
* Corresponding author.
E-mail address: abwhite@ascension.org

Obstet Gynecol Clin N Am 48 (2021) 449–466
https://doi.org/10.1016/j.ogc.2021.05.002
0889-8545/21/© 2021 Elsevier Inc. All rights reserved.

Important material properties of synthetic midurethral slings include a macroporous pore size, weave, and appropriate elasticity. Integration of the device requires collagen in-growth and capillary permeability. The device must allow permeability of both bacteria and host defense cells, including macrophages and lymphocytes, to prevent infection. Optimal material properties of the device must discourage long-term complications and maintain efficacy.

BACKGROUND

Ulmsten and Petros postulated that stress urinary incontinence occurred because of the pubococcygeal muscle's inability to elevate the anterior vaginal wall, resulting in a lack of urethral closure against the pubourethral ligament.[5] They referred to this mechanism of continence and resulting incontinence as the integral theory. The first described midurethral sling procedure (TVT, Gynecare, Ethicon, Somerville, NJ) was hypothesized to strengthen the interface between the pubococcygeal muscle and the anterior vaginal wall at the midurethra, thereby addressing the Integral Theory.

Although the originally described device involved the passage of synthetic tape from a vaginal route through the retropubic space, subsequent modifications in technique showed similar efficacy via a transobturator approach. Initially described by Delorme in 2001,[5] the transobturator approach was designed to avoid the inherent risks of retropubic hematoma formation and bladder perforation associated with trocar passage through the retropubic space. As opposed to passage through the retropubic space, the transobturator trocar was designed to pass from the outside-in, through the groin and obturator foramen. In 2003, the technique was further modified to an inside-out approach by de Leval.[6] The transobturator approach was associated with an increased rate of groin pain as compared with the retropubic approach.[7]

RETROPUBIC SLING

As originally described, the TVT device was placed in a bottom-up fashion, beginning with trocar passage through the bilateral periurethral tunnels, subsequently through the retropubic space, and finally exiting through the abdominal fascia and bilateral suprapubic skin incisions[8] (**Fig. 1**). The initial outcomes were first defined in a prospective multicenter study of 6 sites in which patients underwent the procedure under local anesthetic. Patients were followed for 1 year and 119 of the 131 treated patients met the definition of cure.[9] Two hematomas and 1 bladder perforation were noted perioperatively, and no mesh extrusion was noted at 1 year.[8] The authors concluded that the retropubic midurethral sling was safe and effective for the minimally invasive treatment of stress urinary incontinence.

After the introduction of the TVT, longer term follow-up at 7 years was published by Nilsson and associates.[8] In a multicenter, prospective, observational cohort design of 90 patients, the authors reported an 81.3% objective and subjective cure rate at a mean of 91 months. Although urinary tract infection (7%) and de novo urinary urgency (6.5%) were somewhat frequent, no other significant complications were noted in the long-term follow-up.[8]

A subsequent modification to the originally described TVT included placement of a retropubic sling through a top-down approach from the suprapubic region through the retropubic space with an exit in the vagina. In a meta-analysis by Ford and colleagues,[9] the bottom-up approach to top-down comparison favored a bottom-up

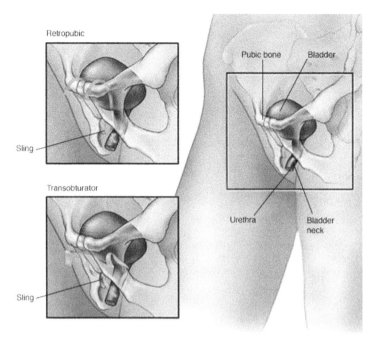

Fig. 1. Retropubic and transobturator slings. (*From* Mayo Foundation for Medical Education and Research; with permission).

approach, citing a higher subjective cure rate, less voiding dysfunction, fewer bladder perforations, and fewer mesh extrusions.

TRANSOBTURATOR SLING

In 2001, Delorme[5] published the results of a case series of the 40 women who underwent sling placement via a transobturator route. Although patients in the series were treated for stress urinary incontinence alone as well as stress urinary incontinence at the time of prolapse repair, 39 of 40 patients were deemed to be continent after the surgery. The most common adverse event was dysuria, which occurred in 5 patients. The authors concluded that the procedure was both safe and effective.[5]

A subsequent modification to the transobturator sling was the direction of trocar passage. Although the procedure was designed to pass the trocar from the outside-in, through the groin and obturator foramen and finally into the vaginal tunnel, de Leval modified the approach in 2003 to traverse inside-out from the vaginal tunnel through the obturator foramen and finally out through the groin (see **Fig. 1**).

de Leval published his perioperative findings on 107 women who underwent this approach using the transvaginal tape obturator inside out.[6] With a mean operative time of 14 minutes and no bladder or urethral perforations, the authors determined the procedure to be feasible.[6] Interestingly, the results were used to discourage the need for urethral evaluation with cystoscopy at the time of transvaginal tape obturator inside out placement, because the urethra and bladder were considered free from risk of injury.[6] Subsequent studies have confirmed that the transobturator approach carries a risk of injury to the urethra and bladder, and cystoscopy is recommended at the time of any midurethral sling placement. Multiple comparative studies have shown similar subjective efficacy between the inside-out and outside-in approaches. However, vaginal perforations were noted to be fewer with an outside-in approach.[9,10]

RETROPUBIC VERSUS TRANSOBTURATOR SLING
Clinical Outcomes

Recent comparative efficacy data were compiled in 55 trials in the 2017 Cochrane Database of Systematic Review's midurethral sling operations for stress urinary incontinence in women.[9] Most trials reported on outcomes at 1 year, although 5 trials reported 1- to 5-year outcomes. Only 1 trial reported the comparative efficacy at more than 5 years. There was no difference in subjective cure at any time point, with subjective cure rates of 62% to 98% in the transobturator sling group and 71% to 97% in the retropubic sling group at 1 year. Overall, subjective cure was maintained with both sling approaches at 5 years. At short, medium, and long-term follow-up, defined by the intervals described elsewhere in this article, no difference in objective cure rates by route of sling placement were observed. At 1 year, the objective cure rate was 85.7% in the transobturator group and 87.2% in the retropubic sling group.[9,10]

Quality-of-life outcomes have been reported inconsistently in comparative trials between retropubic and transobturator slings. Ford and colleagues noted variable outcome measures reported in 33 of 55 comparative trials using 16 different validated measurement tools. In all measures, condition-specific quality of life improved significantly postoperatively, with no difference between groups. At 6 to 24 months, sexual function improved significantly with no difference between groups. Although the quality-of-life outcome reporting continues to be heterogeneous, more recent trials have more consistently reported on condition-specific symptom and sexual function outcomes.[9]

Complications and Concerns

The adverse event profile for midurethral slings depends on the route of sling placement. Although there are some adverse events that occur independent of sling route, there are many important differences. Retropubic placement is associated with an increased risk of bleeding and major vascular injury, bladder perforation (4.5 vs 0.6%), and postoperative voiding dysfunction.[10–12] Interestingly, do novo urgency (8%) and mesh extrusion rates (2%–3%) seem to be similar between groups. Groin pain is significantly greater in patients undergoing transobturator sling placement (6.5% vs 1.5%).[10]

SINGLE INCISION SLING

Although the transobturator approach was initially developed to decrease morbidity, a high rate of groin and hip pain, up to 12%, as well as a 1% reoperation rate encouraged the development of the single incision sling.[13] Both retropubic and transobturator approaches were developed. The sling incision sling was designed to use a much smaller mesh length placed into the obturator internus muscle or obturator membrane, using the transobturator approach, or to anchor into the retropubic space without transversing it. By avoiding the extent of the obturator foramen and groin structures, this less invasive approach was thought to decrease complications, including groin pain, visceral injury, and vascular injury.

Discussion

One early single incision sling, the TVT-Secur (Gynecare, Bridgewater, NJ), was widely studied and shown to be inferior to traditional full-length midurethral slings in several randomized studies. In 4 of 5 randomized trials comparing the single incision sling TVT-Secur with bottom-up retropubic slings, women were more likely to have persistent urinary incontinence after single incision sling surgery. The device was thus withdrawn from clinical use.[14] Nonetheless, Nambiar's Cochrane review of single incision slings noted that TVT-Secur was inferior to full-length midurethral slings, but that single incision slings with an obturator approach may be more cost effective than full-length transobturator slings based on 1 year of follow-up.[14]

Summary

Clinical outcomes

Subsequent single incision slings with anchors have demonstrated comparable efficacy to transobturator slings. Recent publications comparing transobturator slings with single incision slings have shown similar objective and subjective cure rates ranging from 81.6% to 96.4% for transobturator slings and 67% to 87% for single incision slings at a mean of 18.6 months.[14] Mostafa and colleagues[15] noted that, when 10 trials involving TVT-Secur were excluded from 26 available trials comparing single incision slings with standard midurethral slings, no significant difference in patient-reported cure (relative risk, 0.94; 95% confidence interval, 0.88–1.00) or objective cure (relative risk, 0.98; 95% confidence interval, 0.94–1.01) were observed. Recent results of the 522-study, a postmarket surveillance study required under Section 522 of the Food, Drugs and Cosmetics Act, comparing the single incision sling Solyx with the transobturator sling Obtryx II (Boston Scientific, Marlborough, MA) noted no difference in treatment success at 36 months (90.4% to 88.9%; $P = .93$).[16]

No differences in quality-of-life measures in 13 comparative trials or in sexual function measures in 5 comparative trials were found between the single incision slings and full-length slings.[14] Perioperative data showed that single incision slings were associated with shorter operative times with a mean difference of 17.33 minutes when compared with retropubic slings.[14] When compared with a transobturator sling, women undergoing single incision sling surgeries also have lower rates of postoperative pain (6% after single incision sling, 23.9% after transobturator sling).[14] Women undergoing single incision sling surgery have been reported to return to normal activities 5 days earlier and to work 7 days earlier than women undergoing standard midurethral sling surgeries.[15]

Complications and Concerns

Differences in complication rates between single incision slings and traditional midurethral slings are varied. However, after excluding TVT-Secur studies, lower urinary tract injury, voiding dysfunction, extrusions, do novo urinary urgency, and worsening of preexisting urgency do not differ between the groups.[14] In a 2020 prospective study comparing the single incision sling Solyx with the transobturator sling Obtryx II, mesh-related complications were similar between groups at 36 months of follow-up (mesh exposure, 2.8% vs 5.0%; $P = .38$). Serious adverse events including pain during intercourse (0.7% vs 0%; $P = 1.00$), pelvic pain (0.7% vs 0%; $P = 1.00$), and urinary retention (2.8% vs 4.3%; $P = .54$) were also similar between groups.[16]

Although the use of synthetic mesh for stress urinary incontinence surgery has remained the source of controversy in the recent decade, as evidenced by worldwide practice patterns including the removal of synthetic mesh slings from the market in the UK in 2018 and increased postmarket surveillance requirements in the United States, the midurethral sling remains a germane option for women seeking a surgical solution to stress urinary incontinence.[2–4]

CLINICS CARE POINTS

- Synthetic midurethral slings placed either via the retropubic or transobturator route are highly effective for the treatment of stress urinary incontinence in women.
- Full-length retropubic slings are associated with a significantly higher risk of bladder perforation and postoperative voiding dysfunction, whereas full-length transobturator slings are associated with a higher incidence of groin pain.
- Women undergoing single incision sling placement have less pain and a quicker return to activity, with similar subjective outcomes as women undergoing other types of midurethral sling placement.

CLINICAL CASE

A 47-year-old G1P1 presents to clinic with complaints of bothersome urinary incontinence, primarily during running and high-impact exercise. She notes that, since the birth of her child 6 years ago, she has been unable to run during the daylight hours, for fear that her leakage will be obvious to those around her. She has no significant past medical or surgical history. On examination, she has a stage 2 anterior vaginal wall prolapse with a positive empty supine stress test during minimal cough. She has a postvoid residual of 5 mL. She strongly desires sling surgery for treatment of her stress urinary incontinence.

1. What type of sling surgery would you recommend and why?

Given leakage on examination with minimal effort, the patient likely has poor urethral closure pressure. Subjective and objective cure rates would be similar should she desire to undergo either a retropubic or transobturator approach. However, retropubic sling placement may optimize outcomes in patients with urethral sphincter compromise.

2. How would you counsel the patient on the need for urodynamic testing before sling placement?

With demonstrable leakage during increased abdominal pressure, as well as a normal postvoid residual, there is no need for urodynamic evaluation before surgery. In the ValUE randomized trial, completing urodynamic evaluation in women with demonstrable stress urinary incontinence did not result in any alteration to the surgeon's treatment plan.[17]

NONMESH APPROACHES

Other surgical treatment options for stress urinary incontinence include autologous fascial slings, retropubic colposuspension and urethral bulking. Patients who are not candidates for surgical treatment with synthetic mesh may consider one of these extensively studied and effective nonmesh surgical approaches.

AUTOLOGOUS SLING
History

The first fascial suburethral sling was described by Price in 1933,[18] with a strip of fascia lata (deep fascia of the thigh) passed beneath the urethra and fixed to the rectus muscles. Aldridge[19] published his modification of the technique in 1942, which involved the transfer of fascial strips from the external oblique aponeurosis (rectus fascia) through the rectus abdominis muscle to the vaginal incision, where they were sutured together to allow for elevation of the urethra and bladder neck. This technique was the most popular for fascial sling for stress incontinence for many years. The method has since undergone multiple modifications, including transition to a combined abdominovaginal approach with the introduction of perioperative antibiotics, the use of a single continuous portion of rectus fascia, complete detachment of the fascia from both ends before passage under the urethra, and the use of a permanent suture bridge on both ends of a fascial sling.[20] Various attachment points of the autologous sling, including the rectus fascia and the pubocervical and periurethral ligaments, have also been suggested.[20] The most popular modern technique was introduced by McGuire and Lytton in 1978.[21]

Discussion

Today, autologous slings are typically harvested from either the rectus fascia (abdominal) or fascia lata (thigh). Rectus fascia harvest may be accomplished via a Pfannenstiel incision, with final fascial strip measurements reported between 1.5 and 2.5 cm in width and 7 and 16 cm in length.[19,22,23] A permanent suture is attached to both ends of the portion of the harvested fascia. A vaginal incision is made over the bladder neck and tunnels are developed with posterolateral dissection to the level of the endopelvic fascia with entry into the retropubic space. The fascial sling is then passed around the urethra at the level of the bladder neck; the permanent sutures are passed through the rectus fascia just above the symphysis pubis using Stamey needles. Cystourethroscopy is performed to rule out bladder or urethral injury, and may also be used to confirm adequate urethral coaptation with sling placement. The ends of the permanent suture tails attached to the fascial sling are then attached to one another in the midline, avoiding tension under the bladder neck, and the abdominal incision is closed (**Fig. 2**). The sling may also be attached to the periurethral fascia using delayed absorbable sutures before closing the vaginal incision.[23,24]

Alternatively, patients may be placed in the lateral decubitus position for harvesting of the fascia lata via an incision on the lateral aspect of either thigh, 4 cm above the knee. A comparison of fascia lata and rectus fascia slings found no difference in

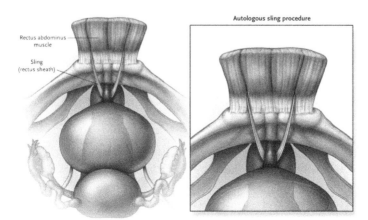

Fig. 2. Autologous sling. (*From* Albo ME, Richter HE, Brubaker L, et al. Burch Colposuspension versus Fascial Sling to Reduce Urinary Stress Incontinence. *N Engl J Med*. 2007;356:2143-55; with permission)

functional outcomes at 1 year postoperatively, with no statistically significant increase in perioperative adverse events.[25] This practice may be preferable in an obese patient, or in the setting of multiple prior abdominal surgeries.[26] A similar width of 1.5 to 2.0 cm and an increased length of 18 to 22 cm may be obtained, often with the aid of a fascial stripper device.[27] The fascia lata is not reapproximated before multilayer incision closure with compression dressing application. The fascial sling is then placed using the technique described elsewhere in this article.

Autologous fascial slings may be considered for women with severe stress urinary incontinence and a fixed urethra, those with a concurrent urethral diverticulum, urethral fistula or history of prior mesh complications, or a patient who strongly desires a nonmesh sling.[28]

Clinical Outcomes

The reported efficacy of the autologous sling for stress urinary incontinence varies in the literature with definition of objective cure. In patients undergoing autologous sling with rectus fascia, 3-year cure rates of 75.6% and patient satisfaction as high as 84.7% have been reported.[23] A randomized controlled trial comparing retropubic colposuspension with autologous slings, which included women with a history of prior anti-incontinence surgery found a similar 5-year patient satisfaction of 83%.[29] Despite this high satisfaction, strictly defined continence (no symptoms on a 3-day bladder diary, no self-reported incontinence and no surgical retreatment) was found to be low at 30.8% after fascial sling.[29] Long-term follow-up at a single institution likewise reported a cure rate of 45% as measured by a 24-hour voiding diary, 24-hour pad test, and patient questionnaire.[26] Patient satisfaction remains high regardless of route of fascial harvest; at the 4-year follow-up after a fascia lata autologous sling surgery, 85% of patients reported being cured or significantly improved.[27]

Patient-reported satisfaction after an autologous fascial sling surgery is high. Validated quality-of-life questionnaires administered to patients 5 years after an autologous sling procedure found a decrease in symptom bother, with no significant difference when compared with patients 5 years after retropubic colposuspension.[29] Clinically important improvements in sexual function have also been reported at 12 and 24 months after autologous fascial sling and did not differ significantly when compared with women undergoing transobturator sling, retropubic sling, or a retropubic colposuspension procedures.[30] A smaller study found no significant postoperative changes in sexual function.[31] Data on sexual function after autologous sling are otherwise scarce.

Complications and Concerns

Intraoperatively, there is a risk of bladder injury of approximately 3.3%; this risk may increase with scarring owing to prior anti-incontinence procedures.[32] Postoperative risks include urinary tract infection (1.1%–11.4%),[31,32] de novo urgency (11%–18.5%),[23,27] de novo urgency incontinence (7.2%),[27] and urinary retention (≤20%).[22] Observation and self-catheterization for at least 3 months postoperatively in anticipation of gradually decreasing sling tension is recommended for the initial management of urinary retention, after which time urethrolysis may be considered.[22] Finally, there is a reported 6.0% to 7.7% risk of wound infection after an autologous sling procedure, which may account for a more significant proportion of complications after rectus fascia harvest as compared with fascia lata.[24,32] Overall, the reoperation rate after autologous sling is reported at 6%.[32]

RETROPUBIC COLPOSUSPENSION
History

A retropubic colposuspension was first described by Dr John C. Burch in 1961 and is today known as the Burch procedure.[33] Although Dr Burch originally published the attachment of paravaginal fascia to the tendinous arch of the fascia pelvis, this process was later modified to attach the paravaginal fascia to Cooper's ligament.[34] In 1978, Dr Emil Tanagho[35] published a further modification of the procedure to include the placement of paravaginal fascia sutures more lateral to the urethra and under less tension, thus describing the current approach to the Burch colposuspension. The procedure was considered the gold standard of stress urinary incontinence treatment before the introduction of the midurethral sling.[34] The Marshall–Marchetti–Krantz procedure was described by Drs Marshall, Marchetti, and Krantz in 1949, involving the fixation of the bladder neck to the symphysis pubis periosteum.[36] There is a risk of osteitis pubis associated with this procedure, and in 2009 the International Consultation on Incontinence Committee determined that there was no evidence for continued use of the Marshall–Marchetti–Krantz procedure.[37]

Discussion

Historically, retropubic colposuspension was performed using an open abdominal incision; in more recent years, a laparoscopic approach has gained popularity. Regardless of the surgical route, the first step is a careful dissection of the retropubic space, followed by the identification of the bladder neck. With the bladder deviated to one side, 2 to 4 stitches are placed in the paravaginal fascia 2 to 3 cm lateral to the urethra from the level of the bladder neck to the proximal one-third of the urethra (**Fig. 3**). These stitches are then anchored to the ipsilateral Cooper's ligament and tied off tension, aided by the elevation of the vagina by an assistant.[38]

Ideal candidates for a retropubic colposuspension include women who strongly desire to avoid synthetic mesh in surgical repair of their stress urinary incontinence, and for whom fascial harvest for autologous sling is not favorable.[28]

Clinical Outcomes

As one of the oldest established surgical procedures for stress urinary incontinence, the success rates and long-term complications of retropubic colposuspension are

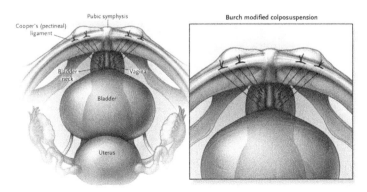

Fig. 3. Retropubic colposuspension. (*From* Albo ME, Richter HE, Brubaker L, et al. Burch Colposuspension versus Fascial Sling to Reduce Urinary Stress Incontinence. *N Engl J Med.* 2007;356:2143-55; with permission)

well-described in the literature. Fifty-five trials involving open retropubic colposuspension with a total enrollment of 5417 women were included in the most recent Cochrane review, which reported an overall cure rate of 68.9% to 88.0%.[39] A Cochrane review of 26 trials involving laparoscopic retropubic colposuspension and a total of 2271 woman found similar cure rates, with decreased morbidity, shorter hospital stays, and fewer postoperative complications given the minimally invasive approach.[40] The efficacy of both open and laparoscopic retropubic colposuspension is reported to decrease from 90% at 1 year to 70% at 10 years.[40] Given the similar reported efficacy of the laparoscopic approach and the minimally invasive midurethral sling procedure, the retropubic colposuspension procedure has been performed less frequently in recent years; however, it may still be offered to index patients undergoing surgery for stress urinary incontinence.[41]

The most recent Cochrane Reviews of both open and laparoscopic retropubic colposuspension encourage future studies of quality-of-life outcomes for patients undergoing these procedures, because data are lacking. Studies that collected validated quality-of-life questionnaires generally reported improvement in patient-reported symptoms or no change when compared with alternative stress urinary incontinence treatment.[39,40] One randomized controlled trial of midurethral sling and colposuspension found that patients undergoing colposuspension reported less improvement in some quality-of-life measures at 6 months and 2 years; however, there was no difference at 5 years of follow-up.[42] Sexual function after retropubic colposuspension is inconsistently reported in the literature, with conflicting results. Coital incontinence is likely to be cured or improved postoperatively,[43] and the addition of colposuspension to sacrocolpopexy in a randomized controlled trial did not adversely affect sexual function.[44] Conversely, a small prospective study comparing colposuspension and midurethral sling found statistically significant decreases in multiple domains of sexual function.[45]

Complications and Concerns

Perioperative complications associated with retropubic colposuspension are listed in **Table 1**. The reported rates of postoperative voiding dysfunction vary widely based on definition; however, up to 25% of patients experience immediate postoperative voiding dysfunction[34] and 22% of patients noted voiding difficulties in a 10- to 20-year postoperative follow-up.[46] De novo detrusor instability may also occur in 5% to 27% of patients.[38] Despite this finding, reoperation after a retropubic colposuspension is reported to be low at 4.2 per 1000 woman-years.[47] An association of retropubic colposuspension with future development of prolapse has been noted with rectocele formation in 11% to 25% and enterocele formation in 4% to 10% of patients, although direct causation has not been demonstrated.[46]

Table 1 Perioperative complications of retropubic colposuspension	
Complication	**Rate of Occurrence (%)**
Bleeding owing to injury of paravaginal veins	2
Bladder injury	0.4–9.6
Ureteral injury	0.2–2.0
Urinary tract infection	4–40
Wound infection	4.0–10.8

Data from Sohlberg EM, Elliott CS. Burch Colposuspension. *Urol Clin North Am.* 2019;46(1):53-59.

Table 2		
Currently available urethral bulking agents and year of introduction or approval		
Generic name	Brand Name	Year
Carbon-coated zirconium oxide beads	Durasphere	1999
Calcium hydroxyl apatite	Coaptite	2001
Polydimethylsiloxane elastomer	Macroplastique	1991
Polyacrylamide hydrogel	Bulkamid	1996

Data from Hussain SM, Bray R. Urethral bulking agents for female stress urinary incontinence. Neurourol Urodyn 2019;38:887-92.

URETHRAL BULKING
History

Urethral bulking was first described at the end of the nineteenth century by Austrian surgeon Dr Robert Gersuny, who pioneered the use of paraffin as an injectable material in a variety of clinical settings, including breast augmentation.[48] In 1914, renowned American gynecologist Dr Howard Kelly cautioned against the use of periurethral paraffin injections, citing the risk of emboli formation with only temporary symptomatic improvement.[49] The use of sclerosing agents in the treatment of stress urinary incontinence was first described by the British obstetrician Dr Bryan Murless in 1938 when he injected sodium morrhuate in the anterior vaginal wall of 20 women. The agent achieved its intended goal by resulting in periurethral tissue scarring.[50] In 1963 Sachse, a German physician, published on the periurethral use of a sclerosing agent named Dondren. Although the treatment was moderately successful, several patients developed pulmonary emboli and Dondren use was halted.[51] A later alternative of polytetrafluoroethylene (Teflon) was introduced in the 1970s, but failed to gain approval from the US Food and Drug Administration owing to reports of granuloma and periurethral abscess formation, with only an 18% 5-year cure rate.[52]

Since the historical use of paraffin and Dondren, a wide variety of materials have since been tested for use in urethral bulking agents, including autologous fat, ethylene vinyl alcohol, and hyaluronic acid. All of these agents were found to have various increased risks, including the reabsorption of fat resulting in pulmonary embolism, urethral erosion (ethylene vinyl alcohol), and sterile abscess formation (hyaluronic acid) and are no longer available for use.[53] The most successful historical urethral bulking agent was glutaraldehyde cross-linked bovine collagen. Collagen was introduced in 1993 with cure rates ranging from 40% to 60%, and rate of both improvement and/or cure as high as 68% to 90%.[54] Although production was discontinued in 2011, these promising reported success rates made collagen the gold standard in the development of new urethral bulking agents.[55]

Discussion

Today, urethral bulking is accomplished with 1 of 4 available urethral bulking agents, each of which optimize cure rates while minimizing adverse events as compared with previous agents (**Table 2**). Insufficient data exist to determine the superiority of one urethral bulking agent over another.[56] Regardless of the material selected, all urethral bulking agents are injected in the clinical setting with the goal of improving urethral mucosal coaptation.[56] The agent of choice is typically injected into the periurethral tissue at the level of the bladder neck and proximal urethra, although at least 1 trial has compared this practice with a midurethral injection and found no significant difference

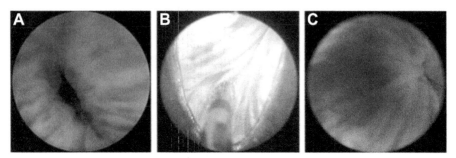

Fig. 4. *A)* A patient with previous urethral injection is noted to have incomplete coaptation of the urethra with residual bulge on the left side of the urethra. (*B*) After injecting the right side of the urethra, (*C*) coaptation is noted. (*From* Li H, Westney OL. Injection of Urethral Bulking Agents. *Urol Clin N Am.* 2019;46:1-15; with permission).

in cure rate.[57] The proceedure may be accomplished with either transurethral or periurethral injection. Urethral bulking is most often performed under direct cystoscopic visualization, although ultrasound guidance and the use of an implantation device have also been used.[58]

In transurethral injection under direct cystoscopic visualization, an injection needle is introduced via cystoscope and used to inject lateral to the urethral meatus, typically at the 3 and 9 o'clock positions. This technique is illustrated in **Fig. 4**. A limited volume of 0.5 mL or less is injected in each site given the limitations of the submucosal space.[55] If performed without or with minimal systemic anesthesia, local anesthetic solution may be injected before injection of urethral bulking agent to enhance patient comfort during injection.

Periurethral injection is also performed under direct cystoscopic visualization and may result in less urethral trauma.[53] In this technique, the injection needle is placed periurethrally through the vaginal epithelium.[56] Urethral insertion devices may be

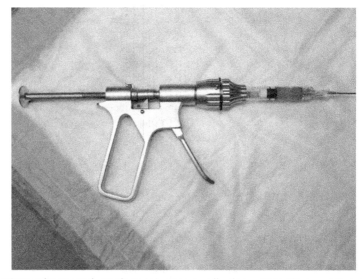

Fig. 5. Syringe adaptor and uroplasty injection needle. (*From* Li H, Westney OL. Injection of Urethral Bulking Agents. *Urol Clin N Am.* 2019;46:1-15; with permission)

used to deliver both silicone and dextronomer preparations of urethral bulking agents to the periurethral tissue, as pictured in **Fig. 5**. The urethral length is first measured to ensure that the device is placed at the appropriate depth before injection. The device allows for passage of 4 needles for injection. Repeat injections are not recommended less than 12 weeks after the prior procedure.[55] Based on gradually diminishing efficacy over time, it is generally accepted that women undergoing urethral bulking will require future repeat injection. Current studies' length of follow-up have not allowed for an established an interbulking interval, although many trials have limited the number of repeat injections to between 3 and 5.[56,59]

The ideal candidates for urethral bulking include women with bothersome stress urinary incontinence who would prefer to avoid the use of synthetic mesh and the need for general anesthesia. The procedure may also be considered in patients who have failed to achieve adequate symptom improvement with surgery, those without urethral mobility, or those who have previously experienced mesh-related complications.[30]

Clinical Outcomes

The reported improvement and objective cure rates vary between types of urethral bulking agents. A meta-analysis of polydimethylsiloxane elastomer (Macroplastique) reported a short-term (<6 months) improvement rate of 75% and long-term (>18 months) 64% improvement.[60] This rate was significantly higher than the cure rate, which ranged from 43% in the short term to 36% in the long term.[60] Carbon-coated zirconium (Durasphere) has reported improvement rates as high as 80% at 1 and 2 years in 2 randomized controlled trials,[61,62] and as low as 21% after 36 months in a prospective cohort study.[63] A multicenter randomized trial involving calcium hydroxyl apatite (Coaptite) reported a 63.4% improvement and 39% cure rate at 12 months.[64] Finally, polyacrylamide hydrogel (Bulkamid) was found in a multicenter prospective cohort study to have a 64% improvement at 2 years after injection.[65] Although these results are promising, the most recent Cochrane review of urethral bulking maintains that there is an unsatisfactory basis for practice, and that bulking cannot be recommended for women who are appropriate candidates for other surgical procedures.[56]

Table 3	
Complications of urethral bulking	
Complication	**Rate of Occurrence (%)**
Urinary retention	8.4
Urinary urgency/Urgency incontinence	7.0
Pain with injection	6.4
Urinary tract infection	5.5
Transient hematuria	3.4
Pseudocyst/Periurethral mass formation	0.7
Urethral erosion	0.3

Data from Li H, Westney OL. Injection of Urethral Bulking Agents. *Urol Clin N Am.* 2019;46:1-15; and Ghoniem G, Boctor N. Update on urethral bulking agents for female stress urinary incontinence due to intrinsic sphincter deficiency. *J Urol Res.* 2014;1:1009; and de Vries AM, Wadhwa H, Huang J, Farag F, Heesakkers J, Kocjancic, E. Complications of Urethral Bulking Agents for Stress Urinary Incontinence: An Extensive Review Including Case Reports. *Female Pelvic Med Reconstr Surg.* 2018;24(6):392-8.

Trials investigating the use of various urethral bulking agents have demonstrated modest improvements on validated quality-of-life measures.[56] Although improvement from baseline quality of life scores is reported by the studies highlighted in the most recent Cochrane review, most demonstrated no significant difference when compared with groups receiving alternative therapies.[56] The only noted exception is a comparison between Macroplastique and home pelvic floor exercises in which patients receiving Macroplastique injections had statistically significant improvement in the Urinary Incontinence Quality of Life Scale.[56] Outcomes specific to sexual function after urethral bulking have not been reported.

Complications and Concerns

Known complications of urethral bulking are listed in **Table 3**. Urethral bulking is generally considered a low-risk procedure, because only 3% of complications require invasive treatment such as abscess incision and drainage or periurethral mass removal.[66] Most complications are managed conservatively with oral antibiotics, anticholinergics, clean intermittent catheterization, an indwelling catheter, or watchful waiting.

SUMMARY

Traditional surgical techniques for the management of stress urinary incontinence are nonmesh approaches, including autologous slings, retropubic colposuspension, and urethral bulking. Autologous slings involve increased morbidity owing to fascial harvest, and are ideal in patients who have failed alternative therapies for stress incontinence or who are not candidates for a synthetic mesh. Retropubic colposuspension is a well-studied technique that may be performed via an open or a laparoscopic approach, with a high reported cure rate. By increasing urethral coaptation with injection of synthetic bulking agents, urethral bulking results in improvement in stress incontinence symptoms without the need for general anesthesia.

CLINICS CARE POINTS

- Autologous slings may be harvested from the rectus fascia (abdominal) or fascia lata (thigh) for placement at the level of the bladder neck in patients with a fixed urethra, a concurrent urethral diverticulum, or with a history of mesh complications.

- Retropubic colposuspension was long considered the gold standard for stress urinary incontinence treatment with high reported improvement and cure rates, despite an increase in postoperative voiding dysfunction.

- Urethral bulking agents may be ideal in the medically frail patient with stress urinary incontinence.

- Although patient satisfaction with urethral bulking is high with few adverse events, efficacy gradually diminishes over time and is low when compared with alternative therapies.

CASE STUDY: MS L

An 87-year-old G1P1 presents with complaints of bothersome urinary incontinence, requiring her to wear briefs as well as 2 to 3 pads daily. Her medical history is significant for atrial fibrillation, chronic kidney disease, congestive heart failure, coronary artery disease and hypertension, with prior cardiac stent ×2. On examination, she has no significant prolapse and a normal postvoid residual volume, with a positive stress test of large volume of urine. She is interested in surgery to manage her incontinence.

3. What type of surgery would you recommend and why?

This patient is an ideal candidate for a urethral bulking procedure, because it may allow her to avoid general anesthesia in the setting of multiple medical comorbidities.

4. The patient returns 1 year later with the complaint of recurrent urinary incontinence, and requests repeat urethral bulking. Can this be safely offered to her?

Yes; although there are limited data on a recommended interval of urethral bulking, efficacy has been noted to gradually decrease over time. The need for repeat injections should be included in the preoperative counseling for urethral bulking.

DISCLOSURE

L. Caldwell.: nothing to disclose. A.B. White: Boston Scientific: investigator (522 Solyx), consultant.

REFERENCES

1. Nager C, Tulikangas P, Miller D, et al. Position statement on mesh midurethral slings for stress urinary incontinence. Female Pelvic Med Reconstr Surg 2014; 20(3):123–5.
2. Anger JT, Weinberg AE, Albo ME, et al. Trends in surgical management of stress urinary incontinence among female Medicare beneficiaries. Urology 2009;74(2): 283–7.
3. Oliphant SS, Wang L, Bunker CH, et al. Trends in stress urinary incontinence inpatient procedures in the United States, 1979-2004. Am J Obstet Gynecol 2009;200(5):521.e1-6.
4. Erekson EA, Lopes VV, Raker CA, et al. Ambulatory procedures for female pelvic floor disorders in the United States. Am J Obstet Gynecol 2010;203(5):497.e1-5.
5. Delorme E. [Transobturator urethral suspension: mini-invasive procedure in the treatment of stress urinary incontinence in women]. Prog Urol 2001;11(6): 1306–13.
6. de Leval J. Novel surgical technique for the treatment of female stress urinary incontinence: transobturator vaginal tape inside-out. Eur Urol 2003;44(6):724–30.
7. Richter HE, Albo ME, Zyczynski HM, et al. Retropubic versus Transobturator Midurethral Slings for Stress Incontinence. N Engl J Med 2010;362:2066–76.
8. Nilsson CG, Falconer C, Rezapour M. Seven-year follow-up of the tension-free vaginal tape procedure for treatment of urinary incontinence. Obstet Gynecol 2004;104(6):1259–62.
9. Ford AA, Rogerson L, Cody JD, et al. Mid-urethral sling operations for stress urinary incontinence in women. Cochrane Database Syst Rev 2017;7(7):CD006375.
10. Schimpf MO, Rahn DD, Wheeler TL, et al, Society of Gynecologic Surgeons Systematic Review Group. Sling surgery for stress urinary incontinence in women: a systematic review and meta-analysis. Am J Obstet Gynecol 2014;211(1):71.e1-7.
11. Barboglio PG, Ann Gormley E. The fate of synthetic mid-urethral slings in 2013: a turning point. Arab J Urol 2013;11(2):117–26.
12. Ulmsten U, Falconer C, Johnson P, et al. A multicenter study of tension-free vaginal tape (TVT) for surgical treatment of stress urinary incontinence. Int Urogynecol J Pelvic Floor Dysfunct 1998;9(4):210–3.

13. Latthe PM, Foon R, Toozs-Hobson P. Transobturator and retropubic tape proced-ures in stress urinary incontinence: a systematic review and meta-analysis of effectiveness and complications. BJOG 2007;114(5):522–31.
14. Nambiar A, Cody JD, Jeffery ST, et al. Single-incision sling operations for urinary incontinence in women. Cochrane Database Syst Rev 2017;7(7):CD008709.
15. Mostafa A, Lim CP, Hopper L, et al. Single-incision mini-slings versus standard midurethral slings in surgical management of female stress urinary incontinence: an updated systematic review and meta-analysis of effectiveness and complica-tions. Eur Urol 2014;65(2):402–27.
16. White AB, Kahn BS, Gonzalez RR, et al. Prospective study of a single-incision sling versus a transobturator sling in women with stress urinary incontinence: 3-year results. Am J Obstet Gynecol 2020;223(4):545.e1-11.
17. Nager CW, Brubaker L, Litman H, et al. Urinary Incontinence Treatment Network. A randomized trial of urodynamic testing before stress-incontinence surgery. N Engl J Med 2012;366(21):1987–97.
18. Price PB. Plastic operation for incontinence of urine and of faeces. Arch Surg 1933;26:1043–53.
19. Aldridge A. Transplantation of fascia for the relief of urinary stress incontinence. Am J Obstet Gynecol 1942;44:398–411.
20. Ghoniem GM, Shaaban A. Sub-Urethral Slings for Treatment of Stress Urinary In-continence. Int Urogynecol J 1994;5:228–39.
21. McGuire EJ, Lytton B. Pubovaginal sling procedure for stress incontinence. J Urol 1978;119:82–4.
22. Mahdy A, Ghoniem GM. Autologous rectus fascia sling for treatment of stress uri-nary incontinence in women: a review of the literature. Neurourol Urodyn 2019;38:S51–8.
23. Blaivas JG, Simma-Chiang V, Gul Z, et al. Surgery for stress urinary incontinence: autologous fascial sling. Urol Clin N Am 2019;46:41–52.
24. Peng M, Sussman RD, Escobar C, et al. Rectus fascia versus fascia lata for autol-ogous fascial pubovaginal sling: a single-center comparison of perioperative and functional outcomes. Female Pelvic Med Reconst Surg 2020;26:493–7.
25. Latini JM, Lux MM, Kreder KJ. Efficacy and morbidity of autologous fascia lata sling cystourethropexy. J Urol 2004;171:1180–4.
26. Blaivas JG, Chaikin DC. Pubovaginal fascial sling for the treatment of all types of stress urinary incontinence: surgical technique and long-term outcome. Urol Clin N Am 2011;38:7–15.
27. Athanasopoulos A, Gyftopoulos K, McGuire EJ. Efficacy and preoperative prog-nostic factors of autologous fascia rectus sling for treatment of female stress uri-nary incontinence. Urology 2011;78:1034–8.
28. Urinary incontinence in women. Practice Bulletin No. 155. American College of Obstetricians and Gynecologists. Obstet Gynecol 2015;126:e66–81.
29. Brubaker L, Richter HE, Norton PA, et al. Five year continence rates, satisfaction and adverse events for Burch urethropexy and fascial sling surgery for urinary in-continence. J Urol 2012;187:1324–30.
30. Glass Clark SM, Huang Q, Sima AP, et al. Effect of surgery for stress incontinence on female sexual function. Obstet Gynecol 2020;135:352–60.
31. Wadie BS, Mansour A, El-Hefnawy AS, et al. Minimum 2-year follow-up of mid-urethral slings, effect on quality of life, incontinence impact and sexual function. Int Urogynecol J 2010;21:1485–90.
32. Chan PTK, Fournier C, Corcos J. Short-term complications of pubovaginal sling procedure for genuine stress incontinence in women. Urology 2000;55:207–11.

33. Burch JC. Urethrovaginal fixation to Cooper's ligament for correction of stress urinary incontinence, cystocele, and prolapse. Am J Obstet Gynecol 1961;81: 281–90.
34. Sohlberg EM, Elliott CS. Burch Colposuspension. Urol Clin North Am 2019; 46(1):53–9.
35. Tanagho EA. Colpocystourethropexy: the way we do it. J Urol 1978;116:751–3.
36. Marshall VF, Marchetti AA, Krantz KE. The correction of stress incontinence by simple vesicourethral suspension. Surg Gynecol Obstet 1949;88(4):509–18.
37. Smith AR, Chand D, Dmochowski R, et al. Committee 14. Surgery for urinary incontinence in women. In: Abrams P, Cardozo L, Khoury S, editors. Incontinence. Plymouth (United Kingdom). Health Publications; 2009. p. 1191–272.
38. Veit-Rubin N, Dubuisson J, Ford A, et al. Burch colposuspension. Neurourol Urodyn 2019;38(2):553–62.
39. Lapitan MCM, Cody JD, Mashayekhi A. Open retropubic colposuspension for urinary incontinence in women. Cochrane Database Syst Rev 2017;7(7):CD002912.
40. Freites J, Stewart F, Omar MI, et al. Laparoscopic colposuspension for urinary incontinence in women. Cochrane Database Syst Rev 2019;12(12):CD002239.
41. Kobashi KC, Albo ME, Dmochowski RR, et al. Surgical treatment of female stress urinary incontinence: AUA/SUFU guideline. J Urol 2017;198:875.
42. Ward KL, Hilton P, on behalf of the UK and Ireland TVT Trial Group. Tension-free vaginal tape versus colposuspension for primary urodynamic stress incontinence: 5-year follow up. BJOG 2008;115:226–33.
43. Baessler K, Stanton SL. Does Burch colposuspension cure coital incontinence? Am J Obstet Gynecol 2004;190:1030–3.
44. Handa VL, Zyczynski HM, Brubaker L, et al. Sexual function before and after sacrocolpopexy for pelvic organ prolapse. Am J Obstet Gynecol 2007;197:629.e1-6.
45. Çayan F, Dilek S, Akbay E, et al. Sexual function after surgery for stress urinary incontinence: vaginal sling versus Burch colposuspension. Arch Gynecol Obstet 2008;227:31–6.
46. Alcalay M, Monga A, Stanton SL. Burch colposuspension: a 10-20 year follow up. Br J Obstet Gynaecol 1995;102:740–5.
47. Fialkow M, Symons RG, Flum D. Reoperation for urinary incontinence. Am J Obstet Gynecol 2008;199:546.e1-e8.
48. Schultheiss D, Höfner K, Oelke M, et al. Historical aspects of the treatment of urinary incontinence. Eur Urol 2000;38(3):352–62.
49. Kelly HA, Dumm WM. Urinary incontinence in women, without manifest injury to the bladder. J Am Coll Surg 1914;18:444–50.
50. Murless BC. The injection treatment of stress incontinence. J Obstet Gynaecol Br Emp 1938;45:521–4.
51. Sachse S. Treatment of urinary incontinence with sclerosing solutions: indications, results, complications. Urol Int 1963;15:225–9.
52. Kiilholma PJ, Chancellor MB, Makinen J, et al. Complications of Teflon injection for stress urinary incontinence. Neurourol Urodyn 1993;12(2):131–7.
53. Hussain SM, Bray R. Urethral bulking agents for female stress urinary incontinence. Neurourol Urodyn 2019;38:887–92.
54. Dmochowski RR, Appell RA. Injectable agents in the treatment of stress urinary incontinence in women: where are we now? Urology 2000;56:32–40.
55. Li H, Westney OL. Injection of Urethral Bulking Agents. Urol Clin N Am 2019; 46:1–15.
56. Kirchin V, Page T, Keegan PE, et al. Urethral injection therapy for urinary incontinence in women. Cochrane Database Syst Rev 2017;7(7):CD003881.

57. Kuhn A, Stadlmayr W, Lengsfeld D, et al. Where should bulking agents for female urodynamic stress incontinence be injected? Int Urogynecol J 2008;19(6): 817–21.
58. Ghoniem G, Boctor N. Update on urethral bulking agents for female stress urinary incontinence due to intrinsic sphincter deficiency. J Urol Res 2014;1:1009.
59. Ziddiqui ZA, Abboudi H, Crawford R, et al. Intraurethral bulking agents for the management of female stress urinary incontinence: a systematic review. Int Urogynecol J 2017;28:1275–84.
60. Ghoniem GM, Miller CJ. A systematic review and meta-analysis of Macroplastique for treating female stress urinary incontinence. Int Urogynecol J 2013; 24(1):27–36.
61. Lightner D, Calvosa C, Andersen R, et al. A new injectable bulking agent for treatment of stress urinary incontinence: results of a multicenter, randomized, controlled, double-blind study of Durasphere. Urology 2001;58(1):12–5.
62. Andersen RC. Long-term follow-up comparison of durasphere and contigen in the treatment of stress urinary incontinence. J Low Genit Tract Dis 2002;6(4): 239–43.
63. Chrouser KL, Fick F, Goel A, et al. Carbon coated zirconium beads in beta-glucan gel and bovine glutaraldehyde cross-linked collagen injections for intrinsic sphincter deficiency: continence and satisfaction after extended followup. J Urol 2004;171(3):1152–5.
64. Mayer RD, Dmochowski RR, Appell RA, et al. Multicenter prospective randomized 52-week trial of calcium hydroxylapatite versus bovine dermal collagen for treatment of stress urinary incontinence. Urology 2007;69(5):876–80.
65. Toozs-Hobson P, Al-Singary W, Fynes M, et al. Two-year follow-up of an open-label multicenter study of polyacrylamide hydrogel (Bulkamid®) for female stress and stress-predominant mixed incontinence. Int Urogynecol J 2012;23(10): 1373–8.
66. de Vries AM, Wadhwa H, Huang J, et al. Complications of urethral bulking agents for stress urinary incontinence: an extensive review including case reports. Female Pelvic Med Reconstr Surg 2018;24(6):392–8.

Accidental Bowel Leakage/ Fecal Incontinence
Evidence-Based Management

Isuzu Meyer, MD, MSPH*, Holly E. Richter, PhD, MD

KEYWORDS

- Accidental bowel leakage • Anal incontinence • Anal sphincter
- Defecatory disorders • Fecal incontinence • Treatment • Surgical treatment

KEY POINTS

- Fecal incontinence, defined as involuntary loss of liquid and/or solid stool, is caused by disruption of the multicomponent continence mechanism.
- Fecal incontinence is a physically and psychosocially debilitating condition. Many women are reluctant to report their symptoms and seek care.
- Management options for fecal incontinence consist of conservative and surgical approaches. More invasive therapies should be reserved for patients with refractory fecal incontinence.
- New devices improve fecal incontinence symptoms without the risks of surgical intervention.
- Sacral neuromodulation has largely replaced sphincteroplasty as the first-line surgical option for women with fecal incontinence remote from delivery.

INTRODUCTION

The prevalence of fecal incontinence (FI), the complaint of involuntary loss of liquid and/or solid stool, varies widely from 2% to 21% and increases with advancing age.[1–3] Epidemiologic studies suggest that up to 70% of patients with FI have not reported their symptoms to health care professionals.[4,5] Thus, the prevalence of FI is often underestimated. The negative consequences of FI include not only physical debilitation, but also social isolation, embarrassment, and loss of employment. FI affects intimate relationships and self-esteem. To reduce the burden of FI, eliminate stigma, and to promote care-seeking, it is important to raise awareness of the condition and various treatment options available. Another obstacle to help-seeking is that

Division of Urogynecology and Pelvic Reconstructive Surgery, Department of Obstetrics and Gynecology, University of Alabama at Birmingham, 1700 6th Avenue South, Suite 10382, Birmingham, AL 35233, USA
* Corresponding author.
E-mail address: imeyer@uabmc.edu
Twitter: @isuzu_meyer (I.M.)

Obstet Gynecol Clin N Am 48 (2021) 467–485
https://doi.org/10.1016/j.ogc.2021.05.003
0889-8545/21/© 2021 Elsevier Inc. All rights reserved.

many providers do not screen for FI because of lack of clinical experience and knowledge about evaluation and management.

FI is caused by the disruption of 1 or more components of the continence mechanism, which depends on anal sphincter function, intact rectal sensation, adequate rectal capacity, compliance, colonic transit time, stool consistency, and cognitive and neurologic factors. Its etiology is commonly multifactorial, with 80% of patients having more than 1 continence factor compromised.[6] We recommend that health care providers routinely ask patients about FI. Using a written questionnaire is helpful, especially at the initial encounter, as women are more likely to report their symptoms on a written questionnaire, compared with disclosing FI to their providers even when directly asked.[7] In addition, women may be more comfortable using the term "accidental bowel leakage" when referring to FI.[8]

MANAGEMENT

Treatment goals focus on restoring continence and improving quality of life (QOL). Clinicians should determine symptom severity, characterizing stool type, the frequency/amount of leakage, and the presence of fecal urgency. Bowel diaries are helpful as they are superior to self-reports for characterizing bowel habits, and can better predict colonic transit.[9] Recognizing FI type based on the awareness of the desire to defecate before leakage can provide clues to underlying pathology. Traditionally, 3 phenotypes characterize FI:

1. Urge incontinence: inability to postpone defecation on urgency, related to external anal sphincter (EAS) dysfunction.
2. Passive incontinence: the loss of stool without the urge to defecate, often attributed to internal anal sphincter (IAS) dysfunction and peripheral neuropathy.
3. Fecal seepage: seepage of stool without awareness, often related to incomplete evacuation and impaired rectal sensation.

Recently, a fourth phenotype, stress FI, has been introduced, which is described as the loss of stool when coughing or sneezing.[10] The underlying pathophysiology associated with stress FI has not been well characterized.

Management of FI consists of conservative and surgical approaches. Conservative treatment includes lifestyle/dietary changes, medications, and pelvic floor muscle exercises with and without biofeedback. Unfortunately, no single approach has been shown to provide consistent, long-term effectiveness with low complication rates. However, symptoms may be alleviated by simple measures.

Dietary Considerations

Avoid offending foods
Patients should be educated on factors contributing to loose stool consistency, including food items containing incompletely digested sugars (fructose, lactose), sweeteners (sorbitol, xylitol, mannitol), carbonated beverages, caffeine, alcohol, cured or smoked meat (sausage, ham, turkey), spicy foods, and fatty and greasy foods. Bowel and food diaries can help identify the individual's offending food items that cause loose stools and incontinence. In the case of diarrhea, patients should be evaluated and treated for any underlying etiology. Fecal impaction should be treated to avoid overflow incontinence.

Fiber supplementation
Fiber supplementation is helpful in women with loose stools or low-volume FI. The mechanisms of dietary fiber depend on stool composition and consistency, which

vary among the types of fiber ingested. Fiber, when fermented but not completely degraded by colonic bacteria, has been shown to increase stool bulk. In addition, fiber with high water-holding capacity allows gel formation that normalizes stool consistency (softens hard stool and firms loose/liquid stool). Insoluble fiber increases fecal water content and bulking; however, accelerates colonic transit rate, thus having a laxative effect. Increasing rectal distension can improve sensory awareness of the need to defecate, which may reduce FI episodes and promote complete evacuation of stool, leaving less in the rectum to leak.[11–13] Compared with constipation, the effects of fiber supplementation on FI are not as robustly described. Commonly used fiber supplements include the following:

1. Psyllium (Metamucil, moderate solubility, fermentable)
2. Methylcellulose (Citrucel, high solubility, nonfermentable)
3. Calcium polycarbophyl (Fibercon, an insoluble hydrophilic fiber)

Fiber is typically available in capsule/tablet (0.4–0.52 g per pill) or powder forms (typically 2 g per tablespoon). A placebo-controlled study compared the effect of different dietary fiber supplements (carboxy-methylcellulose, gum arabic, and psyllium) in subjects with loose/liquid stool associated FI. After the 32-day treatment period, psyllium significantly decreased FI episodes compared with the placebo or other fiber groups.[11]

Recommended *total* daily fiber intake ranges depending on age from 21 to 30 g for adult women. Fiber should be added to the diet slowly to avoid bloating. Fiber's stool-bulking impact may exacerbate FI symptoms in women with decreased rectal compliance secondary to radiation, prior surgery, or proctitis.

Medications

Oral medications aim to optimize stool consistency and reduce frequency of bowel movements. Antidiarrheal medications improve diarrhea-associated FI. Loperamide (Imodium) is a synthetic opioid that inhibits intestinal peristalsis, increasing oral-cecal transit time and resting anal sphincter tone. In addition, it improves rectal perception and compliance.[14] Compared with placebo, loperamide was more effective for reducing urgency FI, with more people achieving full continence, improved symptoms, and fewer FI episodes.[15] Loperamide has fewer central nervous system side effects compared with diphenoxylate/atropine (Lomotil).[16] In a randomized, double-blind, placebo-controlled crossover trial examining the effectiveness of loperamide versus psyllium for reducing FI episodes, a significant reduction in FI episodes per week was found in both groups compared with baseline (loperamide 7.9–4.1, $P<.001$; psyllium 7.3–4.8, $P = .008$). Both interventions improved symptom severity and QOL with similar overall rates of adverse events; constipation was seen more in the loperamide group (29% loperamide vs 10% psyllium).[17]

A recent randomized controlled trial compared the use of loperamide to oral placebo and the use of anal sphincter exercise training with biofeedback to usual care (basic education with pamphlet) in 300 women with at least monthly FI (CAPABLe: Controlling Anal incontinence by Performing Anal Exercises with Biofeedback or Loperamide).[18] In the trial, there were 4 treatment arms: (1) oral placebo plus education only, (2) placebo plus anorectal manometry assisted biofeedback and pelvic floor muscle exercises, (3) loperamide plus education, and (4) loperamide and biofeedback/exercises. Using symptom severity and QOL impact changes from baseline to 24 weeks as the primary outcome, no significant differences were noted in the loperamide or manometry-directed biofeedback groups alone or in combination.[18] A planned secondary analysis of the CAPABLe trial demonstrated that greater baseline

FI symptom severity, being overweight, drug adherence, and FI subtypes were associated with treatment outcomes.[19]

Cholestyramine (2–6 g daily), a bile acid sequestrant, can be helpful as an adjunct therapy in patients with bile salt malabsorption or history of cholecystectomy. The medication is in a powder form, taken by mixing with 4 to 6 ounces of liquid at mealtime. Although not supported by placebo-controlled trials, clinical experience suggests anticholinergic medications such as hyoscyamine 0.125 to 0.25 mg, taken 30 to 60 minutes before meals, may be helpful in postprandial bowel leakage.[20] Given dose-dependent adverse events related to anticholinergics (dry mouth, dizziness, and blurred vision, fatigue, constipation), this medication should be avoided in older adults.

Amitriptyline prolongs colon transit time by decreasing rectal contractions in patients with idiopathic FI.[21,22] Clonidine, an α-2 adrenergic agonist, 0.1 mg twice daily, has been also used for the treatment of FI. However, a randomized controlled trial (RCT) on urgency-predominant FI reported that clonidine did not affect bowel symptoms, fecal continence, or anorectal functions, compared with placebo. Among patients with diarrhea, clonidine increased stool consistency and decreased diarrheal episodes, but not FI frequency.[23] The currently available supplements/medications and their level of evidence on the treatment of FI are listed in **Table 1**.

Pelvic Floor Muscle Exercises and Biofeedback

Pelvic muscle exercises and biofeedback alleviate FI symptoms by improving contraction of the pelvic floor muscles, sensory-motor coordination required for continence, and enhancing the ability to perceive rectal distension.[24] Pelvic floor muscle training is recommended for nearly all patients with FI, but no consensus exists on exercise regimen and the data are less established compared with urinary incontinence. Biofeedback is performed using anorectal manometry or surface electromyography (EMG). Biofeedback therapy focuses on 3 main targets:

1. Rectal sensitivity training: gradually distending a rectal balloon with air or water to help patients determine the sensation of rectal filling. In patients with higher

Table 1
Current evidence on medical treatment of fecal incontinence

Medication	Suggested Dose	Level of Evidence[a]	Recommendation Grade[b]
Fiber supplementation	2–6 g[c]	II	B
Loperamide	2–4 mg per dose up to 16 mg/d	II	B
Diphynoxylate (with atropine)	2.5-5 mg (0.025 mg) per dose up to 20 mg/d	II	B
Cholestyramine	2–6 g/d	III	C
Hyoscyamine	0.125–0.25 mg before meal	III	C
Amitriptyline	20 mg nightly	II	B
Clonidine	0.1 mg twice daily	II	C

[a] I: ≥1 properly randomized controlled trail available; II: evidence based on well-designed cohort or retrospective case-controlled studies; III: the evidence based on expert opinion or descriptive studies, case reports.
[b] A: strongly recommended; B: recommended; C: evidence is not sufficient to recommend for or against the therapy.
[c] Suggested total daily intake for adults is 25 to 35 g.

threshold, the training should focus on feeling the distention at lower volume to give a signal to get to the toilet sooner or squeeze muscles to prevent leakage. If the patient has a low threshold (low capacity, hypersensitive rectum), the goal is to focus on tolerating larger volumes.
2. Strength training: visual or auditory signals are used to aid in the muscle isolation and improve squeeze pressures.
3. Coordination training: focusing on coordinating rectal distention and anal sphincter contraction.

A lack of biofeedback standardization treatment likely contributes to a wide range in reported success rates of exercises ± biofeedback, from 38% to as high as 100%.[6,18,25–27] More recent RCTs with robust study designs have favored the addition of biofeedback to pelvic floor muscle training.[25,28–31] The current consensus among professional societies, such as the American College of Gastroenterology and the American Gastroenterological Association, is that biofeedback is a safe and effective approach and should be used especially in patients with weak sphincters and/or impaired rectal sensation.[6,26] The National Institutes of Health state of the science summary concluded that there is a need for long-term data for the benefit of biofeedback as well as standardizing therapy protocols.[13]

Devices and Office-Based Procedures

Anal plugs
Anal plugs are designed to temporarily occlude the anal canal to prevent stool leakage. Although existing studies suggest anal plugs may be difficult to tolerate based on a considerably high dropout rate (35%) for use, they may alleviate symptoms particularly in patients with impaired anal-rectal sensation and those who are institutionalized or immobilized. The Renew Insert is a disposable silicone anal insert, designed for self-insertion with an applicator and natural expulsion with a bowel movement, and may be better tolerated than prior anal inserts (**Fig. 1**). In a cohort of 91 subjects who intended to use the insert, 73 (80%) completed all 12 weeks of treatment ("completers"), whereas 85 (93%) completed at least 1 week of treatment (modified intention-to-treat [mITT] cohort). The study showed a significant reduction

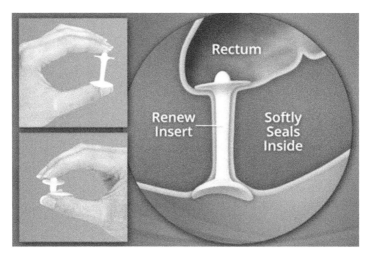

Fig. 1. Anal plug (renew insert). (*Courtesy of* Renew Medical, Foster City, CA.)

in FI frequency, 0.9 FI episodes per day at baseline to 0.2 episodes at 12 weeks (P<.001) in the mITT cohort. A ≥50% reduction in FI frequency was seen in 62% and 78% of the ITT and mITT cohorts, respectively. A significant reduction in the Wexner scores (16.2 baseline vs 10.9 with treatment, P<.001) was observed. Adverse events were seen in 51%; 98% of events were mild, such as anorectal urgency, irritation, gastrointestinal discomfort, gas, or hemorrhoids. Subjectively, 78% of completers were very or extremely satisfied with the device.[32]

Vaginal bowel control system

A vaginal bowel control system (Eclipse System) has been designed to provide a low-risk, effective, and easily reversible treatment for women with FI. The device consists of a silicone-coated base with an inflatable balloon and a hand-held pressure-regulated pump. The system is inserted into the vagina, like a pessary, with the balloon directed posteriorly. When the balloon is inflated, the vaginal wall occupies rectal space, preventing unwanted stool passage. Deflating the balloon allows stool passage, allowing patients to control their own bowel movements (**Fig. 2**). A prospective open-label study evaluated its effectiveness and safety. Of 110 subjects, 61 were

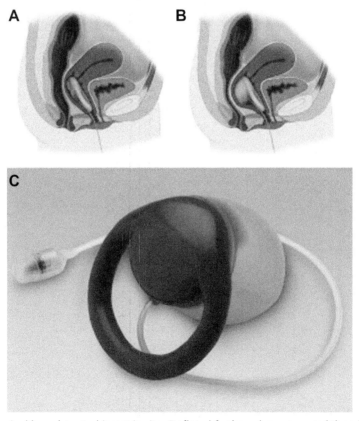

Fig. 2. Vaginal bowel-control insert in situ. Deflated for bowel movements (A) and inflated to prevent accidental passage of stool (B). Eclipse System (C). (*From* Pelvalon, Inc. The illustration was published in Obstetrics and Gynecology, Vol 125 (3), Richter HE Matthews CA, Takase-Sanchez MM, et al. A vaginal bowel-control system for the treatment of fecal incontinence, 540-7, Copyright: Wolters Kluwer Health, Inc. (2015); with permission.)

successfully fitted with the device and subsequently proceeded with a 4-week treatment period, during which 79% (ITT) and 86% (per protocol) reported a $\geq$50% reduction in FI episodes. Subjectively, 86% reported their bowel symptoms were very much or much better and a significant improvement in QOL was demonstrated using validated instruments. Mild to moderate adverse events (pelvic discomfort or pain, urinary symptoms, vaginal spotting or irritation) were observed in 47 of 110 participants, most during the fitting period. During the treatment period, adverse event rates were less common.[33] In an extended follow-up study (LIBERATE study), the primary outcome of 50% or greater reduction in baseline FI episodes at 3 months was 73% (ITT) and 84% (per protocol). Satisfaction rate remained high: 92% at 3 months, 90% at 6 months, and 94% at 12 months. On the Patient Global Impression of Improvement, 77% of patients at 3 months, 78% at 6 months, and 80% at 12 months reported that they were "very much" or "much better."[34]

Perianal injectables
Perianal injection of a bulking agent to increase the resting anal sphincter tone was first described in 1993. Before injectable therapy was available, the treatment for passive incontinence and IAS dysfunction was limited. Bulking materials into the submucosa or intersphincteric space increase the tissue volume in the high-pressure zone, especially in the proximal sphincter canal, creating a tighter seal at rest, and can target defective areas of the IAS, if present, to create canal symmetry. Of the bulking agents, non-animal stabilized hyaluronic acid/dextranomer (NASHA Dx, **Fig. 3**) has been most extensively studied for the treatment of FI refractory to conservative therapy (approved by the US Food and Drug Administration [FDA] in 2011). In the lithotomy, left-lateral, or prone position, 1 mL is injected into the deep submucosa through an anoscope at 4 sites (typically, 3, 6, 9, and 12 o'clock), slightly above the dentate line targeting the proximal part of the high-pressure zone. When the response is not satisfactory, a repeat injection can be administered after 4 weeks. Given the minimally invasive technique, this therapy is typically offered as an office procedure with significantly low morbidity.

A double-blinded RCT evaluating the short-term efficacy of NASHA Dx versus sham injections for FI demonstrated that 52% in the NASHA Dx group and 31% in the sham group achieved a $\geq$50% reduction in FI episodes. At 12 months, the treatment response increased to 69% in the NASHA Dx group. Interestingly, no difference was observed between the 2 groups at 3 months, suggesting a strong placebo effect for this population.[35,36] The study was extended to 36 months evaluating the long-term efficacy. Of the 136 patients randomized to the NASHA Dx group in the initial study, 82% (112 of 136) were available for the long-term assessment. Success rates (a $\geq$50% reduction in FI episodes) were sustained at 52.2% at 36 months of follow-up. Complete continence was seen in 13.2% at 36 months, increased from 6% at 6 months. Most patients (82% in the original study, 87% in the long-term follow-up study) received a second injection after 4 weeks from their initial treatment. No patients received further injections.[37] Common treatment-related adverse events were transient and minor bleeding, pain, and discomfort, mostly self-resolved. Of the 136 patients, only 2 had serious adverse events (abscesses) within 6 months, which were treated with antibiotics or surgical intervention. Adverse events unique to long-term follow-up (6–36 months) are injection site nodules seen in 2%.[35,36] Contraindications include active inflammatory bowel disease, previous anorectal radiation, full-thickness rectal prolapse, and anorectal malformations.

Although complete continence may not be achieved, perianal bulking therapy may be an effective and safe option to alleviate symptoms, especially in patients with mild to moderate passive FI.

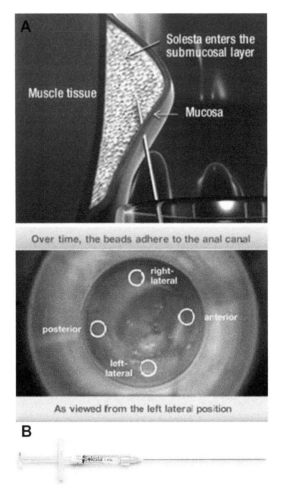

Fig. 3. (*A*) Dextranomer-microspheres in sodium hyaluronate gel injection (Solesta) and (*B*) injection syringe. (*Courtesy of* Palette Life Sciences, Santa Barbara, CA.)

Surgical Management

Innovative changes in the surgical treatment of FI have emerged over the past decade. Existing studies vary in the definition of treatment response (continence, frequency and number of incontinence episodes, symptom severity, and condition-specific QOL via questionnaires) making the interpretation and comparison of the results challenging. In general, surgery should be offered to patients who have failed a credible attempt of conservative therapies.

Sacral neuromodulation

Sacral neuromodulation (SNM) was first introduced in Europe in 1995 as a minimally invasive treatment for FI, and was approved by the FDA for chronic refractory FI in April 2011. The electrode is typically inserted in the S3 foramen to provide low-amplitude electrical current via a battery-operated stimulator. Proposed mechanisms of action include that SNM acts through a somato-visceral reflex pathway to reduce colonic activity, a direct effect on the anal sphincter complex to increase sphincter tone, reduce spontaneous sphincter relaxation, and change rectal sensitivity or compliance through afferent nerve modulation.[38–41] SNM is effective in patients with disrupted anal sphincters, including previously failed sphincteroplasty. Treatment outcomes appear to be independent of sphincter defect size, although the results are less predictable, and sample sizes are smaller in these studies.[42–45] SNM efficacy in patients with neurogenic bowel (FI due to nerve injury or neurologic conditions), appears to be good, although long-term data are lacking.[46,47]

SNM is a 2-step procedure: (1) testing phase with a temporary external neurostimulator, and (2) placement of a battery-operated implantable pulse generator (IPG). For the testing phase, the "staged trial" technique with a permanent lead placement is typically preferred to the percutaneous nerve evaluation (PNE) using a temporary monopolar lead. Although the PNE approach can be done in the office with local anesthesia, it is prone to incorrect lead placement and lead migration, especially in obese or active patients, and does not usually stay in place for the testing period (14 days) often required for patients with FI. Studies have shown high progression rates to IPG implantation with the staged procedure using a permanent lead.[48]

In the pivotal US multicenter trial including 133 patients undergoing SNM procedures for FI in 2010, 90% had a successful test stimulation and proceeded to the permanent implantation. At 12 months, 83% of the patients achieved therapeutic success, and 41% had complete continence. Incontinence episodes decreased from 9.4 episodes per week at baseline to 1.9 at 12 months, and 2.9 at 24 months.[49] In a sample of patients from this trial, FI episodes per week remained low (1.7) at 5 years, with 89% of the subjects having ≥50% symptomatic improvement and 36% achieving complete continence.[50] Sustained clinical benefit of up to 14 years has been demonstrated in more than 80% of SNM subjects.[51] The efficacy of medium-term to long-term follow-up studies are summarized in **Table 2**.

Most SNM adverse events (67%) occur within the first year of implantation, and most required none to minimal interventions such as medications. Common device-related adverse events are implant site pain (28%), paresthesia (15%), and changes in the sensation of stimulation (12%).[52] A meta-analysis of existing data has shown the rate of implant site pain to be much lower (6%).[53] Pain is usually managed conservatively by reprogramming the device, medication, or no treatment. In some cases, revision or explantation of the IPG and/or the lead may be required.[52–55] With advancements in the lead design and techniques, infection rates are generally low (3%–11%)[49,52,56] and explantation of the device is rarely necessary (3%–4%).[53,57] Because of its minimally invasive surgical technique, high success rates, and minimal morbidity, SNM is the preferred surgical approach for FI treatment.[42,56,58,59]

Most SNM efficacy and safety data on FI treatment are from InterStim (Medtronic, Inc., Minneapolis, MN), the first SNM system approved for the treatment of refractory chronic FI, and the second-generation, InterStimII. The original InterStim systems were not compatible with MRI and had some issues related to durability and size of IPG. To overcome these challenges, a new miniaturized rechargeable SNM system was introduced by Axonics (Axonics Modulation Technologies, Inc., Irvine, CA) in September 2019. Compared with the InterStim system (InterStimII, model 3058), which only allowed for head MRI scan (1.5-T horizontal closed bore with radiofrequency transmit head coil only), the Axonics rechargeable SNM system allows full-body MRI (1.5 T and 3 T). In August 2020, Medtronic also obtained the FDA clearance for their miniature rechargeable version of the InterStim (InterStim Micro) as well as the new lead (InterStim SureScan), which allows full-body MRI like the Axonics system. A summarized comparison of the SNM systems (**Fig. 4**) is shown in **Table 3**.

Table 2
Sacral neuromodulation efficacy in medium-term to long-term follow-up studies

Author, Year	Median Follow-up	Number of Subjects	FI Episodes per Week		≥50% Reduction in FI Episodes (%)		Complete Continence (%)	
			Baseline	Post-Therapy	Per Protocol	ITT*	Per Protocol	ITT
Matzel et al,[55] 2004	24	30	16	2	88	81	35	32
Gourcerol et al,[47] 2007	12	29	5	1	69	33	21	10
Tan et al, 2007	12	53	10	3	—	—	—	—
Holzer et al,[46] 2007	35	29	2	1	—	—	—	—
Melenhorst et al, 2007	36	33	10	2	79	59	—	—
Melenhorst et al, 2007	48	15	10	2	—	—	—	—
Melenhorst et al, 2007	60	10	10	2	—	—	—	—
Tjandra et al, 2008	12	53	10	3	71	63	47	42
Munoz-Duyos et al, 2008	36	29	1	0	86	58	48	33
El-Gazzaz et al, 2009	28	24	5	2	77	53	—	—
Govaert et al, 2009	35	169	—	—	—	—	—	—
Dudding et al, 2009	51	18	6	0	94	—	39	—
Altomare et al, 2009	74	52	4	1	—	—	18	10
Matzel et al,[51] 2009	118	9	9	0	78	58	44	33
Wexner et al,[49] 2010	12	106	9	1	83	66	—	—
Koch et al, 2010	24	35	11	2	—	—	21	11
Michelsen et al, 2010	24	126	8	1	—	—	—	—
Oom et al, 2010	32	37	9	0	81	65	5	4
Ratto et al,[44] 2010	33	10	26	1	—	—	—	—
Lombardi et al, 2010	46	11	5	1	100	—	27	—
Boyle et al, 2011	17	37	7	1	73	54	46	40
Hollingshead et al, 2011	33	86	9	1	83	—	—	—

Mellgren et al,[52] 2011	36	77	9	2	86	59	40	26
Uludağ et al, 2011	85	50	8	0	84	—	—	—
Santoro et al, 2012	18	16	14	0	—	—	68	68
Duelund-Jakobsen et al, 2012	46	147	6	1	75	—	36	—
Devroede et al, 2012	48	77	9	2	87	50	34	20
George et al, 2012	114	23	9	2	—	—	52	48
Hull et al,[50] 2013	60	72	9	2	89	—	36	—

Abbreviation: ITT, intention to treat.

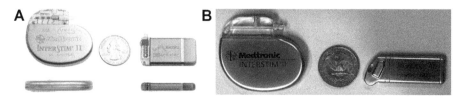

Fig. 4. (A) InterStim II IPG (non-rechargeable, left) and Axonics rechargeable SNM (right). (B) InterStim II IPG (non-rechargeable, left) and InterStim Micro (rechargeable, right). ([A] From Neurourol Urodyn. 37(S2), Elterman DS, A novel Axonics® rechargeable sacral neuromodulation system: Procedural and technical impressions from an initial North American experience, S1-8, Copyright (2018), with permission from John Wiley and Sons.)

SNM safety and efficacy in pregnancy has not been established. SNM data on use in pregnancy are derived from retrospective studies or case series with a small number of women with urinary complaints.[60,61] Due to lack of evidence, women who are attempting conception or are pregnant are advised to turn off their neurostimulator.

Sphincteroplasty

FI may result from anal sphincter disruption, often noted in the anterior segment following obstetric trauma.[62] Obstetric anal sphincter injury should be recognized and repaired at the time of delivery. The existing data comparing overlapping versus end-to-end repair of third-degree and fourth-degree obstetric laceration repairs at the time of delivery are conflicting. For immediate repair with no scar present, most studies show that the 2 approaches do not differ in surgical outcomes.[63,64] More recently, a randomized trial by Farrell and colleagues[65] reported that end-to-end repairs of complete third-degree and fourth-degree obstetric lacerations are associated with significantly lower rates of anal incontinence at 12 months. However, no differences were observed over 3 years.

Chronic sphincter disruptions can result from unrecognized injuries at the time of childbirth, perineal repair breakdown, or persistent injuries after the primary repair.[66] Sphincter plication is effective in the short-term, with 70% to 80% of patients reporting

Table 3			
Comparison of currently available sacral neuromodulation (SNM) products			
Manufacturer	Medtronic		Axonics
Product Name	InterStim II with Sure Scan lead	InterStim Micro	Rechargeable SNM system
FDA approval	August 2020		September 2019
Rechargeable	No charging needed	Yes	Yes
Charging time	None	Weekly to monthly	Weekly to monthly
Battery life	5+ y	15+ y	15+ y
Implant weight size	22g	7g	11g
Volume	14 mL	3mL	5mL
Amplitude control	Voltage controlled		Constant current
MRI	1.5 T and 3 T head full body		1.5 and 3 T[a] head full body

[a] Initial approval was 1.5 T only, subsequently approved for both 1.5 T and 3 T in July 2020.

symptom improvement, but success rates generally deteriorate over time, with most studies demonstrating improvement in less than 50% (as low as 10%–14%) over 5 years.[62–64,67] Existing data on the long-term efficacy of sphincteroplasty from a systematic review are shown in **Fig. 5**. The most common complication is wound infection (2%–35%), and deep infection results in poor long-term outcomes.[67–69] Other factors associated with long-term failure include advanced age at the time of repair, duration of FI symptoms, and pudendal neuropathy, although the link between pudendal neuropathy and FI is controversial.[68,69]

The current consensus regarding surgical repair of sphincter disruption remote from delivery[6,42] is as follows:

1. Obvious anatomic defects, such as cloacalike deformity with severe perineal body defect or fistula should be corrected.
2. Sphincteroplasty may be offered to symptomatic patients with a defined defect of the EAS to restore the circumferential anatomy.
3. Repeat sphincter reconstruction after a failed overlapping sphincteroplasty should generally be avoided.
4. Preoperative anorectal manometry has a limited role in predicting surgical success.
5. Diagnosis of a sphincter defect on imaging studies, most commonly with endoanal ultrasound, is recommended before surgical correction.

The traditional sphincteroplasty is performed via a curvilinear incision made in the perineum on the outer edge of the EAS in the plane between the rectum and vagina. To avoid pudendal nerve injury posteriorly, care should be taken not to extend the dissection laterally beyond 180° circumference of the anus. The sphincter muscles are typically divided through scar anteriorly if present, then plicated in an overlapping fashion to narrow the canal. When disrupted, both internal and external sphincters are mobilized en bloc to create the overlapping repair. Separate dissection of the internal and external sphincters does not provide better function postoperatively and should be avoided.[70,71] Levator muscle plication or posterior colporrhaphy are often performed at the time of sphincteroplasty to restore the anatomy.

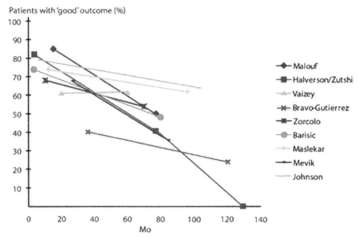

Fig. 5. Long-term efficacy outcomes of sphincteroplasty. (*From* Diseases of the Colon & Rectum, Vol 55, Glasgow SC and Lowry AC, Long-term Outcomes of Anal Sphincter Repair for Fecal Incontinence: A Systematic Review, 482-490, Copyright: Wolters Kluwer Health, Inc. (2012); with permission.)

Artificial bowel sphincter

The artificial bowel sphincter consists of an inflatable cuff implanted around the anal canal with a pressure-regulating balloon placed in the prevesical space and a pump in the labia connecting the cuff and balloon. Patients can inflate the cuff to prevent stool passage and deflate to allow defecation. These devices, although effective in some patients, have high rates of complications requiring surgical intervention (80%–90%) and are removed in approximately 50% of patients.[72–75] The most common reason for surgical revision is device malfunction, such as micro-perforation or cuff leak; device erosion and infection are the most common reasons for device removal.[75]

Fecal diversion

A colostomy or ileostomy is a definitive option when other treatments have failed or are unsuitable. Early discussion regarding treatment options, including diversion, is helpful to cope with possible lifestyle changes in patients with severe FI. People with an ostomy can be very active in their social and professional lives. Most activities, including sports, can be performed with minimal modifications. Ostomy does not appear to affect sexual function. Both general and disease-specific QOL improve after colostomy, including improvement in social function, coping, embarrassment, lifestyle, and depression.[76] Those patients with FI who opt for a stoma feel positively about having a stoma and have high satisfaction with the stoma (median score of 9 on a scale of 0–10). Most (83%) reported the stoma restricted their life "a little" or "not at all" with significant improvement from their previous incontinence.[77] Fecal diversion via laparoscopy is a safe and effective option with decreased morbidity, such as reduced postoperative pain, ileus, and the length of hospital stay.[6,78,79] Although considered a last resort, diverting ostomy can ameliorate symptoms and improve QOL in women with severe refractory FI.

Other Treatments: Experimental Therapies

Other treatment options have been described and evaluated for the treatment of FI, but have lack of evidence to support their use or are not approved for use by the FDA. These therapies include posterior tibial nerve stimulation, radiofrequency ablation, anal sling, magnetic anal sphincter, and dynamic graciloplasty.

SUMMARY

FI is a physically and psychosocially debilitating condition that negatively impacts QOL. Despite a high prevalence rate, many women are reluctant to report symptoms and seek care, and feel that there is little to do for their condition. Health care providers often fail to screen for FI because of their limited awareness of its prevalence and lack of clinical experience evaluating and treating it.

FI etiology is often multifactorial, and conservative measures improve symptoms for many. Prevention and early intervention should focus on eliminating potential modifiable risk factors and identifying women suffering from FI at earlier stages to avoid worsening symptoms. Management consists of conservative and surgical approaches, and more invasive therapies are reserved for patients with refractory conditions. Traditionally, treatment options were limited once patients failed conservative therapies. FI surgery was considered invasive with high complication rates, and the success rates deteriorated over time. However, recent research has provided additional data on existing treatments as well as the development of less invasive options and new investigational treatments. Further RCTs evaluating long-term efficacy and safety of each modality, as well as well-designed comparative studies of available options, and the effectiveness of combination therapies are still needed to solidify a management algorithm for FI. Future research should focus on the cost-effectiveness of current therapies, as direct and indirect costs associated with FI are substantial. The optimal FI treatment regimen is often a combination of various conservative and surgical approaches. Health care providers should individualize FI management using evidence-based practice.

CLINICS CARE POINTS

- FI, or accidental bowel leakage, is a highly prevalent and debilitating condition associated with profound psychosocial consequences.
- As many women are reluctant to report their accidental bowel leakage symptoms to health care professionals, it is important to screen for FI.
- FI is often multifactorial, thus the management should be individualized based on the patient's clinical history and goals of therapy.
- Conservative approaches including dietary modification and pharmacologic treatment are quite effective, and can be offered without extensive diagnostic testing.
- More research is needed to solidify a management algorithm for FI, including conservative, pharmacologic, and surgical approaches.

FINANCIAL DISCLAIMER/CONFLICT OF INTEREST

I. Meyer: nothing to disclose. .H.E. Richter: Renovia-research funding.

REFERENCES

1. Ng KS, Sivakumaran Y, Nassar N, et al. Fecal incontinence: community prevalence and associated factors–a systematic review. Dis Colon Rectum 2015;58: 1194–209.
2. Menees SB, Almario CV, Spiegel BMR, et al. Prevalence of and factors associated with fecal incontinence: results from a population-based survey. Gastroenterology 2018;154:1672–81.e3.
3. Matthews CA, Whitehead WE, Townsend MK, et al. Risk factors for urinary, fecal, or dual incontinence in the Nurses' Health Study. Obstet Gynecol 2013;122: 539–45.
4. Dunivan GC, Heymen S, Palsson OS, et al. Fecal incontinence in primary care: prevalence, diagnosis, and health care utilization. Am J Obstet Gynecol 2010; 202:493.e1-6.
5. Johanson JF, Lafferty J. Epidemiology of fecal incontinence: the silent affliction. Am J Gastroenterol 1996;91:33–6.
6. Rao SS, Committee ACoGPP. Diagnosis and management of fecal incontinence. American College of Gastroenterology Practice Parameters Committee. Am J Gastroenterol 2004;99:1585–604.
7. Cichowski SB, Dunivan GC, Rogers RG, et al. Patients' experience compared with physicians' recommendations for treating fecal incontinence: a qualitative approach. Int Urogynecol J 2014;25:935–40.
8. Brown HW, Wexner SD, Segall MM, et al. Accidental bowel leakage in the mature women's health study: prevalence and predictors. Int J Clin Pract 2012;66: 1101–8.

9. Saad RJ, Rao SS, Koch KL, et al. Do stool form and frequency correlate with whole-gut and colonic transit? Results from a multicenter study in constipated individuals and healthy controls. Am J Gastroenterol 2010;105:403–11.

10. Hoke TP, Meyer I, Blanchard CT, et al. Characterization of symptom severity and impact on four fecal incontinence phenotypes in women presenting for evaluation. Neurourol Urodyn 2020;40(1):237–44.

11. Bliss DZ, Savik K, Jung HJ, et al. Dietary fiber supplementation for fecal incontinence: a randomized clinical trial. Res Nurs Health 2014;37:367–78.

12. Eswaran S, Muir J, Chey WD. Fiber and functional gastrointestinal disorders. Am J Gastroenterol 2013;108:718–27.

13. Whitehead WE, Rao SS, Lowry A, et al. Treatment of fecal incontinence: state of the science summary for the National Institute of Diabetes and Digestive and Kidney Diseases Workshop. Am J Gastroenterol 2015;110:138–46.

14. Read M, Read NW, Barber DC, et al. Effects of loperamide on anal sphincter function in patients complaining of chronic diarrhea with fecal incontinence and urgency. Dig Dis Sci 1982;27:807–14.

15. Omar MI, Alexander CE. Drug treatment for faecal incontinence in adults. Cochrane Database Syst Rev 2013;6:CD002116.

16. Palmer KR, Corbett CL, Holdsworth CD. Double-blind cross-over study comparing loperamide, codeine and diphenoxylate in the treatment of chronic diarrhea. Gastroenterology 1980;79:1272–5.

17. Markland AD, Burgio KL, Whitehead WE, et al. Loperamide versus psyllium fiber for treatment of fecal incontinence: The Fecal Incontinence Prescription (Rx) Management (FIRM) Randomized Clinical Trial. Dis Colon Rectum 2015;58:983–93.

18. Jelovsek JE, Markland AD, Whitehead WE, et al. Controlling faecal incontinence in women by performing anal exercises with biofeedback or loperamide: a randomised clinical trial. Lancet Gastroenterol Hepatol 2019;4:698–710.

19. Richter HE, Jelovsek JE, Iyer P, et al. Characteristics associated with clinically important treatment responses in women undergoing nonsurgical therapy for fecal incontinence. Am J Gastroenterol 2020;115:115–27.

20. Trinkley KE, Nahata MC. Medication management of irritable bowel syndrome. Digestion 2014;89:253–67.

21. Ehrenpreis ED, Chang D, Eichenwald E. Pharmacotherapy for fecal incontinence: a review. Dis Colon Rectum 2007;50:641–9.

22. Wang JY, Abbas MA. Current management of fecal incontinence. Perm J 2013;17:65–73.

23. Bharucha AE, Fletcher JG, Camilleri M, et al. Effects of clonidine in women with fecal incontinence. Clin Gastroenterol Hepatol 2014;12:843–51.e842 [quiz: e844].

24. Byrne CM, Solomon MJ, Young JM, et al. Biofeedback for fecal incontinence: short-term outcomes of 513 consecutive patients and predictors of successful treatment. Dis Colon Rectum 2007;50:417–27.

25. Norton C, Cody JD. Biofeedback and/or sphincter exercises for the treatment of faecal incontinence in adults. Cochrane Database Syst Rev 2012;7:CD002111.

26. Madoff RD, Parker SC, Varma MG, et al. Faecal incontinence in adults. Lancet 2004;364:621–32.

27. Parker CH, Henry S, Liu LWC. Efficacy of biofeedback therapy in clinical practice for the management of chronic constipation and fecal incontinence. J Can Assoc Gastroenterol 2019;2:126–31.

28. Norton C, Chelvanayagam S, Wilson-Barnett J, et al. Randomized controlled trial of biofeedback for fecal incontinence. Gastroenterology 2003;125:1320–9.

29. Heymen S, Scarlett Y, Jones K, et al. Randomized controlled trial shows biofeedback to be superior to pelvic floor exercises for fecal incontinence. Dis Colon Rectum 2009;52:1730–7.

30. Solomon MJ, Pager CK, Rex J, et al. Randomized, controlled trial of biofeedback with anal manometry, transanal ultrasound, or pelvic floor retraining with digital guidance alone in the treatment of mild to moderate fecal incontinence. Dis Colon Rectum 2003;46:703–10.

31. Bols E, Berghmans B, de Bie R, et al. Rectal balloon training as add-on therapy to pelvic floor muscle training in adults with fecal incontinence: a randomized controlled trial. Neurourol Urodyn 2012;31:132–8.

32. Lukacz ES, Segall MM, Wexner SD. Evaluation of an anal insert device for the conservative management of fecal incontinence. Dis Colon Rectum 2015;58: 892–8.

33. Richter HE, Matthews CA, Muir T, et al. A vaginal bowel-control system for the treatment of fecal incontinence. Obstet Gynecol 2015;125:540–7.

34. Richter HE, Dunivan G, Brown HW, et al. A 12-month clinical durability of effectiveness and safety evaluation of a vaginal bowel control system for the nonsurgical treatment of fecal incontinence. Female Pelvic Med Reconstr Surg 2019;25: 113–9.

35. Maeda Y, Laurberg S, Norton C. Perianal injectable bulking agents as treatment for faecal incontinence in adults. Cochrane Database Syst Rev 2013;2: CD007959.

36. Graf W, Mellgren A, Matzel KE, et al. Efficacy of dextranomer in stabilised hyaluronic acid for treatment of faecal incontinence: a randomised, sham-controlled trial. Lancet 2011;377:997–1003.

37. Mellgren A, Matzel KE, Pollack J, et al. Long-term efficacy of NASHA Dx injection therapy for treatment of fecal incontinence. Neurogastroenterol Motil 2014;26(8): 1087–94.

38. Patton V, Wiklendt L, Arkwright JW, et al. The effect of sacral nerve stimulation on distal colonic motility in patients with faecal incontinence. Br J Surg 2013;100: 959–68.

39. Uludağ O, Koch SM, van Gemert WG, et al. Sacral neuromodulation in patients with fecal incontinence: a single-center study. Dis Colon Rectum 2004;47:1350–7.

40. Kenefick NJ, Vaizey CJ, Cohen RC, et al. Medium-term results of permanent sacral nerve stimulation for faecal incontinence. Br J Surg 2002;89:896–901.

41. Vaizey CJ, Kamm MA, Turner IC, et al. Effects of short term sacral nerve stimulation on anal and rectal function in patients with anal incontinence. Gut 1999;44: 407–12.

42. Matzel KE. Sacral nerve stimulation for faecal incontinence: its role in the treatment algorithm. Colorectal Dis 2011;13(Suppl 2):10–4.

43. Melenhorst J, Koch SM, Uludag O, et al. Is a morphologically intact anal sphincter necessary for success with sacral nerve modulation in patients with faecal incontinence? Colorectal Dis 2008;10:257–62.

44. Ratto C, Litta F, Parello A, et al. Sacral nerve stimulation is a valid approach in fecal incontinence due to sphincter lesions when compared to sphincter repair. Dis Colon Rectum 2010;53:264–72.

45. Jarrett ME, Dudding TC, Nicholls RJ, et al. Sacral nerve stimulation for fecal incontinence related to obstetric anal sphincter damage. Dis Colon Rectum 2008;51:531–7.

46. Holzer B, Rosen HR, Novi G, et al. Sacral nerve stimulation for neurogenic faecal incontinence. Br J Surg 2007;94:749–53.
47. Gourcerol G, Gallas S, Michot F, et al. Sacral nerve stimulation in fecal incontinence: are there factors associated with success? Dis Colon Rectum 2007; 50:3–12.
48. Baxter C, Kim JH. Contrasting the percutaneous nerve evaluation versus staged implantation in sacral neuromodulation. Curr Urol Rep 2010;11:310–4.
49. Wexner SD, Coller JA, Devroede G, et al. Sacral nerve stimulation for fecal incontinence: results of a 120-patient prospective multicenter study. Ann Surg 2010; 251:441–9.
50. Hull T, Giese C, Wexner SD, et al. Long-term durability of sacral nerve stimulation therapy for chronic fecal incontinence. Dis Colon Rectum 2013;56:234–45.
51. Matzel KE, Lux P, Heuer S, et al. Sacral nerve stimulation for faecal incontinence: long-term outcome. Colorectal Dis 2009;11:636–41.
52. Mellgren A, Wexner SD, Coller JA, et al. Long-term efficacy and safety of sacral nerve stimulation for fecal incontinence. Dis Colon Rectum 2011;54:1065–75.
53. Tan E, Ngo NT, Darzi A, et al. Meta-analysis: sacral nerve stimulation versus conservative therapy in the treatment of faecal incontinence. Int J Colorectal Dis 2011;26:275–94.
54. Tjandra JJ, Lim JF, Matzel K. Sacral nerve stimulation: an emerging treatment for faecal incontinence. ANZ J Surg 2004;74:1098–106.
55. Matzel KE, Kamm MA, Stösser M, et al. Sacral spinal nerve stimulation for faecal incontinence: multicentre study. Lancet 2004;363:1270–6.
56. Tan EK, Vaizey C, Cornish J, et al. Surgical strategies for faecal incontinence–a decision analysis between dynamic graciloplasty, artificial bowel sphincter and end stoma. Colorectal Dis 2008;10:577–86.
57. Chiarioni G, Palsson OS, Asteria CR, et al. Neuromodulation for fecal incontinence: an effective surgical intervention. World J Gastroenterol 2013;19:7048–54.
58. Wong MT, Meurette G, Rodat F, et al. Outcome and management of patients in whom sacral nerve stimulation for fecal incontinence failed. Dis Colon Rectum 2011;54:425–32.
59. Brown SR, Nelson RL. Surgery for faecal incontinence in adults. Cochrane Database Syst Rev 2007;(2):CD001757.
60. Wiseman OJ, v d Hombergh U, Koldewijn EL, et al. Sacral neuromodulation and pregnancy. J Urol 2002;167:165–8.
61. Khunda A, Karmarkar R, Abtahi B, et al. Pregnancy in women with Fowler's syndrome treated with sacral neuromodulation. Int Urogynecol J 2013;24:1201–4.
62. Anandam JL. Surgical management for fecal incontinence. Clin Colon Rectal Surg 2014;27:106–9.
63. Tjandra JJ, Han WR, Goh J, et al. Direct repair vs. overlapping sphincter repair: a randomized, controlled trial. Dis Colon Rectum 2003;46:937–42 [discussion: 942–3].
64. Garcia V, Rogers RG, Kim SS, et al. Primary repair of obstetric anal sphincter laceration: a randomized trial of two surgical techniques. Am J Obstet Gynecol 2005;192:1697–701.
65. Farrell SA, Flowerdew G, Gilmour D, et al. Overlapping compared with end-to-end repair of complete third-degree or fourth-degree obstetric tears: three-year follow-up of a randomized controlled trial. Obstet Gynecol 2012;120:803–8.
66. Bradley CS, Richter HE, Gutman RE, et al. Pelvic floor disorders N: risk factors for sonographic internal anal sphincter gaps 6-12 months after delivery complicated by anal sphincter tear. Am J Obstet Gynecol 2007;197:310 e311–315.

67. Sung VW, Rogers ML, Myers DL, et al. National trends and costs of surgical treatment for female fecal incontinence. Am J Obstet Gynecol 2007;197:652.e1-5.
68. Glasgow SC, Lowry AC. Long-term outcomes of anal sphincter repair for fecal incontinence: a systematic review. Dis Colon Rectum 2012;55:482–90.
69. Oom DM, Gosselink MP, Schouten WR. Anterior sphincteroplasty for fecal incontinence: a single center experience in the era of sacral neuromodulation. Dis Colon Rectum 2009;52:1681–7.
70. Oberwalder M, Dinnewitzer A, Baig MK, et al. Do internal anal sphincter defects decrease the success rate of anal sphincter repair? Tech Coloproctol 2006;10: 94–7 [discussion: 97].
71. Wexner SD, Marchetti F, Jagelman DG. The role of sphincteroplasty for fecal incontinence reevaluated: a prospective physiologic and functional review. Dis Colon Rectum 1991;34:22–30.
72. van der Wilt AA, Breukink SO, Sturkenboom R, et al. The artificial bowel sphincter in the treatment of fecal incontinence, long-term complications. Dis Colon Rectum 2020;63:1134–41.
73. Wong MT, Meurette G, Wyart V, et al. The artificial bowel sphincter: a single institution experience over a decade. Ann Surg 2011;254:951–6.
74. Mundy L, Merlin TL, Maddern GJ, et al. Systematic review of safety and effectiveness of an artificial bowel sphincter for faecal incontinence. Br J Surg 2004;91: 665–72.
75. Hong KD, Dasilva G, Kalaskar SN, et al. Long-term outcomes of artificial bowel sphincter for fecal incontinence: a systematic review and meta-analysis. J Am Coll Surg 2013;217:718–25.
76. Colquhoun P, Kaiser R, Efron J, et al. Is the quality of life better in patients with colostomy than patients with fecal incontinence? World J Surg 2006;30:1925–8.
77. Norton C, Burch J, Kamm MA. Patients' views of a colostomy for fecal incontinence. Dis Colon Rectum 2005;48:1062–9.
78. Ludwig KA, Milsom JW, Garcia-Ruiz A, et al. Laparoscopic techniques for fecal diversion. Dis Colon Rectum 1996;39:285–8.
79. Lyerly HK, Mault JR. Laparoscopic ileostomy and colostomy. Ann Surg 1994;219: 317–22.

Telemedicine in Urogynecology

Miriam C. Toaff, MD, MS[a], Cara L. Grimes, MD, MAS[b],*

KEYWORDS

- Telemedicine • Telehealth • Urogynecology • FPMRS • COVID-19
- Mobile applications

KEY POINTS

- Telemedicine makes care accessible and can provide a high standard of care to patients of all ages.
- There are many diagnoses that can be managed appropriately via telemedicine.
- Even with diagnoses that do require in-person care, telemedicine can be used to collect new patient and historical data before an in-person visit.

INTRODUCTION

Telehealth is becoming increasingly more prominent in United States health care. Spurred by necessity at times, such as during the coronavirus disease 2019 (COVID-19) pandemic or in rural settings, care through telehealth addresses the need for more cost-effective, patient-centered care.[1] It is estimated that telehealth could save $4 million annually in health care costs in the United States.[2] Additionally, telehealth may minimize referrals to specialists, decrease the burden of chronic disease, and streamline care for patients of all types.[2]

DEFINITIONS

The terms telehealth, telemedicine, and virtual care generally refer to the exchange of medical information from one site to another through electronic communication to improve a patient's health.[3] Although often used interchangeably, telehealth, telemedicine, and virtual care are different (**Box 1**). Telehealth, a broader term, refers to the use of virtual platforms to facilitate patient care, education, monitoring, and prevention. It includes many digital platforms that can be used by clinicians and patients for education, wellness, and decision-making, in addition to platforms that allow remote education and meetings.[4] Telemedicine more specifically refers to direct patient care that

[a] PGY-3, Obstetrics and Gynecology, New York Medical College, 19 Bradhurst Avenue, Hawthorne, NY 10532, USA; [b] Obstetrics and Gynecology and Urology, New York Medical College, 19 Bradhurst Avenue, Hawthorne, NY 10532, USA
* Corresponding author.
E-mail address: caragrimesmd@gmail.com

Obstet Gynecol Clin N Am 48 (2021) 487–499
https://doi.org/10.1016/j.ogc.2021.05.004
0889-8545/21/© 2021 Elsevier Inc. All rights reserved.
obgyn.theclinics.com

Box 1
Definitions

- *Telehealth*: The use of virtual technology in medicine with a wide range of clinical objectives, including, but limited to, patient care, remote monitoring, education, health information management, and clinical decision-making.
- *Virtual care*: The interactions between providers and patients using virtual platforms to facilitate consistent and effective patient care.
- *Telemedicine*: The direct provision of care using virtual technology to connect to patient and provider.

---

uses electronic interfaces to connect provider and patient.[2] Virtual care, another broad term, refers to any interaction between providers and patients using virtual communication or technology to improve the quality and effectiveness of patient care. Virtual care includes messaging between patient and provider, remote monitoring of patients, and communication between all members of the health care team to provide continuity and accessibility of care.[5]

This article discusses the use of telemedicine in female pelvic medicine and reconstructive surgery. These patients are typically older, often have more comorbidities than other groups of patients, and may have limited access to transportation, making them an ideal population to care for with telemedicine. During the COVID-19 pandemic, they represented a population vulnerable to infection with COVID-19; telemedicine decreases their exposure to COVID.[6] Because the management of many pelvic disorders is considered elective, during times where travel for care is not recommended, it is essential to use resources effectively and determine how patients can be best served. Telemedicine services can typically be provided via 3 modalities (**Table 1**).[1,2,6,7]

REGULATORY, REIMBURSEMENT, AND ETHICAL CONCERNS
Licensure

The Interstate Medical Licensure Compact, which launched in 2017, was an agreement among multiple states allowing physicians who are licensed in their states and meet specific qualifications as defined by the compact to gain eligibility for licensure in the other states in the compact. Twenty-nine states participated in the Interstate Medical Licensure Compact, which streamlined licensing for providers to treat across state lines while maintaining individual state laws with which providers were required to comply in the state their patient was located. However, in response to the COVID-19 pandemic, the majority of states have revised their policies and allow providers to offer telemedicine services to patients in any state.[8,9] How long these revised policies will continue varies among states, and providers should seek guidance from their specific state medical board.

Reimbursement

On March 17, 2020, the Centers for Medicare and Medicaid Services released a Medicare Telemedicine Health Care Provider fact sheet that provides some guidance on providing telehealth services. Under Waiver 1135, Medicare can pay for office, hospital, and other visits furnished via telehealth across the country and including in patient's places of residence starting on March 6, 2020.[3] The Center for Medicare and Medicaid Services recognizes 3 types of telemedicine services: Medicare telehealth visits, virtual check-in, and e-visits (**Table 2**).

Table 1
Three telemedicine modalities

	Synchronous	Asynchronous	Remote Monitoring
Definition	Phone/video technology to have real-time interactions with patients located at a distance	"Store and forward" method in which one site has diagnostic equipment, and collects images, laboratory tests, videos, etc, which are transmitted to a remote provider	Evaluation of patient via review of laboratory tests, imaging, and clinical data from wearable patient monitoring systems (such as continuous glucose monitor or Holter monitor)/through direct streaming video of patients
Benefits	Interactions similar to in- person visits, resembling "physician- patient" relationship Decrease cost Decreases time Comfortable visits in at-home space	Improve access to specialists "Match" specialty providers to patients with complex medical issues Reduce delays in care Easier scheduling Decrease language and cultural barriers	Allows providers to review a range of clinical information, as opposed to just a "snapshot" in time No scheduling coordination between provider and patient needed Information can be accessed at providers convenience
Drawbacks	Requires fast/secure connections Key health measurements may be missed Patient's may seek unnecessary care owing to ease of access	No established quality standards for transmission of video, images, and audio No real-time communication with provider and patients	No real-time communication with patient If clinically significant data are encountered, it requires provider to communicate with the patient urgently, which may not be immediately feasible

Medicaid reimbursement remains under control of the state law. In response to the pandemic, many states have expanded their Medicaid coverage to reimburse telemedicine at standard rates; however, the amount of compensation and the type of services that can be compensated for is variable.[8] Unfortunately, significant variability among private insurers exists as well. Telehealth parity laws that ensure equal compensation for analogous services provided via telemedicine only exist in 22% of the states. Some states, such as California, have enacted new telehealth parity laws; however, they did not go into effect until January 2021.[10,11]

There are a number of additional modifications that Medicare, many states' Medicaid, and private insurers have made in response to the COVID-19 pandemic. In the past, some payers required that patients have an established relationship before offering telemedicine. However, many have now allowed providers to virtually establish new relationships with patients.[8,9] Additionally, many states had policies that limited reimbursement based on the form of telemedicine provided. In efforts to increase accessibility, many payers are now offering reimbursement for a variety of

Table 2
Telemedicine services recognized by Medicare

Type of Service	Definition	Patient-Provider Relationship	Reimbursement
Medicare telehealth visits	Use of telemedicine modalities, including both audio and videos, for office, hospital visits and other in-person services	New/established patients (previously limited to established patient; however, the 1135 waiver will not conduct audits on claims submitted during the COVID-19 pandemic)	HCPCS/CPT codes, reimbursed the same as in-person visit
Virtual check-in	A 5- to 10-minutc check in with provider via telephone or exchange of images through video/ photographs to decide if in person or telemedicine visit is warranted	Established patients must be educated on the availability of this type of service beforehand	HCPCS codes depending on what is transmitted (recorded videos/images or brief communication) Bill only if unrelated to a previous visit within the last 7 d and does not lead to a visit within the next 24 h
E-Visits	Patient-initiated communication via a patient portal for evaluation/ management of patient concerns	Established patients must be educated on the availability of this type of service beforehand	CPT codes used to bill for cumulative time used in digital evaluation over a period of 7 d

Abbreviations: CPT, Current Procedural Terminology; HCPCS, Healthcare Common Procedure Coding System.

modalities, including audio and video. Finally, Medicare, many state Medicaid programs, and many private insurers have increased their flexibility regarding cost sharing with patients, allowing providers to choose to reduce or waive cost sharing (copays, coinsurance, and deductibles) for telemedicine services.[3,12]

Privacy

In response to the COVID-19 pandemic, the federal government changed the restrictions on the types of applications that can be used for telemedicine. Providers are encouraged to use platforms that are compliant with the Health Insurance Portability and Accountability Act of 1996, such as Doxy.me and Zoom for Healthcare. However, to improve access, the Office for Civil Rights has liberalized their enforcement of the Portability and Accountability Act of 1996 through the provision of telemedicine services in good faith. Providers are now permitted to use any "non-public–facing" platform—video, voice, and texting platforms—that allow the sharing of information without access to the general public. **Table 3** provides examples of these platforms.[12]

Equity and Accessibility

Concerns exist that some patients will not have the technology or the technological literacy to access telemedicine services. The populations in the United States more likely to have this "digital barrier" may include older adults, patients with low socioeconomic statuses, racial/ethnic minorities, patients who live in rural areas, and those with

Table 3	
Non-public facing communication platforms (acceptable for telemedicine)	
Video	**Text**
Apple FaceTime	iMessage
Google Hangouts	WhatsApp
Skype	Jabber
Facebook Messenger	Signal
Zoom	Facebook Messenger

limited health literacy and limited English proficiency.[13] The development of educational programs and training may help those with limited digital proficiency.[1]

PRIOR EXPERIENCE WITH TELEMEDICINE

Telehealth has been used successfully in many settings. Across a broad range of specialties, both patients and providers report high levels of satisfaction with the convenience and cost saving of virtual follow-up visits.[14]

Within the field of gynecology, the use of text message notifications has been useful in improving continuation rates with the use of birth control, including DepoProvera and oral contraceptive pills. Additionally, patient notification of abnormal sexually transmitted infection testing was more successful when text messages accompanied a phone call, versus a text or phone call alone.[15]

Telemedicine has proven useful for transitions of care after hospital admission. In a randomized controlled trial of patients discharged from the hospital, patients who were randomized to the telehealth group (including remote patient monitoring and video visits) were 7 times more likely to adhere to their medications when compared with the traditional transition of care group. Patients also reported enthusiasm and confidence that telehealth could improve their health care.[16]

One common misconception is that telemedicine cannot be implemented easily with an elderly population. However, there is a growing body of literature that suggests the contrary. The hallmarks of care in most elderly populations is monitoring and management of chronic diseases. This factor often requires frequent visits, which may be challenging, considering mobility and transportation issues this population may encounter. A large review has found that telemedicine is superior to in- person visits for many diagnoses including cancer care, congestive heart failure, dementia, hypertension, diabetes, and pain by decreasing emergency room visits, hospitalizations, and complications, and improving quality of life.[17] Another systematic review found that older adults find ambulatory telemedicine acceptable and feasible, with outcomes similar to those of in-person visits.[18]

EXPERIENCE WITH THE CORONAVIRUS DISEASE 2019 PANDEMIC AND TELEMEDICINE

Despite barriers to the widespread use of telemedicine services, the pandemic has catapulted many into the rapid adoption of these services. In New York City, an epicenter of the pandemic, a large health system with a preexisting telemedicine infrastructure, was able to see more than 70% of their ambulatory care volume via virtual visits. Although this expansion included many providers who were virtually inexperienced, patient satisfaction with telemedicine remained high.[19] In a global, cross-section survey of 620 urologists, a large expansion of telemedicine services was noted in response to the pandemic, with telemedicine use at 15.4% during the COVID-19 clinical practice era expanding to 46.1% during the pandemic. Of the urologists who did use telemedicine, 80.9% were interested in incorporating virtual visits into their routine practice.[20]

Despite this rapid expansion, it is important to recognize that not all patients are ready for telemedicine. A study by Lam and colleagues[21] found that 38% of patients older than 65 years of age were unready for video visits; unready was defined as difficulty hearing, speaking, or making themselves understood and/or seen, not having any Internet-ready device, and/or being unsure how to use them, no use of email, texting, Internet in the last months, or dementia.

TELEMEDICINE IN UROGYNECOLOGY

Our current understanding of the use of telemedicine in urogynecology has developed over the last 1 to 2 years. Before the COVID-19 pandemic led to worldwide shut downs and slow downs, a few urogynecology-specific articles were published.[22–24] Further, review articles (including a systematic review) and society statements were published in the early months of the pandemic to help guide us.[25–27] Urogynecologists and their patients became more comfortable with the use of telemedicine and this new literature forms the bedrock of our understanding of the use of telemedicine in Urogynecology.[6]

One concern worthy of addressing is the impact telemedicine will have on the patient–physician relationship. There is a human touch to medicine, especially in the treatment of quality-of-life diseases. Some providers are concerned that this will factor this be lost with telemedicine. Data are promising that patient satisfaction remains strong with telemedicine. In a study of virtual visits on pelvic organ prolapse between interns and simulated patients, the quality of doctor–patient communication, as indicated by information exchange, interpersonal relationship building, and shared decision-making, did not differ significantly between Web-based and face-to-face consultations.[28]

Overall, the virtual management of female pelvic medicine and reconstructive surgery conditions should emphasize behavioral and conservative counseling while still following current management paradigms. Further, telemedicine offers the opportunity for patient education and adjuvant tools for conservative therapy. There are some situations that may require alternate management but can be conducted via telemedicine; however, to conduct these visits virtually, we must be confident that the benefit of a virtual visit including timely access to care, decreasing exposure in a pandemic or flu season, exceeds the potential risks of adverse events and/or missed diagnoses. Finally, there are certain situations that will require in-person management.[29]

Conditions that Follow Current Management Paradigms (Behavioral, Conservative)

Many visit types are appropriate for telemedicine. The ideal telemedicine visit is a patient encounter that can be conducted without deviations from how they would be conducted in the office and/or diagnoses that benefit from behavioral counseling. Examples are listed in **Table 4**.

For patients new to the practice desiring a consultation for incontinence or prolapse, an in-person visit is likely most appropriate if there are associated complaints of new or worsening severe pain, persistent infections such as urinary tract infections (UTI), an inability to void easily, and concern for retention and mesh complications. Only 10% to 20% of women will have a change in prolapse stage over 2 years; therefore, most patients can be reassured regarding delay in surgical or pessary management for symptoms associated with pelvic organ prolapse.[30–33]

Table 4
Visit types to consider for telemedicine

	Appropriate	Inappropriate
Established patients	Medication efficacy and side effect evaluation 3-month Pessary checks/screening for symptoms	Pessary visits greater than 6–12 mo interval
Surgical patients	Preoperative counseling visits Postoperative patients who do not have any concerning symptoms such as urinary retention	Physical examination before surgery Serious postoperative complications
Postoperative	Midurethral slings with no incontinence Prolapse repairs with native tissue Postoperative call to screen for adverse events	De novo incontinence
New patients	Expressed desire for conservative management of prolapse or incontinence Initial intake to establish history and review symptoms and records	New pain Concern for fistula Unable to void Bleeding
Existing patients awaiting surgery or office treatments	Treatment with conservative options while awaiting surgery Home Kegels Behavioral counseling Continence supplies/skin care Incontinence devices Bowel regimen Anticholinergic medication (instead of Botox, or percutaneous tibial nerve stimulation)	New signs/symptoms: bleeding, retention, new pain.

Even for patients who will be seen in person, telemedicine can be used as an adjunct for history taking and administration of questionnaires, or providing bladder or bowel diaries. This practice will allow providers to triage patients and assess for the urgency of symptoms, in addition to decreasing the time that will be spent face to face.

Pessary Management

Many of our patients conservatively manage their prolapse with pessaries. Although self-care should be encouraged, many of our patients cannot perform self-care and rely on outpatient visits for cleaning and assessing vaginal epithelial integrity. Accepted intervals for pessary maintenance varies between 1 and 12 months, but is generally accepted to be 3 months.[29] Grimes and colleagues[25] performed a meta-analysis of 4 studies and estimated the following risks with continuous pessary use continuous pessary use with no interval cleaning or examination between 6 and 24 months with the following results: vaginal erosion or bleeding, 5.0% (95%

confidence interval [CI], 1.9–9.0), vaginal discharge 5.8% (95% CI, 3.6–8.5), vaginitis 1.8% (95% CI 0.2–4.6), voiding dysfunction 4.7% (95% CI, 1.4–9.8), and fistula 0% (95% CI, 0–1.1). These data are reassuring and further support a recent randomized controlled trial that demonstrated the safety of extending pessary follow-up visits to 6 months.[34] Thus, telemedicine could be appropriately used for in-between 6-month pessary visits to screen for warning signs.

Postoperative Visits

Telephone visits are useful in the postoperative period. Postoperative calls to screen for adverse events has been shown to decrease patient-initiated calls in the immediate 6-week postoperative period.[22] Further, in a randomized controlled trial comparing virtual postoperative visits for pelvic surgery via telemedicine versus in-person visits, patient satisfaction was similar between the groups. This practice was not accompanied by increased adverse events, emergency room visits, or primary care visits.[23] Another study demonstrated high patient satisfaction with postoperative virtual visits, although it was acknowledged that recurrent stress incontinence was hard to distinguish from de novo urgency incontinence on a telephone visit and tape extrusions and erosions after sling surgery were not detected during a virtual visit.[29]

Urinary Tract Infections

Empiric treatment of UTIs is often reasonable and this lends itself to a telemedicine visit. If the patient's symptoms are dysuria, worsening frequency or urgency, gross hematuria, and lack of vaginal symptoms such as vaginal discharge or itching, these symptoms are predictive of UTI. Empiric treatment should align with the International Guidelines from the Infectious Disease Society of America and European Society for Microbiology and Infectious Disease guidelines.[35] Additionally, any prior culture results within the last year should be reviewed because they often correspond with subsequent cultures and sensitivities and are useful to guide antibiotic therapy. In uncomplicated UTIs, good first-line choices of antibiotics include fosfomycin (once), bactrim (3–7 days), or nitrofurantoin (Macrobid) for (7 days). If the patient has risk factors such as age greater than 65 years, immunosuppression, diabetes mellitus, catheter use, UTIs in the last year, or recent exposure to antibiotics an alternative antibiotic may be more appropriate, such as ciprofloxacin.[25]

Table 5
Resources for virtual patient education

Type of Resource	Organization/Professional Society	Website(s)
Informational leaflets on a variety of conditions	International Urogynecological Association (IUGA)	www.yourpelvicfloor.org/leaflets/
	American Urogynecological Society (AUGS)	www.augs.org/patient-fact-sheets/
	Voices for Pelvic Floor Disorders	https://www.voicesforpfd.org/resources/fact-sheets-and-downloads/
	National Association for Continence	www.nafc.org/learning-library
Videos	Society of Gynecologic Surgeons A Guide to Female Clean Intermittent Self Catheterization.	https://vimeo.com/261183016

Table 6
Examples of mobile applications

Purpose	Applications	Features
Education/guidance for pelvic floor exercises	Squeezy	Exercise tutorials Cues exercises Reminders
	KegelTrainer	Exercise tutorials Reminders to perform exercises
Education/tracking for incontinence	LeakFreeMe	Bladder diary Monitoring of behavioral modifications
	Urolog	Track intake, voids, and accidents
Dietary guidance for irritable bowel syndrome/interstitial cystitis	Fodmap Swapp	Offers alternatives for patients following diet
	ICN Food List	Food list to identify trigger foods
Education for clean intermittent catheterization	StopUTI	Advice for catheterization technique Prevention of UTIs Education regarding bladder/bowel habits

Patient Education and Adjuvant Tools

Most urogynecologists use websites, handouts, diagrams, and videos in the counseling and follow-up care of their patients (**Table 5**). These adjuvant tools for patient education and counseling are also meaningful when supplementing virtual visits. Various applications exist for educating patients about conservative treatments including tracking and monitoring symptoms, guiding pelvic floor exercise at home, and other behavioral modifications. **Table 6** highlights some examples that have been found to be accurate and practical.[36,37]

Table 7
Potential reasons for urgent visits in female pelvic medicine and reconstructive surgery clinic during a pandemic

Reason	Explanation
Chronic pain with acute flare Pelvic floor myalgia Interstitial cystitis	Rule out unrelated pathology Acute treatment - trigger point injections or bladder instillations
Undertreated or untreated infection UTI Vaginitis	Rule out systemic or widespread infection (pyelonephritis) Need for culture
Postoperative concerns or complications	Acute issue needing immediate treatment (retention, bleeding, cuff dehiscence) Mesh complications
Acute retention	Need for catheter management
New pain Pessary patients Postoperative patients	Evaluate and treat acute issue
Other	Hematuria Suspected fistula

Complaints that Require In-Person Management

Various complaints likely inappropriate for telemedicine and that may warrant in-person evaluation include patients with known chronic pain with acute flares; untreated or undertreated infections such as refractory or relapsing UTI; patients with symptoms concerning for pyelonephritis, persistent vaginitis, or vulvitis despite initial treatment; postoperative concerns; acute retention or new pain; or other conditions such as hematuria, suspected fistula, or mesh complications (**Table 7**).

SUMMARY

Telemedicine has the striking ability to improve equity and accessibility in health care. Instances when in-person medical care is warranted exist; however, telemedicine can be used to triage these patients and assess the risk–benefit ratio of coming to the hospital versus staying home. By virtually evaluating and treating appropriate patients, providers can help to combat the care debt that accumulates as patients defer seeking care and elective surgeries are canceled when access to in-person health care is limited.[38] As we continue to develop our knowledge and use of telemedicine, further research should focus on the quality and outcomes of virtual care. Despite the challenges and uncertainties, telemedicine is here to stay, and urogynecologists and patients alike will ultimately benefit from this rapidly evolving, accessible mode of care.

CLINICS CARE POINTS

- Establish a clearly defined workflow for all members of the team participating in the televisit, including the provider, nurse or medical assistant, and scheduler.
- Be flexible with your use of various platforms; what works for some patients, will not work for others.
- Manage telemedicine visits as you do in-person visits; have a nurse or medical assistant do their routine assessment and review of information.
- Use telemedicine for brief patient encounters such as medication checks, postoperative visits in patients with no complaints, results review, and UTI follow-ups to maximize efficiency for providers and patients.
- Consider telemedicine for initial appointments for stress urinary incontinence and overactive bladder.
- Consider use of a platform that allows screen share, ancillary websites, or handouts that can be mailed to patients so you do not lose the valuable educational component of in-person visits.
- Offer telemedicine to both young and elderly patients.
- Enlist family members, caregivers, or friends to join virtual visits if a patient would typically bring them along to an in-person visit.

DISCLOSURE

C.L. Grimes: Consultant Provepharm, Inc., Expert Witness Johnson and Johnson, M.C. Toaff: no disclosures to report.

REFERENCES

1. Schwamm LH. Telehealth: seven strategies to successfully implement disruptive technology and transform health care. Health Aff 2014;33(2):200–6.

2. Mechanic OJ, Persaud Y, Kimball AB. Telehealth systems. [Updated 2020 Sep 18]. In: StatPearls [Internet]. Treasure Island (FL): StatPearls Publishing; 2021. Available at: https://www.ncbi.nlm.nih.gov/books/NBK459384/.

3. Medicare telemedicine health care provider fact sheet. Centers for Medicare & Medicaid Services. 2020. Available at: https://www.cms.gov/newsroom/fact-sheets/medicare-telemedicine-health-care-provider-fact-sheet. Accessed October 1, 2020.

4. Bashshur RL, Reardon TG, Shannon GW. Telemedicine: a new health care delivery system. Annu Rev Public Health 2000;21:613–37.

5. Jamieson T, Wallace R, Armstrong K, et al. Virtual care: a framework for a patient-centric system. Toronto: Women's College Hospital Institute for Health Systems Solutions and Virtual Care; 2015.

6. Serna-Gallegos T, Ninivaggio CS. A lasting impression: telemedicine in urogynecology during the coronavirus disease 2019 pandemic. Curr Opin Obstet Gynecol 2020;32(6):456–60.

7. About Telehealth. Public health institute center for connected health policy. Available at: https://www.cchpca.org/about/about-telehealth. Accessed October 1, 2020.

8. U.S. States and Territories Modifying Requirements for Telehealth in Response to COVID-19. Federation of state medical boards. 2020. Available at: https://www.fsmb.org/siteassets/advocacy/pdf/states-waiving-licensure-requirements-for-telehealth-in-response-to-covid-19.pdf. Accessed October 1, 2020.

9. Telehealth Parity Laws. Health affairs health policy brief, August 15, 2016. Health Affairs, Bethesda, MD. DOI: 10.1377/hpb20160815.244795.

10. Baumann BC, MacArthur KM, Michalski JM. The importance of temporary telehealth parity laws to improve public health during COVID-19 and future pandemics. Int J Radiat Oncol Biol Phys 2020;108(2):362–3.

11. American Medical Association Council on Medical Service. Established patient relationships and telemedicine: CMS report 1-i-19. Available at: https://www.ama-assn.org/system/files/2019-12/i19-cms-report1-patient-relations-telemedicine.pdf. Accessed October 1, 2020.

12. Policy changes during the COVID-19 public health emergency. Department of Health and Human Services. Available at: https://telehealth.hhs.gov/providers/policy-changes-during-the-covid-19-public-health-emergency/?section=1,2,4,6. Accessed October 1, 2020.

13. Nouri S, Khoong EC, Lyles CR, et al. Addressing equity in telemedicine for chronic disease management during the COVID-19 pandemic. NEJM Catal Innov Care Deliv 2020;1(3). https://doi.org/10.1056/CAT.20.0123.

14. Donelan K, Barreto EA, Sossong S, et al. Patient and clinician experiences with telehealth for patient follow-up care. Am J Manag Care 2019;25(1):40–4.

15. DeNicola N, Grossman D, Marko K, et al. Telehealth interventions to improve obstetric and gynecologic health outcomes: a systematic review. Obstet Gynecol 2020;135(2):371–82.

16. Noel K, Messina C, Hou W, Schoenfeld E, Kelly G. Tele-transitions of care (TTOC): a 12-month, randomized controlled trial evaluating the use of Telehealth to achieve triple aim objectives. BMC Fam Pract 2020;21(1):27.

17. Merrell RC. Geriatric telemedicine: background and evidence for telemedicine as a way to address the challenges of geriatrics. Healthc Inform Res 2015;21(4):223–9.

18. Batsis JA, DiMilia PR, Seo LM, et al. Effectiveness of ambulatory telemedicine care in older adults: a systematic review. J Am Geriatr Soc 2019;67(8):1737–49.

19. Mann DM, Chen J, Chunara R, Testa PA, Nov O. COVID-19 transforms health care through telemedicine: evidence from the field. J Am Med Inform Assoc 2020; 27(7):1132–5.

20. Dubin JM, Wyant WA, Balaji NC, et al. Telemedicine usage among urologists during the COVID-19 pandemic: cross-sectional study. J Med Internet Res 2020; 22(11):e21875.

21. Lam K, Lu AD, Shi Y, Covinsky KE. Assessing telemedicine unreadiness among older adults in the united states during the COVID-19 pandemic. JAMA Intern Med 2020;180(10):1389–91.

22. Iwanoff C, Giannopoulos M, Salamon C. Follow-up postoperative calls to reduce common postoperative complaints among urogynecology patients. Int Urogynecol J 2019;30(10):1667–72.

23. Thompson JC, Cichowski SB, Rogers RG, et al. Outpatient visits versus telephone interviews for postoperative care: a randomized controlled trial. Int Urogynecol J 2019;30(10):1639–46.

24. Jefferis H, Muriithi F, White B, Price N, Jackson S. Telephone follow-up after day case tension-free vaginal tape insertion. Int Urogynecol J 2016;27(5): 787–90.

25. Grimes CL, Balk EM, Crisp CC, et al. A guide for urogynecologic patient care utilizing telemedicine during the COVID-19 pandemic: review of existing evidence. Int Urogynecol J 2020;31(6):1063–89.

26. Huang Z, Wu S, Yu T, Hu A. Efficacy of telemedicine for urinary incontinence in women: a systematic review and meta-analysis of randomized controlled trials. Int Urogynecol J 2020;31(8):1507–13.

27. Guidance for the Management of Urogynecological Conditions During the Coronavirus (COVID-19) Pandemic. 2020. Available at: https://www.iuga.org/news/message-from-the-president-guidance-for-the-management-during-covid-19. Accessed November 30, 2020.

28. Tates K, Antheunis ML, Kanters S, Nieboer TE, Gerritse MB. The effect of screen-to-screen versus face-to-face consultation on doctor-patient communication: an experimental study with simulated patients. J Med Internet Res 2017;19(12): e421.

29. Balzarro M, Rubilotta E, Trabacchin N, et al. A prospective comparative study of the feasibility and reliability of telephone follow-up in female urology: the patient home office novel evaluation (PHONE) study. Urology 2020;136:82–7.

30. Khaja A, Freeman RM. How often should shelf/Gellhorn pessaries be changed? A survey of IUGA urogynaecologists. Int Urogynecol J 2014;25(7):941–6.

31. Bradley CS, Zimmerman MB, Qi Y, Nygaard IE. Natural history of pelvic organ prolapse in postmenopausal women. Obstet Gynecol 2007;109(4):848–54.

32. Gilchrist AS, Campbell W, Steele H, Brazell H, Foote J, Swift S. Outcomes of observation as therapy for pelvic organ prolapse: a study in the natural history of pelvic organ prolapse. Neurourol Urodyn 2013;32(4):383–6.

33. AUGS best practice statement: evaluation and counseling of patients with pelvic organ prolapse. Female Pelvic Med Reconstr Surg 2018;24(3):256.

34. Propst K, Mellen C, O'Sullivan DM, Tulikangas PK. Timing of office-based pessary care: a randomized controlled trial. Obstet Gynecol 2020;135(1):100–5.

35. Neal CM, Kus LH, Eckert LO, Peipert JF. Noncandidal vaginitis: a comprehensive approach to diagnosis and management. Am J Obstet Gynecol 2020;222(2): 114–22.

36. Sudol NT, Adams-Piper E, Perry R, Lane F, Chen KT. In search of mobile applications for patients with pelvic floor disorders. Female Pelvic Med Reconstr Surg 2019;25(3):252–6.
37. Barnes KL, Dunivan G, Jaramillo-Huff A, Krantz T, Thompson J, Jeppson P. Evaluation of smartphone pelvic floor exercise applications using standardized scoring system. Female Pelvic Med Reconstr Surg 2019;25(4):328–35.
38. Wosik J, Fudim M, Cameron B, et al. Telehealth transformation: COVID-19 and the rise of virtual care. J Am Med Inform Assoc 2020;27(6):957–62.

Recurrent Urinary Tract Infections
Diagnosis, Treatment, and Prevention

Julie Peck, MBBS, BAO*, Jonathan P. Shepherd, MD, MSc

KEYWORDS

- Recurrent urinary tract infection • Women • Uncomplicated UTI • UTI prevention

KEY POINTS

- Uncomplicated recurrent urinary tract infections are common in women.
- Antibiotics are the first-line treatment for recurrent urinary tract infections, but urine cultures should be obtained and quinolones should be avoided.
- First-line antibiotic treatment options for recurrent urinary tract infections are nitrofurantoin, trimethoprim/sulfamethoxazole, and fosfomycin.
- Prevention of recurrent urinary tract infections includes vaginal estrogen in postmenopausal women and behavioral modifications, 6- to 12-month antibiotic suppression, postcoital antibiotic suppression, and lactobacilli supplementation.

INTRODUCTION

Primary care and obstetrician/gynecologist physicians frequently see female patients with urinary tract infections (UTI). These infections affect approximately 1 out of 2 women in their lifetime.[1,2] The term UTI refers to both upper and lower genital tract infections but, it is most commonly used to refer to acute cystitis.[3,4] The discomfort that may occur with UTI can affect quality of life, and rare sequelae, such as pyelonephritis or urosepsis, may occur in susceptible populations such as elderly, immunosuppressed, or pregnant patients. Recurrent UTI (rUTI) is also common and occurs in up to 50% of women who have a UTI.[3,5] The definition of rUTI is not fully agreed upon, but general consensus over the past decade uses a definition of 2 or more culture-proven UTIs in 6 months or 3 or more UTIs in 1 year, occurring a minimum of 2 symptom-free weeks from each other.[3,6] This definition does not cover complicated UTIs, which are infections arising from structural or anatomic changes, such as neurogenic alterations, repeated catheter use, pregnancy, or immunocompromised states.[2–4,7] The purpose of this article is to aggregate the most recent research

St Francis Hospital Trinity Health, 114 Woodland Street, OB Administration 43, Hartford, CT 06105, USA
* Corresponding author.
E-mail address: Julie.michele.peck@gmail.com

Obstet Gynecol Clin N Am 48 (2021) 501–513
https://doi.org/10.1016/j.ogc.2021.05.005
0889-8545/21/© 2021 Elsevier Inc. All rights reserved.

and consensus statements on the prevention, diagnosis, and treatment of uncompli-cated rUTI in women.

Recent research has described the bladder microbiome and particularly the bacte-rial community that it comprises.[7–10] Little research had previously been done on this topic because it was presumed that the bladder was sterile in the absence of UTI.[9] It had also been presumed that the urethra would have similar bacterial composition to that of the vagina, but Price and colleagues[9] note the urethra and bladder microbiome have some differing bacterial species than the vagina. With further description of the healthy versus nonhealthy bladder microbiome, nonpharmacologic prophylactic inter-ventions as treatment for rUTI have increased.[1,11,12]

EPIDEMIOLOGY AND RISK FACTORS

Assessing UTI incidence is difficult, because UTIs can be incorrectly diagnosed, over-diagnosed, or underdiagnosed. Multiple methods are used to assess UTI incidence. Medina and Castillo-Pino[13] noted that UTI increases in frequency with age, with a pri-mary bimodal peak in women from age 14 to 25. In the United States, the prevalence of UTI is 11% in the overall population and 50% to 60% of women will have at least 1 UTI in their lifetime.[13] Recurrence is seen in about 25% to 50% of women after a UTI.[3–5,14] UTI is a highly burdensome condition that affects every age, race, ethnicity, socioeconomic status, and sexual orientation, and leads to almost $2 billion worth of expenses on diagnosis and treatment annually.[4,14]

UTI risk factors are variable, but the primary ones are a low estrogen state in post-menopausal women, UTI before 15 years of age, spermicide use, and a maternal history of rUTIs.[1,6,14–17] A number of common sense risk factors are not supported by evi-dence. These include wiping from back to front, multiple sexual partners, not voiding after intercourse, douching, tampon use, inadequate hydration, high body mass index, use of hot tubs and/or bubble baths, and wearing certain underwear types.[1,6,14–16]

PATHOPHYSIOLOGY

In general, the main causative organism of UTI is *Escherichia coli*, which is responsible for 70% to 95% of UTIs and more than 50% of rUTI.[1,3,6] Other common causative or-ganisms include *Klebsiella pneumoniae*, *Proteus mirabalis*, and *Escherichia faeca-lis*.[1,3,7] It is presumed that UTIs begin when gastrointestinal tract bacteria are introduced to the periurethral space and subsequently migrate via the urethra to the bladder.[1,7] This migration requires flagella and pili, which use adhesins to adhere to the bladder epithelium.[7] Uropathogenic *E coli* invade the bladder epithelium and secrete toxins and proteases to incite host cells to release nutrients and siderophores, allowing for iron release.[7] These factors make *E coli* a pervasive and successful bac-terium for UTI.

Evidence supports that increased UTI vulnerability can be associated with the vaginal microbiome.[10] Although seemingly a common sense concept, proof can be seen after intervention with topical estrogens in postmenopausal women and, to a lesser extent, the introduction of lactobacilli supplementation.[10] Shen and col-leagues[18] showed that postmenopausal women had higher levels of lactobacilli in the vagina. They also noted that women with low levels of lactobacilli in the vagina more frequently contained vaginal *E coli*.[10] It is unclear how vaginal organisms interact with the bladder microbiome, but these authors hypothesize that there are 3 possibil-ities: (1) the vaginal introitus is the reservoir for *E coli*, (2) less common uropathogens are found in the vagina, and (3) there is episodic exposure of the urinary tract from vaginal organisms that can prime or trigger the urinary tract for rUTI.

Although academic medical societies have generally agreed on *E coli* as the predominant causative organism for UTI, previously undiagnosed or commensal organisms may also be causative agents. Currently, the gold standard of a midstream clean catch sample sent for urinary culture is skewed by the culture medium used, leading to decreased growth of organisms outside of those normally cultured.[19] Neugent and colleagues[19] noted the presence of bacteria in 90% of cultures formerly read as "no growth" when 16S rRNA amplicon sequencing and enhanced quantitative urine culture was used instead of standard culture media. These investigators concluded that a healthy bladder community consists of *Firmicutes*, *Bacteroides*, *Actinobacteria*, *Fusobacteria*, and *Proteobacteria*, but there is large variability in the microbial inhabitants both among individuals and within a single person over time, including during periods of menstruation or after menopause.[9,19]

DIAGNOSIS

Frequently, UTIs are diagnosed based on clinical symptoms, but when there is concern for rUTI, urine culture is the gold standard. Urine culture allows for review of causative organisms to better tailor therapy, as well as to confirm the presence of microbiota.[4] Obtaining a urinalysis has proven to have 95% sensitivity and 70% specificity, but ensuring that patients can provide a noncontaminated midstream urine catch is the limiting factor.[2,4] Because urinalysis is generally processed with greater alacrity than urine culture and can highlight the existence of pyuria, it continues to be standard practice and is still recommended during an rUTI workup.[2,4,6] The main symptoms of UTI are dysuria, frequent voiding, hematuria, and suprapubic pain — with dysuria being the most common symptom.[3,16] Some of these symptoms overlap with other pathology, such as overactive bladder, hence the preference for culture to confirm the diagnosis when rUTI is suspected. We strongly prefer catheterized cultures in our practice owing to difficulty with obtaining a clean catch specimen and other contamination issues, which can obscure results. Fever, chills, back pain, nausea, and vomiting are more concerning for pyelonephritis and the workup should be more extensive.[3,16] The pyelonephritis workup includes urinalysis and urine culture, but will also include a renal ultrasound examination. The rapid diagnosis of pyelonephritis and further assessment of whether the patient will require in-patient versus out-patient treatment depends on clinical judgment and objective assessment. With aging, symptoms can change or diminish. Sudden incontinence, new-onset urgency, or increased frequency can all be signs of a UTI. For intellectually impaired patients or patients who are unable to verbalize symptoms, an altered mental status or a change in energy level may indicate a UTI.[3]

A physical examination is essential because it can delineate between UTI and anatomic or extravesical problems that may lead to similar symptoms. Uncomplicated UTI refers to an acute process, involving the lower urinary tract, most commonly the bladder, that has not led to pyelonephritis or urosepsis and was not caused by a possible reversible factor outside of infection including prolapse, other altered anatomy, neurogenic bladder, or pregnancy.[1,3,5,6]

A urine dipstick can be used as a first-line test to rule out acute UTI; in patients who are low risk with positive features on dipstick, UTI is considered.[3] Women with rUTI will most likely have a positive value on dipstick and thus this test is not as useful for patients with rUTI.[3] Urinalysis with microscopy functions similarly to the urine dipstick, because limited data assist in interpretation in the setting of rUTI. Benefits accrue in the setting of pyelonephritis as pyuria can be seen on microscopy[3] (**Table 1**).

Table 1 Diagnostic modalities and their uses			
Diagnostic Modality	Uncomplicated UTI[3,4]	rUTI	Pyelonephritis
Point-of-care urine dipstick	Useful first step, but not required because the diagnosis can be made with symptoms alone.[2]	Not recommended	Not recommended
Urinalysis	Not recommended	Recommended in conjunction with urine culture[2–4]	Useful for diagnosis of pyuria[3]
Urine culture	Not recommended	Recommended	Recommended
Imaging: Renal ultrasound imaging, computed tomography urogram	Not recommended	Recommended when no resolution of symptoms with appropriate treatment after 72 h or concern for genitourinary tract anomalies[3]	Renal ultrasound imaging or computed tomography urogram are recommended for further workup.[2] computed tomography urogram is useful for repeat episodes.[2]

As stated elsewhere in this article, urine culture is the gold standard for diagnosing UTI and rUTI, but how many colony forming units (cfu)/mL are needed to diagnose UTI vary. The standard diagnosis is based on a clean catch with 100,000 cfu/mL, but the European Association of Urology guidelines allow for 1000 cfu/mL with symptoms and the Canadian OBGYN Society allows for 100 cfu/mL with symptoms.[3,15] Of note, current culturing techniques are only for the highest incidence organisms including E coli, Proteus, Klebsiella, Staphylococcus saprophyticus, and Enterococcus.[3,19,20] No cost-effective or time-efficient way exists to perform testing outside of agar plates and traditional culture methods.[9,17] Both 16S rRNA amplicon sequencing and expanded quantitative urine culture have been shown to be more specific and sensitive, but are currently only relevant to research.[9,19] Ackerman and Chai[8] hope that one day we may use more expansive testing, such as those listed, to better understand individual urinary microbiomes to treat and prevent pathology. The hope is that one day we will discriminate between virulent and commensal organisms with relative ease in an accessible test.[19] Beyond urine cultures, imaging studies including cystoscopy and computed tomography cystogram are not recommended for the initial workup of uncomplicated rUTI, but could be useful if there was concern for pyelonephritis, obstruction, or another complicating factor.[2,3,6] There is no consensus on when to perform imaging for rUTI, but it is a reasonable next step when multiple forms of non-antimicrobial treatments have been attempted and failed to improve recurrence.[3]

TREATMENT

We recommend that acute cystitis from a UTI be treated with a short course of first-line antibiotics. Some physicians prescribe longer antibiotic dose courses of first-line agents, but little evidence or research currently supports the efficacy or need for longer dosing.[3] If resolution of symptoms occurs after the initial treatment, and culture-proven UTI with symptoms then returns, the patient is again treated with first-line antibiotics. At that point, rUTI suppression, prophylaxis, or another intervention should be considered. Some literature suggests that 50% of UTIs are relieved on their own after symptomatic treatment with nonsteroidal anti-inflammatory drugs and monitoring of symptoms for up to 48 hours.[2] This guideline is controversial; some authors maintain that no research supports the use of nonsteroidal anti-inflammatory drugs alone.[2,3]

The mainstay of UTI treatment in the acute phase is antibiotics.[1–3,5,6,13,14] First-line antibiotic choices may be made based on local microbial resistance in your community, but for most areas in the United States, first-line treatment with nitrofurantoin, trimethoprim-sulfamethoxazole (TMP-SMX), or fosfomycin is recommended. If local antimicrobial resistance rates are greater than 20% for TMP-SMX, we recommend switching to other, less resistant methods of treatment.[19] Second-line antibiotics include the β-lactams (amoxicillin) and fluoroquinolones.[1,3–6,14,21] Fluoroquinolones may be efficacious in a 3-day dosing regimen, but owing to data showing high and increasing resistance, these agents are not recommended as first-line treatment.[3,22] A long tradition exists for prolonged dosing regimens for rUTI, but in recent years, research has shown that prolonged therapy (7–14 days) is no more successful than a shorter standard course (3–6 days).[3,4] Dosing varies by institution and by region, and recommendations are given in **Table 2**. Risks and side effects associated with antibiotic use include but are not limited to drug resistance, gastrointestinal intolerance, and hepatic and pulmonary toxicity[1] (**Table 3**). In recent years, concerns for nitrofurantoin use in the elderly has emerged. As always, patients' comorbidities must be considered when prescribing antibiotics.

The usual strategy is to treat with a normal course for acute rUTI. Self-treatment with antibiotics has been used in reliable patients with rare episodes of UTI; we do not endorse this treatment method. We have seen too many women referred for rUTI

Table 2
Dosing regimens for acute and suppression treatment

	Acute Cystitis Regimen	Suppression Therapy	Postcoital Suppression
First-line antibiotics			
Nitrofurantoin	100 mg twice daily × 5 d[2,3]	50–100 mg/d or 3×/week for 6 mo[2,18]	50–100 mg 30 min after coitus, once[2]
TMP-SMX	160/800 mg twice daily × 3 d[2,3]	40/200 mg/d or 40/2000 mg 3×/week for 6 mo	40/200 mg 30 min after coitus, once[2]
Fosfomycin	3 g once[2,3]	3 g every 7–10 d for 6 mo[9]	N/A
Second-line antibiotics			
Ciprofloxacin	500 mg twice daily × 3 d[2]	N/A	N/A
Amoxicillin or amoxicillin/ clavulanic acid	1 g twice daily × 7 d[2]	N/A	N/A
Cefuroxime	500 mg twice daily × 3–5 d[2]	N/A	N/A

Abbreviation: N/A, not applicable.

Table 3
Side effects and contraindications of antibiotic therapy

Antibiotic	Side effects[1,2,20]	Contraindications
Nitrofurantoin	Hepatotoxicity Pulmonary toxicity Neuropathy[1]	Creatinine clearance <30 mL/min Pyelonephritis

TMP-SMX	GI side effects (nausea,
	  vomiting, diarrhea)
	Steven–Johnson syndrome
	Jaundice
	Iatrogenic lupus
	Leukocytopenia and
	  thrombocytopenia
	Lowers levels of oral
	  contraceptives[2]
		Glucose 6 phosphate
		dehydrogenase
		deficiency

Fosfomycin	GI side effects (nausea, vomiting, diarrhea)[2]	Pyelonephritis
Ciprofloxacin	Prolonged QT interval Tendon rupture (rare) Tendonitis Exacerbates symptoms of myasthenia gravis[5]	Women trying to conceive[1]
β-Lactams	GI side effects (nausea, vomiting, diarrhea) Headache Rash	

Abbreviation: GI, gastrointestinal.

who were self-treating multiple infections each year. Cultures ultimately revealed they did not actually have rUTI. In general it is noted that self-treatment is not as effective as prolonged antibiotic suppression but it can be used in patients who are either incapable of using or do not wish to use long-term suppression therapy.[1,3] Treatment should cover the most common uropathogens, antibiotics and duration are highlighted in **Table 2**, and rarely include fluoroquinolones or β-lactams as they are not recommended owing to their resistance profile and cost.[3]

TREATMENT IN DIABETICS

For many years, diabetic women with UTI have been deemed to have complicated UTI.[22–24] Increasing evidence supports that well-controlled diabetes is associated with uncomplicated UTI cases.[22] It is important to acknowledge that those with diabetes, especially when diabetes is poorly controlled, have a higher rate of infection.[25] In general, diabetics have higher rates of antibiotic use and higher prevalence of multidrug-resistant bacteria.[25] The uncomplicated UTI treatment regimen for diabetics has historically been longer in duration, but without evidence to support the extended timeframe.[22] Still controversial is whether females with controlled diabetes, who have otherwise uncomplicated UTIs, should receive the same acute antibiotic regimen.[22,24] Nitzan and colleagues[25] recommend a similar antibiotic regimen for diabetics with uncomplicated UTI with the caveat that they have a higher risk of complications and require closer follow-up. For diabetics, antibiotic prophylaxis includes those agents outlined for nondiabetics, but therapy also includes tight glycemic control and assessment for signs of complicating comorbidities such as pregnancy, genitourinary malformations, and indwelling catheters.[22,25]

PREVENTION

After primary treatment for rUTI is administered and the acute infection is treated, prophylaxis should be considered. The primary method should target the underlying cause. Behavioral changes can also be targeted, to help decrease other external factors that may be easily controlled.[1,3,4] Pharmacologic and nonpharmacological treatments can be used for prevention. The subsequent portion of this article outlines preventative measures for rUTI.

Behavioral Changes

Evidence supports that cessation of spermicide use decreases the incidence of rUTI; Shira and colleagues note that the odds of UTI is twice as likely when using condoms with spermicide than using condoms without spermicide.[1,2,14,17] Some studies have examined the relationship of hydration to UTI. Hooton and colleagues[15] noted that increased water intake by 1.5 L daily in premenopausal women led to 47% decrease in UTIs in a 12-month time period. Although limited evidence supports personal hygiene measures such as wiping front to back and voiding after coitus, these are suitable pragmatic actions that may decrease UTI frequency.[1,2,14] The frequency of urination, especially when delaying voiding, is an active correction that may decrease the risk of infection.[1,2,14] The use of tampons during menstruation, particularly protracted use, can be advised against if there is an increased frequency of UTI during the patient's menstrual period.[1,2,14] Generally, behavioral changes are important first-line actions that a patient can adopt with minimal effort to impact their quality of life.

Daily Antibiotic Suppression

Low-dose daily antibiotic suppression has proven effective for prevention of rUTI. Multiple studies note decreases ranging from 92% to 99% from placebo versus prophylactic antibiotics.[14,24–28] Bergamin and colleagues support prolonged antibiotic use with up to 95% decreased rate of infection.[2] Both nitrofurantoin and TMP-SMX have shown to be efficacious and can be tolerated for up to 12 months.[2,14] However, symptoms generally return after antibiotic prophylaxis has ceased, which limits their long-term effectiveness.[2,14] **Table 2** displays the recommended dosing regimen for suppression.

Postcoital Antibiotic Dosing

Single-dose postcoital antibiotics for UTI prophylaxis have been shown, in the correct setting, to be quite effective. If the exacerbating factor is sexual intercourse, a single postcoital prophylactic antibiotic dose has been shown to decrease rUTI with an efficacy similar to daily regimens (risk reduction by 98.8% and 99.0%, respectively).[2,3] The regimen can be nitrofurantoin or TMP-SMX within 30 minutes after coitus (**Table 2**).[2,3] Fosfomycin and second-line agents are not recommended as 1-time postcoital dosing.[2,3]

Cranberry Juice or Extract

Contradictory evidence exists for cranberry juice as prophylaxis or treatment for UTI. Cranberries contains type A pro-antho-cyanidins, which are broken down to metabolites that interfere with bacterial adhesion.[1,2,25] Multiple authors have assessed the use of cranberry products and have not reported successful prevention of rUTI.[11,14,29-33] However, multiple small trials support cranberry juice or cranberry extract use.[14,33,34] Wawrysiuk and associates[33] and Takahashi and colleagues[34] saw a 20.1% decrease in relapse of rUTI among women over 50 year old. A meta-analysis by Jepson and colleagues[11] observed a nonsignificant risk reduction for infection in the cranberry juice/extract group versus the placebo group. Heterogeneity of dosing regimens across different trials inhibits our ability to recommend specific cranberry consumption for prophylaxis.[11,29] However, in our practice we feel that it is reasonable to try this intervention given the ease of availability, reasonable costs, and minimal risks of emerging antibiotic resistance or other side effects.

Estrogen

In postmenopausal women, the hypoestrogenic state alters the genitourinary tract and leads to tissue atrophy.[1,10] Long term, this leads to multiple vaginal issues, including vaginitis and dyspareunia, as well as an increased rate of cystitis.[10] Topical vaginal estrogens were shown to be efficacious in a 2007 Cochrane review, where with their use the occurrence of UTI went from 5.9 to 0.5 episodes per year.[1,35] Estrogen creams are most often prescribed, but estrogen pessaries may also be used.[1,35] Increased estrogen in postmenopausal women leads to increased lactobacilli colonies and decreased E coli colonies.[1,10,35] Systemic estrogen has not been shown to be as effective for UTI reduction.[1,35] Unlike some benign prophylaxis, estrogens, even topical agents, have side effects that need to be weighed against relief and alteration to quality of life.[1,35] The side effects of estrogen use include breast tenderness, vaginal bleeding, discharge, and irritation.[1,35] Estrogens have their own risk profile and clinical judgment must be used to consider comorbidities such as breast cancer, coronary artery disease, and any history of deep vein thrombosis, pulmonary embolism, or stroke. However, given the lower rates of these side effects with topical compared with systemic estrogens, we use estrogen creams liberally in our postmenopausal population with both vaginal atrophy and rUTI.

Methenamine Hippurate

Methenamine hippurate (MH) is an acidifying agent used for decades to prophylactically treat UTIs.[1,2,14,36,37] The mechanism of action is acidification and sterilization of the urine via the production of formaldehyde from the hexamine.[1,14,36] There is still no clear evidence as to whether the direct bacteriostatic effects or the acidification of the urine is the main mechanism for UTI reduction, but in the most recent Cochrane review there seems to be a decrease of 44% (95% confidence interval, 0.07–0.89) of symptomatic UTI in subgroup analysis.[36,37] The recommended dosing regimen is 1 g twice daily.[36] The side effect profile of MH is minimal and includes gastrointestinal disturbances, rash, transaminitis, and dysuria.[37-40] Bergamin and colleagues[1,2] note that some studies have explored the damage formaldehyde has on the urothelium of rat bladders with concern for the development of urothelial malignancy with long-term use. However, MH is considered safe in long-term courses with minimal side effects and no drug resistance yet noted.[14,36,37]

Lactobacilli

Probiotics, many of which contain lactobacilli, have been studied as an antibiotic-free prophylaxis for rUTI.[41] Probiotic supplementation leads to decreased attachment of bacteria to epithelium, decreases pH, and leads to cytokine production within epithelial cells.[1,10,41] Lactobacilli are prevalent in the vaginal flora and are important organisms within the vaginal microbiome.[1,8,10,24] Considering the interconnected role of the vagina, urethra, and bladder, a healthy vaginal microbiome theoretically permits a healthy urethra and bladder.[10,24] In general, the lactobacilli used in research are rarely the strains found in the bladder microbiome.[10,14] Some research has shown a 55% decrease in the recurrence of infection with intravaginal probiotic use, specifically *Lactobacillus crispatus*, in premenopausal women.[1,19,25] Intravaginal dosing has been more effective than oral dosing, further supporting the theory that a healthy vaginal microbiome leads to a healthy bladder.[1,10,14] Supporting the use of probiotics can be difficult when the word probiotic is used commercially and represents a myriad of products.[25] Conventionally, probiotics have been more beneficial for both gastrointestinal and vaginal interventions. For patients with an overlap of these other comorbidities, current probiotic regimens may be useful. In reports to date, insufficient evidence supports the use of oral probiotics specifically for rUTI prophylaxis.[2,14]

Vaccines

The development of vaccines is seen as highly valuable for the prevention of rUTI. No vaccines are yet approved by the US Food and Drug Administration, but there are 3 vaccines currently available in Europe: Uro-Vaxom, SolcoUrovac, and ExPEC4V.[42,43] Forsyth and colleagues[42] describe Uro-Vaxom as a vaccine comprising 18 *E coli* uropathogen extracts given as a daily oral tablet. SolcoUrovac contains heat-killed uropathogenic bacteria. In trials, Uro-Vaxom showed a 49% decrease and Solco-Urovac showed a 19% decrease in rUTI; the greatest benefit was seen when boosters were received monthly.[17] ExPEC4V showed no decrease when looking at specific serotypes but showed a 55% decrease in UTIs caused by all *E coli* serotypes versus the placebo group.[17] Forsyth and colleagues[42,43] argue for Uro-Vaxom use owing to its once-a-day dosing and side effect profile. Because this area of research is burgeoning, vaccines have been based on the multiple virulent factors of uropathogens, including siderophores and siderophore receptors on the outer membranes, the O antigen, and portions of fimbria and alpha hemolysin.[7,42,43] A recent study using a mouse model showed the intranasal route decreased the median bacterial burden in the bladder by 2-fold in 58% of combined testing, with the dmLT adjuvant yielding the most protection against *E coli* colonization.[42] Expansion to humans will be key in proving that mucosal vaccines can be an effective and less invasive option to protect against rUTI.

Intravesical Installation

Intravesical instillation of hyaluronic acid and chondroitin sulfate has been used to prevent rUTI with the goal of improvement of symptoms and quality of life.[1,12] In a retrospective cohort adjusting for other characteristics, Ciani and colleagues[12] describe a 49% risk reduction that was unfortunately not statistically significant in total incidence rate or hazard ratio. Damiano and colleagues[44] instilled hyaluronic acid weekly for 4 weeks and then monthly for 5 months with a 77% mean difference (95% confidence interval, 72.3–80.8; $P = .0002$) compared with placebo. Improvements cannot be correlated with instillation because most studies do not have sufficient power or are case studies. Although an intriguing option, urinary instillation is primarily reserved for a small subset of patients (multidrug-resistant infections, difficult to treat rUTI, etc) and is not standard care for uncomplicated rUTI.[1] However, as a long-term treatment for decreasing the overall burden of chronic UTI, these treatments are sustainable and safer than antibiotics, thus warranting further research.[1,3,14]

Other Therapies

A variety of nontraditional medicine has been loosely studied throughout the years as both treatment and prophylaxis for UTI. Most notable are the use of Chinese herbs, D-mannose, acupuncture, and vitamin C.[1,3,14] D-Mannose attaches to the adhesins at the end of the pili on *E coli* and inhibits binding to the urothelium.[2,17,37] Huang Lin is a Chinese herbal remedy that interferes with bacterial activity and has some anti-inflammatory effects.[17] Another Chinese herbal medicine is Compound Salvia Plebeia Granules that leads to decreased adherence of *E coli* onto urothelium.[17] Acupuncture has been shown to decrease rUTIs, but no mechanism of action is clear.[14] Vitamin C leads to reduced urinary pH, which may lead to bacterial dysfunction.[1]

Minimal available research supports the use of these methods.[3] Depending on the patient population, following and understanding these nontraditional medical approaches may benefit some patients.

POSSIBILITIES FOR FUTURE RESEARCH

1. Vaginal probiotics that use vaginal- and bladder-directed lactobacilli could effectively aid in the reduction of rUTI through optimization of the vaginal and bladder microbiome. The vaginal probiotics are preferred as their side effect profile is easier to tolerate.[41]
2. Improved, expanded, and faster culture mediums will allow for an improved understanding of virulent microbes leading to UTI and rUTI. Our perspective is currently limited by culture media selective for specific bacteria. Further investigation of virulent microbes and improved detection rates of these microbes will supply important information.
3. Vaccines are the goal for any area of infectious disease prevention. The creation of a sustainable and affordable vaccine will help to decrease emergency department visits, antibiotic use, and poor quality of life. With prolonged use, vaccination could lead to the minimization of rUTIs and could possibly be extended to those with an increased UTI incidence, such as pregnant, immunosuppressed, and diabetic patients.
4. Further understanding the bladder microbiome can aid this research as well as provide generalized knowledge about the pathogens behind a very common disease. Understanding the physiologic interactions within the bladder and the delineation of virulent and commensal organisms (or how one becomes the other) will lead to improved treatment and prophylaxis.

SUMMARY

The worldwide burden of rUTIs requires improved treatment and prevention plans. We recommend obtaining urine cultures and using antibiotic sensitivities to guide treatment. Many prophylactic methods can be used to help decrease rUTIs in women. Estrogen use in postmenopausal women is efficacious and focused, and is our first choice for prevention as long as there are no contraindications to its use. MH is a safe long-term prophylaxis and we recommend this agent in addition to estrogen if symptoms persist. Maintenance antibiotic suppression therapy has been successful in decreasing recurrence rates, but with little prolonged efficacy after the treatment regimen is stopped. In general, if symptoms do not resolve with estrogen and MH, we continue vaginal estrogen, stop MH, and start antibiotic suppression. Generalized lifestyle modifications are of uncertain value, but may be easy to implement and may improve quality of life.

Many research opportunities are now available to understand the bladder microbiome as well as the virulence factors of certain microbes. Vaccines are also an exciting but challenging project, but as yet, no optimal product has been created.

CLINICS CARE POINTS

- rUTIs affect up to 50% of women with UTI.
- rUTI is diagnosed after 2 or more culture-proven UTIs in 6 months or 3 or more UTIs in 1 year, with each UTI separated by a minimum of 2 weeks from the next.
- Nitrofurantoin, TMP-SMX or fosfomycin are all effective first-line antibiotic treatments for UTIs. Fluoroquinolone use is discouraged in absence of allergy or resistance to first-line antibiotics.
- *E coli* is the most prevalent causative organism of UTI and rUTI in women.
- Prevention is key for women with rUTI including antibiotic suppression therapy, postcoital antibiotics, estrogen for postmenopausal women, MH, behavioral changes, and lactobacilli supplementation.
- Novel vaccines may be on the horizon for the long-term prevention of rUTIs.

DISCLOSURE

We have nothing to disclose and have no affiliations other than above listed employment.

REFERENCES

1. Bergamin PA, Kiosoglous AJ. Non-surgical management of recurrent urinary tract infections in women. Transl Androl Urol 2017;6(Suppl 2):S142–52.
2. Betschart C, Albrich WC, Brandner S, et al. Guideline of the Swiss Society of Gynaecology and Obstetrics (SSGO) on acute and recurrent urinary tract infections in women, including pregnancy. Swiss Med Wkly 2020;150:w20236.
3. Brubaker L, Carberry C, Nardos R, et al. American urogynecologic society best-practice statement: recurrent urinary tract infection in adult women. Female Pelvic Med Reconstr Surg 2018;24:321–35.
4. Anger J, Lee U, Ackerman AL, et al. Recurrent uncomplicated urinary tract infections in women: AUA/CUA/SUFU Guideline. J Urol 2019;202:282–9.
5. Gupta K, Trautner BW. Diagnosis and management of recurrent urinary tract infections in non-pregnant women. BMJ 2013;346:f3140.
6. Arnold JJ, Hehn LE, Klein DA. Common questions about recurrent urinary tract infections in women. Am Fam Physician 2016;93:560–9.
7. Flores-Mireles AL, Walker JN, Caparon M, et al. Urinary tract infections: epidemiology, mechanisms of infection and treatment options. Nat Rev Microbiol 2015;13:269–84.
8. Ackerman AL, Chai TC. The bladder is not sterile: an update on the urinary microbiome. Curr Bladder Dysfunct Rep 2019;14:331–41.
9. Price TK, Wolff B, Halverson T, et al. Temporal dynamics of the adult female lower urinary tract microbiota. mBio 2020;11:e00475-20.
10. Lewis AL, Gilbert NM. Roles of the vagina and the vaginal microbiota in urinary tract infection: evidence from clinical correlations and experimental models. GMS Infect Dis 2020;8:Doc02.

11. Jepson RG, Williams G, Craig JC. Cranberries for preventing urinary tract infections. Cochrane Database Syst Rev 2012;10(01):CD001321.

12. Ciani O, Arendsen E, Romancik M, et al. Intravesical administration of combined hyaluronic acid (HA) and chondroitin sulfate (CS) for the treatment of female recurrent urinary tract infections: a European multicentre nested case-control study. BMJ Open 2016;6:e009669.

13. Medina M, Castillo-Pino E. An introduction to the epidemiology and burden of urinary tract infections. Ther Adv Urol 2019;11. 1756287219832172.

14. Smith AL, Brown J, Wyman JF, et al. Treatment and prevention of recurrent lower urinary tract infections in women: a rapid review with practice recommendations. J Urol 2018;200:1174–91.

15. Hooton TM, Vecchio M, Iroz A, et al. Effect of increased daily water intake in premenopausal women with recurrent urinary tract infections: a randomized clinical trial. JAMA Intern Med 2018;178:1509–15.

16. Kodner CM, Thomas Gupton EK. Recurrent urinary tract infections in women: diagnosis and management. Am Fam Physician 2010;82:638–43.

17. Shira N, Goodman A, Zakri R, et al. Nonantibiotic prevention and management of recurrent urinary tract infection. Nat Rev Urol 2018;15(12):750–76.

18. Shen J, Song N, Williams CJ, et al. Effects of low dose estrogen therapy on the vaginal microbiomes of women with atrophic vaginitis. Sci Rep 2016;6:1–10.

19. Neugent ML, Hulyalkar NV, Nguyen VH, et al. Advances in understanding the human urinary microbiome and its potential role in urinary tract infection. mBio 2020; 11:e00218–20.

20. Gupta K, Hooton TM, Naber KG, et al. International clinical practice guidelines for the treatment of acute uncomplicated cystitis and pyelonephritis in women: a 2010 update by the Infectious Diseases Society of America and the European Society for Microbiology and Infectious Diseases. Clin Infect Dis 2011;52:e103–20.

21. Rich SN, Klann EM, Almond CR, et al. Associations between antibiotic prescriptions and recurrent urinary tract infections in female college students. Epidemiol Infect 2019;147:e119.

22. Grigoryan L, Zoorob R, Wang H, et al. Less workup, longer treatment, but no clinical benefit observed in women with diabetes and acute cystitis. Diabetes Res Clin Pract 2017;129:197–202.

23. Holm A, Cordoba G, Møller Sørensen T, et al. Effect of point-of-care susceptibility testing in general practice on appropriate prescription of antibiotics for patients with uncomplicated urinary tract infection: a diagnostic randomised controlled trial. BMJ Open 2017;7:e018028.

24. Erdem I, Kara Ali R, Ardic E, et al. Community-acquired lower urinary tract infections: etiology, antimicrobial resistance, and treatment results in female patients. J Glob Infect Dis 2018;10:129–32.

25. Nitzan O, Elias M, Chazan B, et al. Urinary tract infections in patients with type 2 diabetes mellitus: review of prevalence, diagnosis, and management. Diabetes Metab Syndr Obes 2015;8:129–36.

26. Nicolle LE, Harding GK, Thompson M, et al. Prospective, randomized, placebo-controlled trial of norfloxacin for the prophylaxis of recurrent urinary tract infection in women. Antimicrob Agents Chemother 1989;33(7):1032–5.

27. Rudenko N, Dorofeyev A. Prevention of recurrent lower urinary tract infections by long-term administration of Fosfomycin trometamol. Arzneimittelforschung 2005; 55(7):420–7.

28. Scheckler WE, Burt RAP, Paulson DF. Comparison of low-dose cinoxacin therapy and placebo in the prevention of recurrent urinary tract infections. J Fam Pract 1982;15(5):901–4.
29. Fu Z, Liska D, Talan D, et al. Cranberry reduces the risk of urinary tract infection recurrence in otherwise healthy women: a systematic review and meta-analysis. J Nutr 2017;147:2282–8.
30. Nicolle LE. Cranberry for prevention if urinary tract infection? Time to move on. JAMA 2016;316(18):1873–4.
31. Barbose-Cesnik C, Brown MB, Buxton M, et al. Cranberry juice fails to prevent recurrent urinary tract infection: results from a randomized placebo-controlled trial. Clin Infect Dis 2011;52(1):23–30.
32. Juthani-Mehta M, Van Ness PH, Bianco L, et al. Effect of cranberry capsules on bacteriuria plus pyuria among older women in nursing homes: a randomized clinical trial. JAMA 2016;316(18):1879–87.
33. Wawrysiuk S, Naber K, Rechberger T, et al. Prevention and treatment of uncomplicated lower urinary tract infections in the era of increasing antimicrobial resistance-non-antibiotic approaches: a systemic review. Arch Gynecol Obstet 2019;300:821–8.
34. Takahashi S, Hamasuna R, Yasuda M, et al. A randomized clinical trial to evaluate the preventive effect of cranberry juice (UR65) for patients with recurrent urinary tract infection. J Infect Chemother 2013;19:112–7.
35. Perrotta C, Aznar M, Mejia R, et al. Oestrogens for preventing recurrent urinary tract infection in postmenopausal women. Cochrane Database Syst Rev 2008;(2):CD005131.
36. Lee BSB, Bhuta T, Simpson JM, et al. Methenamine hippurate for preventing urinary tract infections. Cochrane Database Syst Rev 2012;10(10):CD003265.
37. Gill CM, Hughes MRS, LaPlante KL. A review of nonantibiotic agents to prevent urinary tract infections in older women. JAMDA 2020;21:46–54.
38. Gerstein AR, Okun R, Gonick HC, et al. The prolonged use of methenamine hippurate in the treatment of chronic urinary tract infection. J Urol 1968;100:767–71.
39. Cronberg S, Welin CO, Henriksson L, et al. Prevention of recurrent acute cystitis by methenamine hippurate: double blind controlled crossover long term study. Br Med J 1987;294:1507–8.
40. Parvio S. Methenamine hippurate ('Hiprex') in the treatment of chronic urinary tract infections: a trial in a geriatric hospital. J Int Med Res 1976;4(2):111–4.
41. Puebla-Barragan S, Reid G. Forty-five-year evolution of probiotic therapy. Microb Cell 2019;6:184–96.
42. Forsyth VS, Himpsl SD, Smith SN, et al. Optimization of an experimental vaccine to prevent Escherichia coli urinary tract infection. mBio 2020;11:e00555-20.
43. Mobley HL, Alteri CJ. Development of a vaccine against Escherichia coli urinary tract infections. Pathogens 2015;5:1.
44. Damiano R, Quarto G, Bava I, et al. Prevention of recurrent urinary trat infections by intravesical administration of hyaluronic acid and placebo-controlled randomised trial. Eur Urol 2011;59(4):645–51.

Update in Transvaginal Grafts

The Role of Lightweight Meshes, Biologics, and Hybrid Grafts in Pelvic Organ Prolapse Surgery

Visha Tailor, MBBS, BSc[a],*, Alex Digesu, MD, PhD[a],
Steven Edward Swift, MD[b]

KEYWORDS

- Lightweight mesh • Biological mesh • Composite mesh • Tissue engineering
- Prolapse

KEY POINTS

- The use of polypropylene mesh for vaginal pelvic organ prolapse (POP) surgery is associated with a higher risk of complications compared with native tissue repair, including mesh exposure, mesh extrusion, pain, and mesh removal surgery.
- The use of lightweight polypropylene mesh for POP surgery may provide better short-term anatomic surgical success compared with native tissue repair.
- The use of lightweight polypropylene mesh may have the advantage of reducing the current known risk of mesh-related complications. Further long-term clinical trials, however, are warranted.
- Although biological mesh grafts do not provide greater anatomic success in the short term compared with native tissue repair, they should not yet be removed from the armamentarium of scaffolds for vaginal mesh surgery without longer-term outcomes reported.
- Based on animal studies, in the future, tissue engineering may hold the key to producing an optimized mesh for vaginal prolapse surgery.

INTRODUCTION AND BACKGROUND

Pelvic organ prolapse (POP) is a common disease in gynecology. It affects up to 40% of women, increasing with age and parity.[1] Although POP rarely leads to significant health morbidity or mortality, it negatively affects quality of life and sexual function, necessitating surgical treatment of many women. The lifetime risk of surgical intervention for POP is 7% to 19%.[2–4] POP surgery can be carried out through a vaginal or abdominal approach. This review focuses exclusively on the vaginal approach for POP surgery.

[a] Department of Urogynaecology, St Marys Hospital, Imperial College Healthcare NHS Trust, Praed Street, London W2 1NY, United Kingdom; [b] Department of Obstetrics and Gynecology, Medical University of South Carolina, Charleston, SC 29425, USA
* Corresponding author.
E-mail address: vishatailor@nhs.net

Obstet Gynecol Clin N Am 48 (2021) 515–533
https://doi.org/10.1016/j.ogc.2021.05.006
0889-8545/21/© 2021 Elsevier Inc. All rights reserved.

Native tissue repair to restore anatomy for vaginal prolapse long has been the most popular method of POP surgery. Unfortunately, there is a high recurrence rate of POP in the same or alternative compartment reported in up to 30% to 50% of women,[2,5] with 13% to 29% of women seeking further surgical correction, at an average of 12 years following the index POP surgery.[2,6] This high recurrence rate of vaginal prolapse and repeat surgery have encouraged the use of surgical scaffolds to support and provide longevity to the prolapse repair. Inspired from their successful use in hernia surgery, scaffolds initially in the form of nonabsorbable dense polypropylene mesh were developed and have been utilized since the 1990s.[7] Subsequently, there has been advancement in mesh materials, sophistication of the insertion process using mesh kits, and research into alternative graft materials.

Awareness and concerns have increased regarding serious complications, including mesh erosion or exposure, chronic pain, dyspareunia, and need for additional surgical procedures.[8,9] In 2008, the US Food and Drug Administration (FDA) issued a public health notice warning of the serious consequences of mesh complications following gynecologic surgery.[10] A total of 2874 adverse events attributed to mesh utilized for POP or incontinence surgery were reported between January 2008 and December 2010,[11] leading to a second US FDA safety communication in 2011.[12,13] Subsequent activation of Section 522 of the Food, Drug and Cosmetic Act allowed the US FDA to order manufacturing companies to provide evidence of mesh efficacy and safety reports for 119 products in January 2012.[14] The reaction of many manufacturing companies (66%) was to voluntarily withdraw their products from the market and discontinue sale of their mesh kits.[14] A further 22% of the devices under US FDA 522 orders changed the indication for device use and only approximately 9% undertook postmarketing studies.[14]

In January 2016, mesh devices were reclassified as class III, therefore requiring a higher standard of a premarket approval application process to be met. In April 2019, the US FDA banned the use of transvaginal mesh for POP surgery. Negative publicity and the ban on the use of transvaginal mesh products for POP in the United States, United Kingdom, Australia, and New Zealand have led to a decline in their use. This decline has encouraged a drive to research alternative mesh products to augment transvaginal POP surgery.

The authors used PubMed, Google scholar, and the Cochrane database for this narrative review and update on the current use of lightweight polypropylene mesh, absorbable synthetic meshes, biological grafts, hybrid mesh grafts, and tissue-engineered vaginal grafts for vaginal POP surgery. Relevant articles from the year 2000 onwards in the English language have been considered. The following search terms were used to evaluate the literature: lightweight mesh and prolapse, lightweight mesh and prolapse, biological mesh and prolapse, and tissue engineering and prolapse. Searches using the names of the commercial lightweight mesh kits also were carried out: Prolift + M, Pelvimesh, Surgimesh, Surelift, IntePro Lite, Uphold lite, Novasilk, Restorelle, Ugytex and Calistar. Studies describing the use of mesh products for abdominal POP surgery, abdominal rectopexy, transperineum and stress urinary incontinence (SUI) procedures were excluded.

LIGHTWEIGHT POLYPROPYLENE MESH

Traditionally, a type 1 synthetic, polypropylene, macroporous, monofilament mesh was the mesh used most commonly for POP surgery. A macroporous mesh allows for better infiltration of macrophages and fibroblasts for angiogenesis and collagen integration.[15] Over the past decade, lightweight polypropylene mesh products for vaginal mesh surgery have been produced in an attempt to reduce mesh complications. Unlike the type 1 heavyweight polypropylene meshes, the lightweight meshes have a lower density of polypropylene and larger pores, which reduces the foreign body load. A typical lightweight polypropylene mesh weighs 16 g/m^2 to 33 g/m^2 compared with up to 100 g/m^2 for heavyweight mesh.[15]

Placement of mesh invokes an inflammatory response commonly involving macrophages, T cells, and mast cells.[16] Excessive inflammatory response to a foreign body can lead to scarring, shrinkage, contraction, decreased graft compliance, and decreased mesh and tissue flexibility.[17] Animal studies comparing the histologic effects of polypropylene meshes demonstrate fewer inflammatory cells and better tissue incorporation when using a lightweight polypropylene mesh compared with heavier polypropylene meshes.[16–18] The lower inflammatory response is thought to decrease the degree of unorganized or reactive scar formation surrounding the mesh[19] and, therefore, improve the mesh compliance and elasticity.[18,19] In addition, there is reduced shrinkage of implanted lightweight mesh (36%), compared with heavy polypropylene mesh (46%),[17] and less degradation over time[20] and lower stiffness, with retained ability to support the same maximum loads at 60 days postinsertion.[21] These properties of lightweight mesh have encouraged its continued use for POP surgery.

The 2017 PROSPECT trial was the largest primary prolapse repair trial to compare a variety of polypropylene (19–44 g/m^2) mesh grafts (n = 435) with native tissue repair (n = 430). The study results echoed those of recent systematic reviews, including a 2016 Cochrane review, which concluded that the use of synthetic mesh offers no additional benefit to POP surgery due to the mesh specific complications.

There are some data to support better anatomic outcomes, a reduced risk of prolapse recurrence (relative risk [RR] 0.40; 95% CI, 0.30–0.53), reduced need for repeat surgery for POP (RR 0.53; 95% CI, 0.31–0.88), and equal patient satisfaction and quality-of-life outcomes when using transvaginal mesh POP surgery compared with native tissue repair.[22–24] No increased risk of postoperative SUI, dyspareunia, or worsening of sexual function with mesh repair is observed.[22,24,25] These positive benefits, however, are overshadowed by the occurrence of mesh-related complications. Mesh exposure or extrusion rates varied between 1.4% and 19%, with 3% to 8% undergoing a mesh revision procedure.[22,26] The PROSPECT trial reported a mesh erosion rate of 12% at 2 years.

Although these reviews and trial are comprehensive and informative, they do not reflect the evolution of the mesh products implanted and the heterogeneous methods to implant them. An upswing of lightweight mesh products came to the market just prior to the US FDA actions, some of which are no longer available (**Table 1**). Several investigators have compared POP surgery outcomes using heavyweight (45 g/m^2 to 55 g/m^2) or lightweight (InterPro Lite, 25 g/m^2) polypropylene mesh kits. No significant difference in anatomic success was demonstrated between the 2 mesh densities; however, significantly lower mesh exposure rates are reported using lightweight mesh kits[27–31] (**Table 2**).

Lightweight polypropylene mesh appears to have less mesh exposure then the more traditional heavyweight polypropylene mesh while maintaining good efficacy. Mesh exposure rates are 1.3% to 4.8% at midterm (2–3 years) follow-up and up to 7.5% in longer term (4–6 years) studies (**Table 3**). The paucity of high-quality studies beyond 36 months to 48 months for these products makes any definitive statement on lightweight polypropylene mesh efficacy and safety premature. Determining if the rate of exposure is acceptable and whether the benefit of utilizing a lightweight polypropylene mesh offers advantage over native tissue repair requires further study.

SYNTHETIC ABSORBABLE MESH

Few randomized controlled trials (RCTs) have been carried out to evaluate the efficacy and safety of synthetic absorbable polyglactin mesh for vaginal POP repair. The

Table 1
Current and previously utilised polypropylene mesh products used for transvaginal prolapse repair

Mesh Marketing Name	Manufacturer	Material	Density (g/m²)	Current Use
Avaulta	C. R. Bard, USA	Polypropylene	100	Discontinued
Marlex	C. R. Bard, USA	Polypropylene	95	Discontinued
Avaulta Plus	C. R. Bard, USA	Collagen coated PP	58[a]	Discontinued
Avaulta Solo	C. R. Bard, USA	Polypropylene	58	Discontinued
Intepro (Apogee, Perigee)	American Medical Systems, USA	Polypropylene	55	Discontinued
Prolift	Ethicon, USA	Polypropylene	45	Discontinued
Calistar A	Promedon, Argentina	Polypropylene	44	Discontinued
Gynemesh PS Prolift	Ethicon, USA	Polypropylene	42	Discontinued
Ugytex	C. R. Bard, USA	Collagen coated PP	38	Discontinued
TiLOOP ® Total 6	PFM Medical, Germany	Titanium coated PP	35	Available
Vypro II	Ethicon, USA	PP + polyglactin	32[a]	Discontinued
Prolift + M	Ethicon, USA	Polypropylene	31	Discontinued
Pelvimesh - light	Herniamesh, Italy	Polypropylene	30	Available
Surgimesh	Aspide Medical, France	Polypropylene	28	Discontinued
Surelift	Neomedic International, Spain	Polypropylene	28	Available
Intepro Lite (Apogee, Perigee, Elevate)	American Medical Systems, USA	Polypropylene	25	Discontinued
Uphold Lite	Boston Scientific, USA	Polypropylene	25	Available
TiLOOP ® PRO Plus A	PFM Medical, Germany	Titanium coated PP	24	Available
Novasilk	Coloplast, Denmark	Polypropylene	22	Available
OPUR	**Abiss, France**	**Polypropylene**	**22**	**Available**
Pelvimesh - ultralight	Herniamesh, Italy	Polypropylene	20	Available
Restorelle Direct Fix	Coloplast, Denmark	Polypropylene	19	Available
Ti-Mesh®	PFM Medical, Germany	Titanium coated PP	16	Available
Calistar S	Promedon, Argentina	Polypropylene	16	Available
Nuvia® SI prolapse repair system	C. R. Bard, USA	Polypropylene		Discontinued

Abbreviation: PP, polypropylene.
[a] Weight of polypropylene excluding composite collagen or polyglactin weight.

polyglactin mesh was designed to provide a temporary scaffold or lattice for new tissue development; by 14 days, it has lost 50% of its support through hydrolysis. The 2016 Cochrane review concluded that there was insufficient evidence to recommend use of an absorbable polyglactin mesh over native tissue repair.[26] Studies reporting 6-month and 24-month results demonstrate no advantage to the use of polyglactin mesh over native tissue repair for anterior vaginal wall surgery with an objective failure rate of 32% reported at 24 months.[28–31]

A composite mesh that is no longer available for transvaginal mesh surgery was made up of 50% absorbable polyglactin 910% and 50% polypropylene (Vypro II, Ethicon, USA). In a retrospective study, there was no difference in the risk of mesh exposure between the composite mesh and a heavyweight polypropylene mesh (7.2% vs

Table 2
Outcomes of lightweight compared with heavy weight polypropylene mesh for transvaginal prolapse surgery

Authors	Study Length	Mesh Density (g/m²)		Surgical Success Rate (%)		Mesh Exposure/Extrusion (%)		Significance
		Heavyweight Polypropylene	Lightweight Polypropylene	Heavyweight Polypropylene	Lightweight Polypropylene	Heavyweight Polypropylene	Lightweight Polypropylene	
Long et al,[33] 2015	12 mo	55	25	93.4	94	11	2	$^{a}P = .05$
Rogowski et al,[35] 2018	18 mo	55	25	90	90	7.7	0	$^{a}P = .02$
Yang et al,[32] 2017	24 mo	45	25	95.5	97.1	11.7	1.5	$^{a}P = .01$
Moore and Lukban,[34] 2012	24 mo	55	25	86.9	87.1	11	6	$P = .12$
Dykes et al,[27] 2020	6.4 y	55	25	80	75.9	40%	5.	$^{a}P < .0001$

Table comparing outcomes for lightweight compared with heavier-weight polypropylene mesh for transvaginal prolapse surgery. There was no significant difference in the anatomic surgical success rates between lightweight versus heavyweight mesh. The lightweight polypropylene mesh appears to have a lower risk of mesh exposure in the short to medium-term follow-up.

[a] Significant *P* value.

Table 3
Outcomes of transvaginal prolapse surgery using lightweight polypropylene mesh

Mesh Marketing Name (Manufacturer)	Mesh Kit Design and Arm-Fixation Site	Compartment Use	PP Density (g/m²)	No. Studies	Months fu	Anatomical Success	Subjective Success	Mesh Erosion	Other Notable Results
Pelvimesh (Herniamesh, Italy)[36]	4 Arm (anterior): transobturator 2 Arm (posterior/apical): Transgluteal	Anterior or Posterior + Apical	30 or 20	1	3	98%	-	1.38%	
Surgimesh (Aspide Medical, France)[37-39]	4 Arm: Transobturator	Anterior	28	3	36	93%–96%	71%–96%	1.3% – 7.6%	5.7% Mesh Contraction, 2% Pain
Surelift (Neomedic International, Spain)[40,41]	6 Arm: 2 SSLF, 4 transobturator	Anterior + Apical	28	2	12–20	88%–97%	92%	4.8% – 11.8%	21% – 47% de novo SUI
Elevate (American Medical Systems, USA)[42-51]	4 self fixing Arms: 2 SSLF, 2 Transobturator	Anterior + Apical	25	>10	12 24 48 60	70%–96% 60%–95% 94% 96%	90% - 93% - 97% 100%	0% – 5.7% 0% - 5.3% 7.5% 3.8%	0%–4% Buttock pain 3%–14% dyspareunia 62% OAB improvement 4%-26% de novo SUI
Intepro Lite (Apogee) (American Medical Systems, USA)[34,52-54]	2 lateral arms traversing illeococcygeus fascia	Posterior + Apical	25	4	12 24	82% - 100%	96% - 100%	0%–6.5% 5.4% - 7.1%	

Device	Technique	Approach	N		Follow-up (mo)				Outcomes
Intepro Lite (Perigee) (American Medical Systems, USA)[34,52,53,55-57]	4 self fixing arms: 2 SSLF, 2 transobturator	Anterior	25	4	12 24	93% - 100% 88%	90%-100% -	4.6% - 5% 4.5% - 4.8%	Apical success 67% at 2 y 4.5% Mesh Arm Pain
Uphold Lite (Boston Scientific, USA)[58-62]	2 Arm: SSLF	Anterior + Apical	25	4	12 26	76%-95% 97%	91%-94% -	0%-2.5% 3.4%	2%-4% re-op rate 4.3% serious complication risk, 2%-5% pain
OPUR Prosthesis (Abiss, France)[63,64]	6 Arm: 2 SSLF, 4 Transobturator	Anterior + Apical	22	2	33-36	97		1.3%-3%	33%-45% SUI improvement 2% Dyspareunia
Novasilk (Coloplast, Denmark)[65]		Anterior	22	1	72	83%	89%	1.7%	1.7% Dyspareunia
Restorelle Direct Fix (Coloplast, Denmark)[66]	4 arm: 2 SSLF, 2 arcus tendinous fascia pelvis	Anterior or Posterior Repair	19	1	12	72%	82%	2.9%	5.7% Chronic Pain 6.3% Revision Surgery
Nuvia® SI prolapse repair system (C.R.Bard, USA)[67]	4 Arm: SSLF	Anterior + apical	-	2	6	93%	94%	5.5%	
Callistar S (Promedon, Argentina)[68-70]	Single incision, self-fixing, attachments to the SSL and obturator internus	Anterior or posterior with apical support	16	3	12 18	90% 94%-97%	91%-93%	4% 3.7% - 5.6%	64% improvement in SUI

Abbreviations: OAB, overactive bladder syndrome; SSLF, sacrospinous ligament fixation; SUI, stress urinary incontinence.

6.9%, respectively; $P = .41$) at 1 year.[71] At 24 months and 36 months, however, 10% and 22% posterior vaginal wall recurrence occurred, respectively, with 11% and 30% mesh exposure rates, respectively.[72,73] Combined with a 27% risk of de novo dyspareunia,[73] further use of this mesh is not encouraged.

BIOLOGICAL MESH

Biological grafts, in the form of human dermal cadaveric allografts or mammalian extracellular matrix xenografts derived most commonly from porcine or bovine sources, are considered to have the advantage of better biocompatibility and ability to integrate with host tissue with fewer graft-related complications.[74,75] The 2016 Cochrane review and a meta-analysis by Schimpf and colleague[22] compared the use of biological grafts for prolapse repair, including 10 RCTs and 13 RCTS, respectively. They concluded that there was insufficient evidence for use of a biological graft for primary or recurrent vaginal POP repair over native tissue repair.[22,26]

A second arm of the 2017 PROSPECT RCT reported on outcomes comparing native tissue repair (n = 367) with biological graft (n = 368) for primary POP surgery.[76] The biological grafts utilized included porcine acellular collagen matrix, porcine small intestinal submucosa (SIS), or bovine dermal grafts. At 2 years' follow-up, no advantage for using a biological graft to improve quality of life or prolapse symptoms was found.[76] The reported rates of severe SUI (approximately 7%), severe dyspareunia (approximately 4%), stage 2 POP recurrence (approximately 40%), and stage 3 (approximately 7%) POP recurrence for the 2 groups were equivocal.

More recently, Wei and colleagues[77] compared lightweight polypropylene mesh (n = 117) with porcine collagen matrix graft or submucosa of porcine small intestine graft (n = 155) for anterior vaginal wall repair as part of an RCT with a 1-year follow up. There were fewer reported complications (18 vs 5, p=0 .005) and mesh exposure (8 vs 0) with equivocal failure rates (8.5% vs 8.7%) for the biological graft group.[77] Similarly, Balzarro and colleagues reported retrospective data comparing native tissue repair (n = 42) with porcine graft (n = 19) or heavyweight polypropylene mesh (n = 48)– augmented anterior vaginal repair with 80 months' to 100 months' follow-up. Outcomes with the use of the porcine graft were superior to polypropylene mesh repair with significantly fewer complications (4.8% native tissue vs 15.8% for porcine graft vs 29.2% for polypropylene mesh), a trend toward lower prolapse recurrence (19% native tissue vs 10% porcine graft vs 17% polypropylene mesh), and greater patient satisfaction (95% native tissue vs 100% porcine graft vs 83% polypropylene mesh).[78] The exposure rates for the porcine graft were 5% versus 17% for the polypropylene mesh.[78]

Biological grafts for vaginal mesh surgery have not and should not be yet removed from the armory. They demonstrate equal if not superior efficacy to native tissue repair in short-term studies and have reduced complication rates compared with polypropylene mesh. There is an unmet need, however, for longer-term studies to fully evaluate the use of biological grafts for vaginal POP surgery.

COMPOSITE MESH
Titanium-coated polypropylene mesh

A composite mesh combines at least 2 materials. Many such meshes developed for hernia repair[15] have been adapted for POP surgery. In animal studies, titanium coating of polypropylene reduced the inflammatory response and mesh shrinkage compared with polypropylene mesh alone.[79] Human trials yield mixed results. A pilot study utilized a titanium-coated lightweight 16-g/m^2 polypropylene mesh (TiMesh, GfE Medizintechnik, Germany) to repair recurrent prolapse in 71 women. At 9 months' following anterior and or posterior repair, 5.6% were found to have mesh erosions and POP recurrence in the anterior compartment and posterior compartment for 36% and 18%, respectively.[80] A more encouraging study by Levy and colleagues describes the use of a similar mesh with no mesh arms but a U-shaped flexible biocompatible frame holding the mesh.[81] In their pilot study of 20 women undergoing mesh insertion for cystocele repair, there were no recurrences of prolapse, no reports of chronic pain or dyspareunia, 1 frame erosion (at 8 months), and 1 de novo SUI case by 24 months.[81]

Cadenbach-Blome and colleagues trialed a 6-arm titanium-coated lightweight polypropylene mesh (TiLOOP PRO A, 25 g/m^2). At 12 months, no mesh erosions occurred with a 4.3% (2/46) recurrence in stage II prolapse.[82] In comparison, at 36 months following implantation of a higher-weight titanium-coated polypropylene mesh (TiLOOP Total 6, 35 g/m^2), Funfgeld and colleagues report 13% mesh exposure, of which 81% (30/37) required intervention under local or general anesthetic. Recurrent cystocele was found in 4.5%, 15% had posterior vaginal wall prolapse recurrence, and 4.8% had apical recurrence.[83] Quality-of-life scores and sexual function scores remained improved from baseline at 36 months. Postoperative de novo dyspareunia occurred in up to 4.5% of women who have undergone POP surgery with the use of titanium-coated polypropylene mesh.[80,83]

Even for the composite mesh products, polypropylene mesh density could have an impact on mesh exposure complications rates. Further studies are warranted to optimize the mesh insertion methods.

COLLAGEN-COATED MESH

Collagen-coated polypropylene meshes with a hydrophilic film of porcine atelocollagen, polyethylene glycol, and glycerol (Ugytex, Covidien, France) were developed with the aim to reduce the inflammatory response induced by the polypropylene on insertion. Histologic analysis in animal studies demonstrate similar inflammatory response to the collagen-coated mesh compared with an uncoated polypropylene mesh (58 g/m^2) with evidence of infection surrounding the collagen-coated mesh and ongoing tissue remodeling at 180 days postimplantation.[84,85] No difference in the mesh contraction and biomechanical properties between the coated and uncoated polypropylene mesh was observed. Mesh exposure occurred in 33% of the ewe models (3/9 collagen-coated vs 1/9 noncoated) at 12 weeks.[85]

In human studies, successful anatomic repair of anterior prolapse was reported in 86% to 92%[86,87] and considered superior to native tissue repair success of 64% ($P = .0006$) at 1 year.[87] Longer-term (4–8 years), 74% to 96% anatomic success[86,88] using collagen-coated polypropylene mesh compared with 33% ($P = .004$) native tissue repair is described.[88] Mesh exposure or extrusion was up to 7.5% at 1 year and 12.5% at 7 years.[88] Other complications secondary to collagen-coated polypropylene mesh include de novo dyspareunia in 4% to 25% (compared with 7% undergoing native tissue repair), pain requiring surgery to transect the transobturator mesh arm, and painful vaginal examination for up to 18%.[87,89] No overall difference in quality-of-life improvement and sexual function between collagen-coated polypropylene mesh and native tissue repair long term was observed.[88]

A similar product with a heavier collagen-coated polypropylene mesh (Avaulta Plus, Bard, USA) demonstrated a high mesh exposure rate of 14% with no subjective benefit compared with native tissue repair in a 3-year RCT.[90] Both of these collagen-coated polypropylene mesh products no longer are available. The long-term outcomes for lighter-weight collagen-coated polypropylene mesh could encourage further studies into the use of this composite mesh.

Polypropylene and polyglecaprone

Another hybrid mesh is a blend of monofilament nonabsorbable polypropylene and absorbable polyglecaprone-25 (Prolift + M), approved for use in 2008. After absorption of the polyglecaprone component by 90 days to 120 days, the mesh density is reduced to 31 g/m^2. It was hypothesized that this composite mesh would be softer, easier to handle, and induce less inflammation. In animal studies, the addition of polyglecaprone did not reduce the risk of mesh exposure or contraction compared with polypropylene alone (45 g/m^2). One-year follow-up from 2 human studies report an anatomic success of 90% and 94%, subjective success of 88% and 89%, and a low mesh exposure rate of 2.2% to 5%. Of note, 2% to 6% reported dyspareunia, and 0.7% to 3.9% reported pelvic or vaginal pain.[91,92] At 24 months' follow-up, compared with native tissue repair, no significant benefit to the use of the hybrid nonabsorbable polypropylene and absorbable polyglecaprone-25 mesh was observed.[93] Mesh exposure was 5.6%, 25% of which underwent surgery for mesh exposure.[93,94] The product since has been withdrawn from the market. Overall, hybrid meshes have not demonstrated any appreciable benefit over nonhybrid meshes or native tissue repairs. There are few of these meshes currently on the market.

TISSUE ENGINEERING

The optimal support scaffold for POP surgery should aim to facilitate new matrix production to reinforce the fascia while minimizing the development of scar tissue. The use of synthetic mesh grafts or biological grafts has not achieved this balance efficiently and the focus has turned to tissue engineering methods in an attempt to develop better scaffolds.

Tissue engineering has led to the exploration of synthetic electrospun scaffold sheets. These are created with electrostatic forces to be ultrafine, hydrophilic, biomimetic nanofibrous scaffolds that represent the extracellular matrix. The fibers are 10-μm wide to create a large surface area–to–volume ratio.[95] They aim to facilitate cellular attachment, proliferation and extracellular matrix deposition for better host tissue integration and mechanical support. They can be aegradable or nondegradable, single polymer, or blended with other materials. Examples investigated alone, blended, or combined with gelatin and nylon include polylactic acid (PLA), polycaprolactone (PCL), poly-L-lactide-co-1-caprolactone (PLCL), polyurethanes (PUs), and poly(lactic-co-glycolic acid) (PLGA).

In vitro studies show successful attachment, proliferation, and development of extracellular matrix to electrospun materials, such as nylon, blended PLGA/PCL, and PCL with gelatin.[96] Animal studies have also yielded promising results. A comparison of PLA mesh with lightweight polypropylene mesh in Wistar rats demonstrated preservation of tensile strength at 90 days with a milder inflammatory host response and more orderly collagen deposition with the PLA mesh.[97] Lightweight polypropylene mesh (19 g/m^2) compared with trilayer PU and single-layer ureidopyrimidinone–polycarbonate implanted to the posterior vaginal wall of ewe models, identified PU as a promising scaffold that maintained stiffness compared with the lightweight polypropylene mesh.[98] The lightweight polypropylene mesh, however, induced the least inflammation and demonstrated less shrinkage.[98]

Although these initial results are encouraging, complications, such as microabscess and hernia formation due to early degradation of a biodegradable PCL graft in rat models, have been reported.[99] To this end, impregnation of grafts with antimicrobial agents have been tested in animal models. Resistance to infection as well as good biocompatibility was proved and will encourage further research.[100]

Electrospun fibers can be seeded with cultivated cells, such as fibroblasts, skeletal muscle cells, mesenchymal stem cells (MSCs), or growth factors, to form a hybrid material. MSCs are multipotent stem cells that typically reside in bone marrow or as endometrial MSCs (eMSCs) or stromal cells and adipose-derived stem cells (ADSCs). One of the challenges in working with stem cells is harvesting and cultivating the stem cells without further spontaneous differentiation into non-clonogenic fibroblasts.[75] This can be overcome with optimization of culture mediums.[101]

MSCs have immune modulation and anti-inflammatory properties, with eMSCs demonstrating the promotion of type 2 macrophages that promote wound healing over type 1 inflammation generating macrophages.[102] Rat model studies comparing a gelatin-coated polyamide knit mesh with and without seeded eMSCs demonstrated significantly more angiogenesis, delayed degeneration of the electrospun scaffold, and fewer macrophages surrounding the eMSCs seeded mesh.[102] ADSCs on a PLA graft also led to stimulation of angiogenesis, collagen formation, and extensive host cell invasion at only 7 days following implantation in rat models.[103] Clinically, it is hoped this research can lead to the development of a hybrid graft that is associated with reduced scarring and contraction during healing with a reduction in undesirable mesh related complications.

There is interest in the concept of autologous transplantation that may 1 day pave the way for individualized bioengineered tissues, for example, autologous muscle fibers seeded to either decellularized matrix from pig SIS or biodegradable PLGA scaffolds. In rat models, these methods have demonstrated ingrowth of new muscle fibers to abdominal grafts and healthy smooth muscle with vaginal tissue repair.[104,105]

Alternative cells for seeding also could include induced pluripotent stem cells from autologous mature somatic cells. Autologous cells could overcome the challenge of immune rejection. This complicated biotechnology is in its infancy and a greater understanding of how these induced cells would behave in vivo particularly with regard to mutation and the risk of tumor formation still is required.[74]

FACTORS AFFECTING SURGICAL OUTCOMES

Outcomes following vaginal POP surgery with mesh or graft scaffolds are widely heterogeneous and surgical complications utilizing mesh/graft implants likely are multifactorial. Some products have arm extensions passing through the obturator foramen or for sacrospinous ligament fixation. These arms were proposed to decrease the risk of mesh migration and contraction,[63] reduce the risk of SUI, or provide apical support.[37] They do carry specific complications, however, such as intraoperative risk of bleeding, hematoma or visceral injury, and postoperative mesh arm tenderness in 4.5% of women[27] or buttock and perineal pain in 11%.[106] Grafts may be sutured or anchored into place or remain unanchored. Failure of an anchoring system over time may encourage failure of the mesh procedure and should be studied separately before clinical trials are undertaken.[107]

Some surgeons have modified their surgical methods in an attempt to reduce the risk of mesh/graft exposure. For example, soaking the mesh implant in betadine prior to insertion may reduce the risk of infection.[37] Avoiding endopelvic fascia plication[86,87] and not trimming excess vaginal mucosa could reduce mesh contraction and mesh exposure.[86,87,108] The use of perioperative vaginal estrogen[37,42,43,82,83,89] may increase collagen deposition to aid vaginal mucosa healing.[109]

Transvaginal POP procedures using additional mesh for SUI procedures, mesh for more than 1 compartment repair, or hysterectomy also can have an impact on long-term outcomes. Concomitant or previous hysterectomy was associated with an increased risk of prolapse recurrence in the posterior compartment and increased risk of mesh exposure.[82,110,111] Mesh exposure risk also increased with more mesh implantation.[112,113] At 1 year, women with transvaginal mesh placement for both POP and SUI had a higher risk of mesh exposure (2.7%–4.5%) than mesh placement for POP (2%) or SUI alone (1.6%).[112,113]

Many studies include and combine analysis for women undergoing primary and secondary prolapse repair.[5,27,42,44] Studies often are single arm in design and retrospective. In addition, a single definition of surgical success or failure is not unanimously accepted. Therefore, with these described variations, study outcomes for different meshes or graft cannot be generalized or compared due to the nature of their individual material properties, scaffold design, implantation methods, surgical techniques, and patient factors. Most mesh manufacturers now produce lightweight mesh; however, not all mesh or mesh kits are created equally.

SUMMARY

The search continues for optimal constructs to augment vaginal POP surgery to prolong outcomes, improve patient satisfaction, and reduce complications. The current available study results generally are of low-quality evidence over relatively short periods of times, making conclusions on outcomes difficult to establish. Prioritizing research to help understand mesh biomechanics and graft constructs will aid the development of an ideal scaffold for POP repair. The development and implementation of core outcome sets could help standardize outcome reporting for future research.[114]

New products for prolapse surgery must be introduced carefully to the market after robust testing in both animal and clinical trials to generate surgeon and patient support and confidence. At present, mesh complication risks do not favor the use of mesh for primary POP surgery. Women at high risk of prolapse recurrence or requiring recurrent prolapse repair may wish to consider the use of transvaginal mesh or grafts. Careful and considered preoperative patient counseling is imperative to empower and support women in their choice of POP management. In the authors' opinion, the individual patient should contribute a decision toward what is an acceptable level of complication risk. Ongoing follow-up and monitoring of these women are required to ascertain long-term outcomes, and the creation of registries supports this challenge.

CLINICS CARE POINTS

- Should the use of polypropylene mesh be utilized for vaginal prolapse surgery, consideration the use of lightweight mesh should be given.

- Preoperative counseling for vaginal prolapse surgery with polypropylene mesh should include an in-depth discussion on the increased risks of complications compared with native tissue repair, including mesh exposure, mesh extrusion, pain, and mesh removal surgery. Patients should be made aware of the long-lasting or late occurring nature of these risks.

- The use of biological grafts for anterior vaginal compartment surgery demonstrates equal if not superior efficacy to native tissue repair in short term studies and have reduced complication rates compared with polypropylene mesh. Their specific role in vaginal prolapse surgery remains unresolved, however, and patients should be informed that the long-term outcomes are not yet fully evaluated.

- Specialists who wish to consider the use of newer composite or tissue engineered mesh are encouraged to do so only as part of regulated clinical trials.

- Due to the insufficient available evidence, the use of mesh grafts made from any material for vaginal surgery should be recorded in a database. Long-term review and reporting of surgical outcomes are encouraged.

FINANCIAL DISCLOSURE/CONFLICT OF INTEREST

None.

REFERENCES

1. Hendrix SL, Clark A, Nygaard I, et al. Pelvic organ prolapse in the Women's health Initiative: Gravity and gravidity. Am J Obstet Gynecol 2002;186(6): 1160–6.
2. Olsen AL, Smith VJ, Bergstrom JO, et al. Epidemiology of surgically managed pelvic organ prolapse and urinary incontinence. Obstet. Gynecol 1997;89:501–6.
3. Smith FJ, Holman CDAJ, Moorin RE, et al. Lifetime risk of undergoing surgery for pelvic organ prolapse. Obstet Gynecol 2010;116:1096–100.
4. Jelovsek JE, Maher C, Barber MD. Pelvic organ prolapse. Lancet 2007;369: 1027–38.
5. Ferry P, Bertherat P, Gauthier A, et al. Transvaginal treatment of anterior and apical genital prolapses using an Ultra lightweight mesh: Restorelle® Direct FixTM. A retrospective study on feasibility and morbidity. J Gynecol Obstet Hum Reprod 2018;47:443–9.
6. Clark AL, Gregory T, Smith VJ, et al. Epidemiologic evaluation of reoperation for surgically treated pelvic organ prolapse and urinary incontinence. Am J Obstet Gynecol 2003;189:1261–7.
7. Julian TM, Grody T. The efficacy of Marlex mesh in the repair of severe, recurrent vaginal prolapse of the anterior midvaginal wall American Journal of Obstetrics and Gynecology. Am J Obstet Gynecol 1996;175(6):1472–5.
8. Shah HN, Badlani GH. Mesh complications in female pelvic floor reconstructive surgery and their management: A systematic review. Indian J Urol 2012;28: 129–53.
9. Lin LL, Haessler AL, Ho MH, et al. Dyspareunia and chronic pelvic pain after polypropylene mesh augmentation for transvaginal repair of anterior vaginal wall prolapse. Int Urogynecol J 2007;18:675–8.
10. FDA Public Health Notification: Serious Complications Associated with Transvaginal Placement of Surgical Mesh in Repair of Pelvic Organ Prolapse and Stress Urinary Incontinence. October 2008. Available at: http://www.amiform.com/web/documents-risques-op-coelio-vagi/fda-notification-about-vaginal-mesh.pdf.
11. Transvaginal Mesh Recalls, Discontinued Products & FDA Regulation. Available at: https://www.drugwatch.com/transvaginal-mesh/recall/.
12. Urogynecologic Surgical Mesh: Update on the Safety and Effectiveness of Transvaginal Placement for Pelvic Organ Prolapse. Available at: https://www.fda.gov/files/medical%20devices/published/Urogynecologic-Surgical-Mesh–Update-on-the-Safety-and-Effectiveness-of-Transvaginal-Placement-for-Pelvic-Organ-Prolapse-%28July-2011%29.pdf.
13. UPDATE on Serious Complications Associated with Transvaginal Placement of Surgical Mesh for Pelvic Organ Prolapse: FDA Safety Communication. Available at: https://2015.iuga.org/wp-content/uploads/workshops/ws29_literature7.pdf.

14. Heneghan CJ, Goldacre B, Onakpoya I, et al. Trials of transvaginal mesh devices for pelvic organ prolapse: A systematic database review of the US FDA approval process. BMJ Open 2017;7:e017125.
15. Bilsel Y, Abci I. The search for ideal hernia repair; mesh materials and types. Int J Surg 2012;10:317–21.
16. Rosch R, Junge K, Schachtrupp A, et al. Mesh implants in hernia repair: Inflammatory cell response in a rat model. Eur Surg Res 2003;35:161–6.
17. Klinge U, Klosterhalfen B, Müller M, et al. Shrinking of polypropylene mesh in vivo: An experimental study in dogs. Eur J Surg 1998;164:965–9.
18. Klinge U, Klosterhalfen B, Birkenhauer V, et al. Impact of polymer pore size on the interface scar formation in a rat model. J Surg Res 2002;103:208–14.
19. Cobb WS, Kercher KW, Heniford BT. The argument for lightweight polypropylene mesh in hernia repair. Surg Innov 2005;12:63–9.
20. Clavé A, Yahi H, Hammou JC, et al. Polypropylene as a reinforcement in pelvic surgery is not inert: Comparative analysis of 100 explants. Int Urogynecol J 2010;21:261–70.
21. Bigozzi MA, Provenzano S, Maeda F, et al. vivo biomechanical properties of heavy versus light weight monofilament polypropylene meshes. Does the knitting pattern matter? Neurourol Urodyn 2017;36:73–9.
22. Schimpf MO, Abed H, Sanses T, et al. Graft and mesh use in transvaginal prolapse repair. Obstet Gynecol 2016;128:81–91.
23. Juliato CRT, do Santos Júnior LC, Haddad JM, et al. Cirurgia com tela para correção de prolapso de parede anterior. Metanálise Rev Bras Ginecol e Obstet 2016;38:356–64.
24. Maher C, Feiner B, Baessler K, et al. Transvaginal mesh or grafts compared with native tissue repair for vaginal prolapse. Cochrane Database Syst Rev 2016;(2):CD012079.
25. Antosh DD, Kim-Fine S, Meriwether KV, et al. Changes in sexual activity and function after pelvic organ prolapse surgery. Obstet Gynecol 2020;136:922–31.
26. Maher C, Feiner B, Baessler K, et al. Surgery for women with anterior compartment prolapse. Cochrane Database Syst Rev 2016;11(11):CD004014.
27. Dykes N, Karmakar D, Hayward L. Lightweight transvaginal mesh is associated with lower mesh exposure rates than heavyweight mesh. Int Urogynecol J 2020; 31:1785–91.
28. Weber AM, Walters MD, Piedmonte MR, et al. Anterior colporrhaphy: a randomized trial of three surgical techniques. Am J Obstet Gynecol ;(6):1299 - 306 2001;185(6):1299–306.
29. Madhuvrata P, Glazener C, Boachie C, et al. A randomised controlled trial evaluating the use of polyglactin (Vicryl) mesh, polydioxanone (PDS) or polyglactin (Vicryl) sutures for pelvic organ prolapse surgery: Outcomes at 2 years. J Obstet Gynaecol (Lahore) 2011;31:429–35.
30. Minassian VA, Parekh M, Poplawsky D, et al. Randomized controlled trial comparing two procedures for anterior vaginal wall prolapse Neurourol. Urodyn 2014;33:72–7.
31. Allahdin S, Glazener C, Bain C. A randomised controlled trial evaluating the use of polyglactin mesh, polydioxanone and polyglactin sutures for pelvic organ prolapse surgery. J Obstet Gynaecol (Lahore) 2008;28:427–31.
32. Yang T-H, Wu L, Chuang F-C, et al. Comparing the midterm outcome of single incision vaginal mesh and transobturator vaginal mesh in treating severe pelvic organ prolapse Taiwan. J Obstet Gynecol 2017;56:81–6.

33. Long C-Y, Wang C-L, Wu M-P, et al. Comparison of clinical outcomes using "elevate anterior" versus "perigee" system devices for the treatment of pelvic organ prolapse. Biomed Res Int 2015;2015:1–7.

34. Moore RD, Lukban JC. Comparison of vaginal mesh extrusion rates between a lightweight type i polypropylene mesh versus heavier mesh in the treatment of pelvic organ prolapse. Int Urogynecol J 2012;23:1379–86.

35. Rogowski A, Bienkowski P, Tarwacki D, et al. Retrospective comparison between the Prolift and Elevate anterior vaginal mesh procedures: 18-month clinical outcome. Int Urogynecol J 2015;26:1815–20.

36. Banach R, Antosiak B, Blewniewska G, et al. Evaluation of safety and effectiveness of pelvic organ prolapse treatment with the use of polypropylene mesh depending on mesh and application technique. Polish Gynaecol 2013;84: 596–602.

37. Fekete Z, Korösi S, Pajor L, et al. Does anchoring vaginal mesh increase the potential for correcting stress incontinence? BMC Urol 2018;18:53.

38. Kdous M, Zhioua F. 3-year results of transvaginal cystocele repair with transobturator four-arm mesh: A prospective study of 105 patients. Arab J Urol 2014;12: 275–84.

39. de Tayrac R, Brouziyne M, Priou G, et al. Transvaginal repair of stage III–IV cystocele using a lightweight mesh: safety and 36-month outcome. Int Urogynecol J Pelvic Floor Dysfunct 2015;26:1147–54.

40. Mateu-Arrom L, Gutiérrez-Ruiz C, Palou Redorta J, et al. Pelvic Organ Prolapse Repair with Mesh: Description of Surgical Technique Using the Surelift® Anterior Repair System. Urol Int 2020;105(1–2):137–42.

41. Lo TS, Ng KL, Huang TX, et al. Anterior-apical transvaginal mesh (surelift) for advanced urogenital prolapse: surgical and functional outcomes at 1 year. J Minim Invasive Gynecol 2020;28(1):107–16.

42. Marschke J, Hengst L, Schwertner-Tiepelmann N, et al. Transvaginal single-incision mesh reconstruction for recurrent or advanced anterior vaginal wall prolapse. Arch Gynecol Obstet 2015;291:1081–7.

43. Buca DIP, Liberati M, Falò E, et al. Long-term outcome after surgical repair of pelvic organ prolapse with Elevate Prolapse Repair System. J Obstet Gynaecol (Lahore) 2018;38:854–9.

44. Huang K-H, Huang L-Y, Chu L-C, et al. Evaluation of the single-incision Elevate system to treat pelvic organ prolapse: follow-up from 15 to 45 months. Int Urogynecol J 2015;26:1341–6.

45. Azaïs H, Charles CJ, Delporte P, et al. Prolapse repair using the ElevateTM kit: prospective study on 70 patients. Int Urogynecol J 2012;23:1421–8.

46. Stanford EJ, Moore RD, Roovers J-PWR, et al. Elevate Anterior/Apical Female Pelvic. Med Reconstr Surg 2013;19:79–83.

47. Moore RD, Mitchell GK, Miklos JR. Single-incision vaginal approach to treat cystocele and vault prolapse with an anterior wall mesh anchored apically to the sacrospinous ligaments. Int Urogynecol J 2012;23:85–91.

48. Castellani D, Galica V, Saldutto P, et al. Efficacy and safety of Elevate® system on apical and anterior compartment prolapse repair with personal technique modification Int. Braz J Urol 2017;43:1115–21.

49. Huang E, Koh WS, Han HC. Five-year outcomes of an anterior mesh kit for severe pelvic organ prolapse in women. Neurourol Urodyn 2021;40(3):910–9.

50. Rapp DE, King AB, Rowe B, et al. Comprehensive evaluation of anterior elevate system for the treatment of anterior and apical pelvic floor descent: 2-year followup. J Urol 2014;191:389–94.

51. Lo T-S, Al-Kharabsheh AM, Tan YL, et al. Single incision anterior apical mesh and sacrospinous ligament fixation in pelvic prolapse surgery at 36 months follow-up. Taiwan. J Obstet Gynecol 2017;56:793–800.

52. Karmakar D, Hayward L, Smalldridge J, et al. Vaginal mesh for prolapse: a long-term prospective study of 218 mesh kits from a single centre. Int Urogynecol J Pelvic Floor Dysfunct 2015;26:1161–70.

53. Kapur K, Dalal V. Mesh repair of vaginal wall prolapse. Med J Armed Forces India 2014;70:105–10.

54. Lukban JC, Roovers J-PWR, VanDrie DM, et al. Single-incision apical and posterior mesh repair: 1-year prospective outcomes. Int Urogynecol J 2012;23:1413–9.

55. Lo T-S, bt Karim N, Cortes EFM, et al. Comparison between Elevate Anterior/Apical system and Perigee system in pelvic organ prolapse surgery: clinical and sonographic outcomes. Int Urogynecol J 2015;26:391–400.

56. Lamblin G, Gouttenoire C, Panel L, et al. A retrospective comparison of two vaginal mesh kits in the management of anterior and apical vaginal prolapse: long-term results for apical fixation and quality of life. Int Urogynecol J 2016;27:1847–55.

57. Lai QY, Yang X, Zhu Y, et al. Prospective study of the Perigee system in the treatment of anterior pelvic organ prolapse]. Zhonghua Fu Chan Ke Za Zhi 2016;51:103–8.

58. Allegre L, Debodinance P, Demattei C, et al. Clinical evaluation of the Uphold LITE mesh for the surgical treatment of anterior and apical prolapse: A prospective, multicentre trial. Neurourol Urodyn 2019;38:2242–9.

59. Lo TS, Pue LB, Tan YL, et al. Anterior-apical single-incision mesh surgery (uphold): 1-year outcomes on lower urinary tract symptoms, anatomy and ultrasonography. Int Urogynecol J 2019;30:1163–72.

60. Altman D, Mikkola TS, Bek KM, et al, Falconer C and For the Nordic TVM group. Pelvic organ prolapse repair using the UpholdTM Vaginal Support System: a 1-year multicenter study. Int Urogynecol J 2016;27:1337–45.

61. Chang CP, Hsu FK, Lai MJ, et al. Uterine-preserving pelvic organ prolapse surgery using the UPHOLD LITE vaginal support system: The outcomes of 291 patients. Medicine (Baltimore) 2019;98:e15086.

62. Renard N, Bartolo S, Giraudet G, et al. Feasibility of vaginal mesh for anterior vaginal wall prolapse in an ambulatory setting: A retrospective case series. J Gynecol Obstet Hum Reprod 2020;49:101684.

63. Duport C, Duperron C, Delorme E. Anterior and middle pelvic organ prolapse repair using a six tension-free strap low weight transvaginal mesh: long-term retrospective monocentric study of 311 patients. J Gynecol Obstet Hum Reprod 2019;48:143–9.

64. Guyomard A, Delorme E. Transvaginal treatment of anterior or central urogenital prolapse using six tension-free straps and light mesh. Int J Gynecol Obstet 2016;133:365–9.

65. Zangarelli A, Curinier S, Campagne-Loiseau S, et al. Cure de cystocèle par prothèse vaginale libre de faible grammage : résultats à 6 ans Progrès en. Urol 2020;30:367–73.

66. Gauthier A, Ferry P, Bertherat P, et al. Transvaginal treatment of anterior and apical genital prolapse using Restorelle® direct fixTM: An observational study of medium-term complications and outcomes. J Gynecol Obstet Hum Reprod 2020;49:101674.

67. Denancé M, Quiboeuf E, Hocké C. Résultats, tolérance et satisfaction des patientes à 6 mois d'une cure de cystocèle par voie vaginale avec pose de prothèse. Prog en Urol 2016;26:582–8.
68. Rogowski A, Kluz T, Szafarowska M, et al. Efficacy and safety of the Calistar and Elevate anterior vaginal mesh procedures. Eur J Obstet Gynecol Reprod Biol 2019;239:30–4.
69. Naumann G, Hüsch T, Mörgeli C, et al. Mesh-augmented transvaginal repair of recurrent or complex anterior pelvic organ prolapse in accordance with the SCENIHR opinion. Int Urogynecol J 2020;32(4):819–27.
70. Sampietro A, Paradisi G, Scambia G, et al. A retrospective comparison of Calistar a vs Calister S. Pelviperineology 2018;38:106–11.
71. Achtari C, Hiscock R, O'Reilly BA, et al. Risk factors for mesh erosion after transvaginal surgery using polypropylene (Atrium) or composite polypropylene/polyglactin 910 (Vypro II) mesh. Int Urogynecol J 2005;16:389–94.
72. El Haddad R, Martan A, Masata J, et al. Long-term review on posterior colporrhaphy with levator ani muscles plication and incorporating a Vypro II mesh Ces. Gynekol 2009;74:282–5.
73. Lim YN, Muller R, Corstiaans A, et al. A long-term review of posterior colporrhaphy with Vypro 2 mesh. Int Urogynecol J 2007;18:1053–7.
74. Wu X, Jia Y, Sun X, et al. Tissue engineering in female pelvic floor reconstruction. Eng Life Sci 2020;20:275–86.
75. Gargett CE, Gurung S, Darzi S, et al. Tissue engineering approaches for treating pelvic organ prolapse using a novel source of stem/stromal cells and new materials. Curr Opin Urol 2019;29:450–7.
76. Glazener CM, Breeman S, Elders A, et al. Mesh, graft, or standard repair for women having primary transvaginal anterior or posterior compartment prolapse surgery: two parallel-group, multicentre, randomised, controlled trials (PROSPECT). Lancet 2017;389:381–92.
77. Wei A-M, Fan Y, Zhang L, et al. Evaluation of clinical outcome and risk factors for recurrence after pelvic reconstruction of pelvic organ prolapse with implanted mesh or biological grafts: a single-blind randomized trial gynecol. Obstet Invest 2019;84:503–11.
78. Balzarro M, Rubilotta E, Porcaro AB, et al. Long-term follow-up of anterior vaginal repair: A comparison among colporrhaphy, colporrhaphy with reinforcement by xenograft, and mesh. Neurourol Urodyn 2018;37:278–83.
79. Scheidbach H, Tamme C, Tannapfel A, Lippert H and Köckerling F K In vivo studies comparing the biocompatibility of various polypropylene meshes and their handling properties during endoscopic total extraperitoneal (TEP) patchplasty An experimental study in pigs Springer
80. Milani AL, Heidema WM, van der Vloedt WS, et al. Vaginal prolapse repair surgery augmented by ultra lightweight titanium coated polypropylene mesh. Eur J Obstet Gynecol Reprod Biol 2008;138:232–8.
81. Levy G, Padoa A, Fekete Z, et al. Self-retaining support implant: an anchorless system for the treatment of pelvic organ prolapse—2-year follow-up. Int Urogynecol J 2018;29:709–14.
82. Cadenbach-Blome T, Grebe M, Mengel M, et al. Significant improvement in quality of life, positive effect on sexuality, lasting reconstructive result and low rate of complications following cystocele correction using a lightweight, large-pore, titanised polypropylene mesh: final results of a national, multicentre observational study. Geburtshilfe Frauenheilkd 2019;79:959–68.

83. Fünfgeld C, Stehle M, Henne B, et al. Quality of life, sexuality, anatomical results and side-effects of implantation of an alloplastic mesh for cystocele correction at follow-up after 36 months. Geburtshilfe Frauenheilkd 2017;77:993–1002.

84. Feola A, Endo M, Urbankova I, et al. Host reaction to vaginally inserted collagen containing polypropylene implants in sheep. Am J Obstet Gynecol 2015;212: 474.e1-e8.

85. Tayrac R, Alves A, Thérin M. Collagen-coated vs noncoated low-weight polypropylene meshes in a sheep model for vaginal surgery. A pilot study. Int Urogynecol J 2007;18:513–20.

86. de Tayrac R, Devoldere G, Renaudie J, et al. Prolapse repair by vaginal route using a new protected low-weight polypropylene mesh: 1-year functional and anatomical outcome in a prospective multicentre study. Int Urogynecol J 2007;18:251–6.

87. de Tayrac R, Cornille A, Eglin G, et al. Comparison between trans-obturator trans-vaginal mesh and traditional anterior colporrhaphy in the treatment of anterior vaginal wall prolapse: results of a French RCT. Int Urogynecol J 2013; 24:1651–61.

88. Allègre L, Callewaert G, Alonso S, et al. Long-term outcomes of a randomized controlled trial comparing trans-obturator vaginal mesh with native tissue repair in the treatment of anterior vaginal wall prolapse. Int Urogynecol J 2020;31: 745–53.

89. Sergent F, Resch B, Al-Khattabi M, et al. Transvaginal mesh repair of pelvic organ prolapse by the transobturator-infracoccygeal hammock technique: Long-term anatomical and functional outcomes. Neurourol Urodyn 2011;30:384–9.

90. Rudnicki M, Laurikainen E, Pogosean R, et al. A 3-year follow-up after anterior colporrhaphy compared with collagen-coated transvaginal mesh for anterior vaginal wall prolapse: A randomised controlled trial. BJOG 2016;123:136–42.

91. Khandwala S. Transvaginal mesh surgery for pelvic organ prolapse female pelvic. Med Reconstr Surg 2013;19:84–9.

92. Milani AL, Hinoul P, Gauld JM, et al. Trocar-guided mesh repair of vaginal prolapse using partially absorbable mesh: 1 year outcomes. Am J Obstet Gynecol 2011;204:74.e1-8.

93. Steures P, Milani AL, van Rumpt-van de Geest DA, et al. Partially absorbable mesh or native tissue repair for pelvic organ prolapse: a randomized controlled trial. Int Urogynecol J 2019;30:565–73.

94. Ozog Y, Mazza E, De Ridder D, et al. Biomechanical effects of polyglecaprone fibers in a polypropylene mesh after abdominal and rectovaginal implantation in a rabbit. Int Urogynecol J 2012;23:1397–402.

95. Vashaghian M, Zaat SJ, Smit TH, et al. Biomimetic implants for pelvic floor repair Neurourol. Urodyn 2018;37:566–80.

96. Vashaghian M, Ruiz-Zapata AM, Kerkhof MH, et al. Toward a new generation of pelvic floor implants with electrospun nanofibrous matrices: A feasibility study. Neurourol Urodyn 2017;36:565–73.

97. de Tayrac R, Oliva-Lauraire MC, Guiraud I, et al. Long-lasting bioresorbable poly(lactic acid) (PLA94) mesh: A new approach for soft tissue reinforcement based on an experimental pilot study. Int Urogynecol J 2007;18:1007–14.

98. Hympánová L, Rynkevic R, Román S, et al. Assessment of electrospun and ultra-lightweight polypropylene meshes in the sheep model for vaginal surgery. Eur Urol Focus 2020;6:190–8.

99. Hansen SG, Taskin MB, Chen M, et al. Electrospun nanofiber mesh with fibroblast growth factor and stem cells for pelvic floor repair. J Biomed Mater Res B Appl Biomater 2020;108:48–55.

100. Liang C, Ling Y, Wei F, et al. A novel antibacterial biomaterial mesh coated by chitosan and tigecycline for pelvic floor repair and its biological performance. Regen Biomater 2020;7:483–90.

101. Gurung S, Williams S, Deane JA, et al. The transcriptome of human endometrial mesenchymal stem cells under TGFβR inhibition reveals improved potential for cell-based therapies. Front Cell Dev Biol 2018;6:164.

102. Ulrich D, Edwards SL, Su K, et al. Human endometrial mesenchymal stem cells modulate the tissue response and mechanical behavior of polyamide mesh implants for pelvic organ prolapse repair. Tissue Eng A 2014;20:785–98.

103. Roman Regueros S, Albersen M, Manodoro S, et al. Acute In Vivo Response to an Alternative Implant for Urogynecology. Biomed Res Int 2014;2014:1–10.

104. Ho MH, Heydarkhan S, Vernet D, et al. Stimulating Vaginal Repair in Rats Through Skeletal Muscle–Derived Stem Cells Seeded on Small Intestinal Submucosal Scaffolds. Obstet Gynecol 2009;114:300–9.

105. Boennelycke M, Christensen L, Nielsen LF, et al. Fresh muscle fiber fragments on a scaffold in rats–a new concept in urogynecology? Am J Obstet Gynecol 2011;205. 235.e10-e14.

106. Hugele F, Panel L, Farache C, et al. Two years follow up of 270 patients treated by transvaginal mesh for anterior and/or apical prolapse. Eur J Obstet Gynecol Reprod Biol 2017;208:16–22.

107. Anding R, Tabaza R, Staat M, et al. Introducing a Method of In Vitro Testing of Different Anchoring Systems Used for Female Incontinence and Prolapse Surgery. Biomed Res Int 2013;2013:1–7.

108. Vinchant M, Bitumba I, Letouzey V, et al. Reoperation rate and outcomes following the placement of polypropylene mesh by the vaginal route for cystocele: very long-term follow-up. Int Urogynecol J 2020;32(4):929–35.

109. Higgins EW, Rao A, Baumann SS, et al. Effect of estrogen replacement on the histologic response to polypropylene mesh implanted in the rabbit vagina model. Am J Obstet Gynecol 2009;201:505.e1-9.

110. De Tayrac R, Faillie JL, Gaillet S, et al. Analysis of the learning curve of bilateral anterior sacrospinous ligament suspension associated with anterior mesh repair Eur. J Obstet Gynecol Reprod Biol 2012;165:361–5.

111. Belot F, Collinet P, Debodinance P, et al. Facteurs de risque des expositions prothétiques après cure de prolapsus génital par voie vaginale Gynecol. Obstet Fertil 2005;33:970–4.

112. Chughtai B, Barber MD, Mao J, et al. Association between the amount of vaginal mesh used with mesh erosions and repeated surgery after repairing pelvic organ prolapse and stress urinary incontinence. JAMA Surg 2017;152:257–63.

113. Lau H-Y, Twu N-F, Chen Y-J, et al. Comparing effectiveness of combined transobturator tension-free vaginal mesh (Perigee) and transobturator tension-free vaginal tape (TVT-O) versus anterior colporrhaphy and TVT-O for associated cystocele and urodynamic stress incontinence. Eur J Obstet Gynecol Reprod Biol 2011;156:228–32.

114. de Mattos Lourenco TR, Pergialiotis V, Duffy JMN, et al. A systematic review on reporting outcomes and outcome measures in trials on synthetic mesh procedures for pelvic organ prolapse: Urgent action is needed to improve quality of research. Neurourol Urodyn 2019;38:509–24.

Urinary Tract Injury During Gynecologic Surgery

Prevention, Recognition, and Management

Ushma J. Patel, MD[a], Christine A. Heisler, MD, MS[a,b],*

KEYWORDS

- Gynecologic surgery complications • Urinary tract injury • Surgical management

KEY POINTS

- Lower urinary tract (LUT) injuries occur in gynecologic surgery because of the close proximity of the reproductive and urologic organs and vary by procedure, surgical route, and indication.
- Early recognition of LUT injuries and immediate management are critical to reduce morbidity.
- LUT injuries diagnosed postoperatively should be managed conservatively initially, and surgical treatment should be performed by an experienced surgeon.

INTRODUCTION

Lower urinary tract (LUT) injuries occur in gynecologic surgery because of the close proximity of the reproductive organs to the urologic organs.[1–3] Prior studies on the incidence of LUT injuries in gynecologic surgery have been single-center, small-scale datasets or limited to laparoscopic hysterectomy, which can make evaluation for risk factors and overall application to clinical practice difficult. One large retrospective cohort study evaluated 101,021 patients undergoing benign hysterectomy between 2010 and 2014. The investigators noted that LUT injury in benign hysterectomy may be higher than previously reported at 2.4%, as this was the incidence of concomitant urologic procedures performed beyond cystoscopy in this cohort.[1] Considering the morbidity associated with LUT injury, prevention must be emphasized, and, in the setting of iatrogenic complications, the aim must be early recognition and treatment. This chapter provides an evidence-based review of lower urinary tract anatomy and

[a] Department of Obstetrics & Gynecology, University of Wisconsin School of Medicine and Public Health, 202 South Park Street, 5E, Madison, WI 53715, USA; [b] Department of Urology, University of Wisconsin School of Medicine and Public Health, 202 South Park Street, 2E, Madison, WI 53715, USA
* Corresponding author. Department of Obstetrics & Gynecology, University of Wisconsin School of Medicine and Public Health, 202 South Park Street, 2E, Madison, WI 53715.
E-mail address: cheisler@wisc.edu

Obstet Gynecol Clin N Am 48 (2021) 535–556
https://doi.org/10.1016/j.ogc.2021.05.007
0889-8545/21/Published by Elsevier Inc.

histology, mechanisms for prevention of injury, and evaluation and management of LUT injury.

ANATOMY

Gynecologic surgeons must understand the intimate anatomic relationship that exists between the reproductive tract and LUT (**Fig. 1**). The urethra, bladder, and distal portions of the ureters are located within the pelvis.

Urethra

The female urethra is an approximately 3-cm long, 6-mm wide fibromuscular tube. The urethra begins at the bladder neck, continues its course fused to the adventitia of the anterior vagina, and terminates at the external urethral meatus in the vulvar vestibule between the clitoris and vaginal opening. Histologically, the urethra has 4 distinct layers: mucosa or epithelium, submucosa, internal urethral sphincter (primarily oblique and longitudinal smooth muscle fibers innervated by autonomic nerves of the pelvic plexus), and striated external urethral or urogenital sphincter innervated by branches of the pudendal nerve.[4–6]

Bladder

The urinary bladder is a hollow, muscular organ that functions as a reservoir for urine. Histologically, the bladder is composed of mucosa or urothelium (consisting of transitional cell epithelium and underlying lamina propria), the detrusor muscle (consisting of interlacing bundles of smooth muscle), and the adventitia. The anterior bladder is extraperitoneal and adjacent to the retropubic space or space of Retzius. The dome of the bladder is contiguous with the anterior abdominal wall parietal peritoneum that posteroinferiorly sweeps off the bladder into the vesicouterine pouch. The remainder of the bladder is retroperitoneal. The base of the bladder rests directly on the anterior vaginal wall (**Fig. 2**) and contains the trigone, a triangular area bound by the internal urethral meatus and the 2 ureteric orifices, which are equidistant from

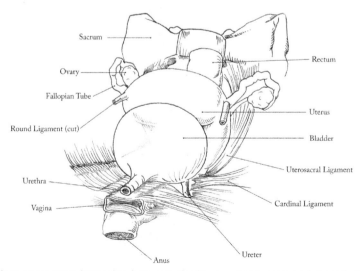

Fig. 1. Close anatomic relationship between the lower urinary tract and reproductive tract. (Illustration by Charlotte Holden.)

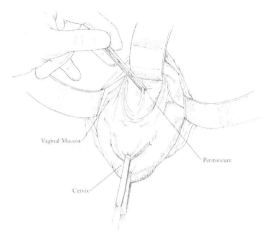

Fig. 2. Transvaginal anatomy. The bladder base rests on the anterior vagina. (Illustration by Charlotte Holden.)

each other with each side of the trigone measuring approximately 3 cm. The superior border of the trigone between the ureteric orifices is the raised interureteric ridge.[4,5]

Ureters

The ureters are 25- to 30-cm long retroperitoneal tubular structures that course from each renal pelvis to the urinary bladder trigone. Histologically, the ureter has one muscular coat of irregular helical muscle bundles that elongate and become parallel to its lumen as it enters the bladder wall. Anatomically divided into pelvic and abdominal components by the pelvic brim, each segment is approximately 12 to 15 cm in length (**Fig. 3**). The ureter enters the pelvis by crossing over the bifurcation of the common iliac artery, initially coursing posterior to the ovarian vessels, attached to the

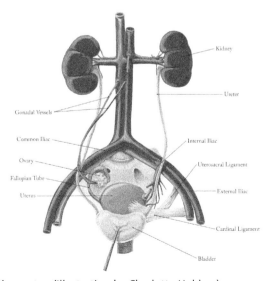

Fig. 3. Course of the ureter. (Illustration by Charlotte Holden.)

peritoneum of the lateral pelvic wall. Proceeding distally, the ureter courses laterally along the uterosacral ligament, descending further into the pelvis within the medial leaf of the broad ligament of the uterus. It passes under the uterine artery, then over the lateral vaginal fornix to enter the anterior bladder pillar (paracervical tunnel of Wertheim), traveling through the wall of the bladder until reaching the trigone. The ureter is 2 to 3 cm lateral to the uterosacral ligament at the level of the ischial spine and 1 cm lateral to the distal uterosacral ligament. The ureter passes under the uterine artery approximately 1.5 cm lateral to the cervix.[4,5,7]

BACKGROUND
Incidence

The risk of injury to the LUT in gynecologic surgery varies with the type of procedure, the surgical approach, and surgeon experience (**Fig. 4**). Factors that increase the risk of LUT injury include altered anatomy, such as pelvic organ prolapse (POP); anomalous anatomy (eg, ureteral duplication, pelvic kidney, or kidney transplantation); pathology (eg, endometriosis or malignancy); and prior surgeries, radiation, or infection causing subsequent scarring.[8–10] The rate of LUT injury in female pelvic surgery has been reported to range from 0.3% to 1.5% for ureteral injury and from 0.2% to 1.8% for bladder injury. More recently published analyses reported a higher rate of 2.4% of patients undergo concomitant urologic intervention secondary to hysterectomy-related LUT injury. Universal cystoscopy in women undergoing benign hysterectomy revealed a cumulative injury rate of 4.3% (bladder injury rate 2.9% and ureteral injury rate 1.8%).[1,8,11–13]

Types of Injuries

Although rare, urethral injuries most commonly occur during surgical correction for urinary incontinence (UI) or POP. The urethra can be injured during dissection of the anterior vagina for midurethral sling placement, anterior colporrhaphy, sacrocolpopexy, or

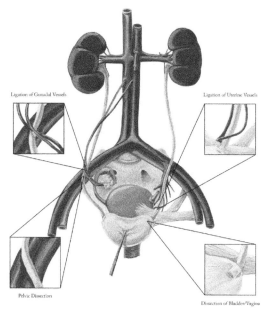

Fig. 4. Common locations of lower urinary injury in gynecologic surgery. (Illustration by Charlotte Holden.)

diverticulum repair. In addition, passage of trocars for midurethral sling placement can perforate the urethra (rates: 1.09%, transobturator; 0.88%, retropubic).[3,9,14] Rarely, patients may present with delayed urethral mesh erosion, although immediate presentations are more typically described.[15,16]

The bladder is the most common site of LUT injury in gynecologic surgery. Bladder injuries include contusion, full or partial thickness injury, devascularization or denervation, and intravesical suture or mesh placement or erosion. Furthermore, bladder injuries can be secondary to incorporation of the bladder into a clamp, sharp dissection, blunt dissection, bladder retraction, or the use of thermal energy devices. Bladder injuries during benign hysterectomies are more common with laparoscopic (1%–1.6%) than abdominal or vaginal routes (0.9% and 0.6%, respectively).[17,18] The cause of cystotomy varies by hysterectomy route: posterior cystotomy occurs during dissection of the bladder from the anterior cervix and proximal vagina in abdominal or laparoscopic hysterectomy and entry into the anterior culdesac in vaginal hysterectomy. Dissection of the bladder from the anterior vagina during anterior colporrhaphy or sacrocolpopexy may result in trigone or bladder neck injury.[3,9] Bladder injury rates during incontinence surgery vary. Bladder perforation with retropubic midurethral sling has been reported to occur in 3% to 5% of cases, although the risk is higher if performed with trainees (**Fig. 5**). The risk of bladder perforation associated with transobturator tape is lower at 0.5%.[14–16,19,20] Although these are viscous injuries, the sequelae are small.

Ureteral injury during gynecologic surgery can occur due to transection, kinking, ligation, laceration, or devascularization.[13] According to ACS NSQIP data from 2005 to 2013, ureteral injuries occurred in 0.48% of minimally invasive (laparoscopic and robotic) hysterectomies, 0.18% of abdominal hysterectomies, and 0.04% of vaginal hysterectomies.[21] Frequently performed vaginally, POP or UI surgery increases the risk of ureteral injury. The most common site of ureteral injury is at the level of the uterine artery.[13] Vaginal reconstructive surgery is associated with a ureteral obstruction rate of 5.1% to 11%, most of which are sustained during uterosacral ligament suspension, proximal McCall culdoplasty, and colpocleisis. Anterior colporrhaphy is associated with a 0.5% to 2% risk of ureteral obstruction.[3]

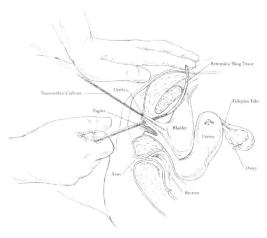

Fig. 5. Proximity of trocar to lower urinary tract during retropubic midurethral sling placement. (Illustration by Charlotte Holden.)

In the United States, the incidence of vesicovaginal fistula (VVF) ranges between 0.13% and 2% and is associated with hysterectomy, pelvic radiotherapy, and malignancy. The association of ureteral injuries with VVF has been variable; however, a large single-center retrospective review of obstetric and gynecologic procedures reported a 3.4% ureteral injury rate.[22,23] Moreover, a recent Cochrane review of benign hysterectomy reported no difference in long-term fistula formation when comparing laparoscopic with other surgical approaches.[24]

PREVENTION

In addition to a thorough understanding of the patient's history, an emphasis must be placed on knowledge of pelvic anatomy in the context of the planned surgical procedure. Routine preoperative imaging has not been shown to reduce the incidence of operative injuries to the lower urinary tract, although cystourethroscopy should be performed if indicated.[3] In addition, with the adoption of electrosurgery, surgeons must have familiarity with operative equipment, as thermal injury accounts for 33% of ureteral injuries, and thermal spread ranging from 1 to 22 mm can lead to delayed injury.[17]

If the bladder is densely adherent, it may be filled through an indwelling catheter to aid delineation of appropriate surgical planes and prevent injury. If the ureter is difficult to identify through the peritoneum, careful retroperitoneal dissection should be performed until it is adequately identified.

Preoperative Ureteral Catheterization

Universal preoperative ureteral catheterization for gynecologic surgery is controversial. Although there is no evidence that stents prevent ureteral injury, they do facilitate immediate recognition of ureteral injury intraoperatively, which decreases the risks of delayed recognition, a second surgery, and associated morbidity.[25,26] However, routine ureteral catheterization is not cost saving until ureteral injury rates approach 3.2%. Although some literature reports that stent placement does not increase operating room time or cause significant complications, colorectal surgery literature reports a 0.5% to 2.2% intraoperative complication rate including perforation or laceration of ureter, infection, and hematuria.[27]

Preoperative Lighted Ureteral Catheterization

Preoperative lighted ureteral catheters are used by some surgeons to assist in identifying the ureters, although their role in LUT injury prevention has not been proved. After insertion, the ureteral stents are illuminated by connecting them to an external power source. Proponents of lighted stents report they are well suited for minimally invasive surgery, as there is no evidence of thermal injury from illumination and ureters can be promptly recognized even in the setting of extensive adhesions and distorted anatomy.[28–31]

Indocyanine Green Administration and Use of Near-Infrared Fluorescence Intraoperatively

Indocyanine green (ICG) is a fluorophore with an excellent safety profile that may be used as a real-time contrast agent to assess ureteral anatomy (**Fig. 6**). Prepared ICG is a cystoscopically injected retrograde into the ureters at the level of the midureter through catheters that are clamped to minimize leakage. After excitation with near-infrared fluorescent light on charge-coupled device cameras, the green luminance of ICG maybe visualized approximately 5 minutes after injection and sustained for greater than 3 hours. ICG may be particularly useful to surgeons operating near the

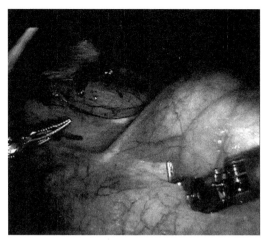

Fig. 6. Indocyanine green used as a real-time contrast agent to assess ureteral anatomy. (Image courtesy of Daniel Eun, MD at Temple University.)

ureter, especially when the ureter deviates from the normal course.[28] Rarely, intravenous ICG has been associated with anaphylactic shock.[32]

ASSESSMENT AND EVALUATION

Early recognition and management of LUT injury are imperative to minimize morbidity for the patient.

Intraoperative

In the event of a suspected LUT injury, dye can be administered intravenously or instilled retrograde into the bladder to assess for extravasation. Findings such as spillage of urine into the surgical field, gas or blood in the indwelling foley catheter bag, or visualization of preoperative ureteral stents or urethral catheters in the dissection field assist intraoperative recognition of LUT injury. Barring these cues, diagnosis is not infrequently delayed to the postoperative period.[3,9,33]

Routine cystourethroscopy is performed in UI and POP repair due to higher risk of LUT injury.[9] However, 40% of LUT injuries occur in the absence of predisposing risk factors, and routine intraoperative cystoscopy may benefit all gynecologic surgery by allowing early diagnosis and repair of injuries, avoiding a secondary surgery, and decreasing risk of renal impairment or loss.[3,9,13] Opponents of routine cystoscopy note increased cost and operating time. A recent cost-effectiveness analysis demonstrated that routine cystoscopy increased hysterectomy cost by $64.59 to 83.99, whereas the cost of selective cystoscopy was lower ($13.20–26.13), although these costs are mitigated with increasing risk or suspicion of injury.[13] However, additional studies report that routine cystoscopy does not increase cost of vaginal surgery and minimally increases cost in all modalities of benign hysterectomy. Importantly, it has been found to be cost saving at ureteral injury rates of 1.5% in abdominal hysterectomy and 2.0% in vaginal hysterectomy. Operative time under anesthesia is not prolonged, and because it increases intraoperative LUT injury detection, those undergoing routine cystoscopy have a shorter time to clinical resolution of injury.[3,11,13,34–37] Although routine cystoscopy increases the intraoperative detection rate of LUT injuries, it does not significantly change postoperative injury detection rates.[11] Despite this, unrecognized iatrogenic ureteral injuries are associated with serious and life-threatening morbidity, and surgeons should maintain a high level of suspicion for injury.[12]

Identification of ureteral injury or patency is completed by assessment of ureteral efflux from each ureteral orifice, and is aided by dyes such as preoperative oral phenazopyridine, intraoperative intravenous methylene blue, indigo carmine, or fluorescein, or by dense distending media such as mannitol or 10% dextrose.[38–40] Because dense distending media may increase the risk of urinary tract infection (UTI), surgeons may choose to administer 200 mg oral phenazopyridine before gynecologic surgery to assist with visualization of ureteral efflux. If cystoscopy equipment is not readily available, and the index of suspicion of ureteral injury warrants evaluation, intentional extraperitoneal cystotomy at the bladder dome allows observation of ureteral jets.[3] In the event that ureteral jets are sluggish or not observed, any object that may be the source of ureteral obstruction should be removed.[9] In addition, some practitioners administer intravenous furosemide 10 mg or fluid boluses. A recent randomized control trial demonstrated that routine intraoperative administration of intravenous furosemide led to a statistically significant decrease in time to confirm ureteral patency in urogynecologic surgery. However, the results were clinically insignificant, and furosemide administration after the start of cystoscopy and delay in ureteral jets was not evaluated.[41]

If ureteral jets remain unsatisfactory, ureteral catheterization can be attempted through cystoscopy or cystotomy. Resistance to passage of the ureteral stent implies kinking or obstruction of the ureter.[3,9] Alternatively, a, retrograde or on-table intravenous pyelography may be performed intraoperatively to evaluate for bladder injury or ureteral obstruction. Radiologic imaging uses contrast medium injected intravenously or into the upper urinary tract through a catheter placed cystoscopically under fluoroscopic guidance.[9,42] Finally, intraoperative ureteroscopy allows direct assessment of the ureters but does independently carry a risk of ureteral injury.[43]

Postoperative

Limited evidence on universal postoperative screening with serum creatinine testing after gynecologic surgery exists, although it does remain an invaluable tool in workup for specific clinical situations among patients with symptoms.[35,44] Patient symptoms should prompt further evaluation in the immediate postoperative period. Intraperitoneal leakage of urine can present with fever, urinary ascites, peritonitis, ileus, wound leakage, flank pain, oliguria, or anuria. A urinoma is diagnosed with elevated fluid collection creatinine. Ureteral obstruction may present as flank or abdominal pain and oliguria or anuria. Finally, LUT injuries can present with ongoing hematuria, urgency incontinence, or abnormal voiding.[9,33]

Most clinical signs and symptoms of iatrogenic LUT injury will present within 48 to 72 hours of the primary procedure. Delayed recognition significantly increases patient morbidity. Long-term consequences of unrecognized LUT injuries include genitourinary fistula formation, ureteral stricture or obstruction, renal failure, mesh erosion, voiding dysfunction, and pain.[9,45–48] Associated symptoms such as hematuria, dysuria, stone formation, urgency, recurrent UTI, UI, or watery vaginal discharge may warrant further evaluation.[9,33] Delayed or undiagnosed ureteral obstruction may result in late diagnosis of a nonfunctioning kidney.[9,43]

When LUT injury is suspected in the postoperative period, various imaging modalities can be used.

Cystography, the instillation of contrast media into the bladder and observation of bladder contour and extravasation via radiographic imaging, is useful in identifying a bladder defect. Addition of computed tomography (CT) to detect extravasation of radiocontrast material from the bladder is helpful if the location of injury is uncertain. It has become the gold-standard diagnostic study for clinically suspected iatrogenic bladder injury with accuracy of 85% to 100%.[9,33,45,46]

In addition, contrast-enhanced CT plays a major role in identifying the source or extent of LUT injury and urine leaks or presence of urinoma (**Fig. 7**). CT urography (or pyelography) has become the most common method for diagnosing missed ureteral injuries over the past 20 years, although there are no published data on sensitivity and specificity.[33,42,46] In the setting of a contraindication to the use of iodine-based contrast, MRI urography with gadolinium-based contrast may be used.[33,42]

Ultrasonography (US) is least specific but remains a quick, noninvasive modality to identify bladder volume and pelvic or abdominal free fluid and fluid collection. US can identify hydronephrosis or absent ureteral jets, suggesting LUT obstruction, and also be helpful in identifying the need for additional imaging.[9,33,42,46]

Cystoscopy can be used to directly evaluate for mesh erosion into the LUT. CT urography is helpful in identifying ureteral stricture or obstruction and can be performed in conjunction with retrograde pyelography to determine the extent of a previous injury.[9] Again, if there is a contraindication to iodine-based contrast, MRI pyelography can be completed.

A genitourinary fistula may be diagnosed through in-office examination and dye testing or through formal imaging. On split speculum examination, granulation tissue or even a small opening may be seen, raising suspicion for a fistulous tract.[9] Because UI is common with genitourinary fistulae, an in-office dye test can distinguish the type of fistula. Oral phenazopyridine is given 1 hour before the study. After complete voiding, dilute methylene blue is instilled into the bladder and a tampon is placed in the vagina. A ureterovaginal fistula is suspected with an orange-stained tampon, prompting evaluation with CT or MRI urography.[3,9,48] Alternatively, if the tampon is stained blue, a vesicovaginal or urethrovaginal fistula should be considered, which may be recognized on cystoscopy. Evaluation with CT or MRI urography is suggested to confirm the diagnosis and exclude concomitant pathology.

Finally, if there is concern for renal impairment or failure, renal nuclear imaging, such as a technetium Tc-99m mertiatide (MAG3) scan, can provide information about renal

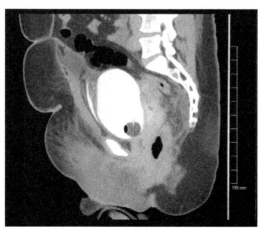

Fig. 7. Computed tomography (CT) scan demonstrating contrast extravasation into the retropubic space. (Image courtesy of Christine Heisler, MD at University of Wisconsin.)

function. Although a MAG3 scan is associated with reduced radiation exposure compared with CT, it is rarely required.[49]

MANAGEMENT AND REPAIR
Intraoperatively Recognized Ureteral Injury

The nature and extent of ureteral injury will determine the route of correction. A partial thickness laceration or ureteral sheath injury may be repaired with interrupted fine absorbable nonreactive material such as polyglactin 910 or poliglecaprone 25. For larger ureteral sheath injuries, ureteral catheters should be placed to facilitate healing and prevent stenosis.[50,51]

With concerns for ureteral kinking or obstruction, the surrounding tissue should be closely observed for inappropriately placed stitches or clamp injuries. Any ligating suture should be removed, or alternatively, a ureteral catheter may be placed and removed after the offending suture has dissolved. Similarly, minor ureteral crush injuries may be managed with catheterization. Significant crush or thermal injuries require excision of devitalized tissue and reanastomosis or reimplantation.[3,9,50,51]

Repair of complete ureteral transections vary with location and the extent of damage. At the level of the pelvic brim, a complete transection may be repaired by performing a ureteroureterostomy (**Fig. 8**). The viable cut ends of each ureteral segment are spatulated approximately 0.5 cm and anastomosed with interrupted 4-0 chromic over a ureteral catheter to bridge the anastomotic site for at least 7 days. An extraperitoneal suction drain is placed to prevent accumulation of fluids in the area and alert to an anastomotic leak; this is typically retained until ureteral stents are removed.[3,9] Regardless of injury location, mobilization of the proximal and distal ends to allow a tension-free repair is paramount.

Because most injuries occur at the distal ureter, ureteroneocystostomy, or ureteral reimplantation, would be indicated (**Fig. 9**). The retropubic space is dissected to mobilize the bladder for a simple reimplantation. The risk of resulting vesicoureteral reflux may be minimized through ureteral submucosal tunneling.[50,52] Tunneling is completed after cystotomy creation by dissecting a submucosal passage approximately 4 cm long and 1 cm wide between the detrusor muscle and mucosa in the direction of

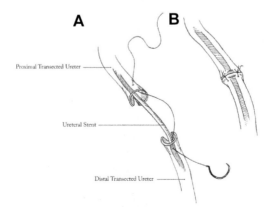

Fig. 8. (*A*) Complete ureteral transection repaired over ureteral stent by first splaying viable transected ends, then proceeding with suture reanastomosis. (*B*) Tension-free ureteroureterostomy over ureteral stent (extraperitoneal suction drain not pictured.) (Illustration by Charlotte Holden.)

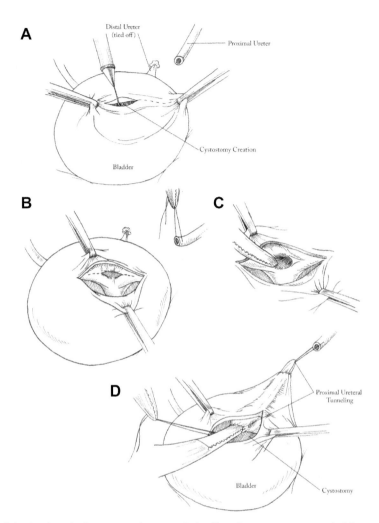

Fig. 9. (*A*) Distal end of transected ureter tied off and cystotomy created. (*B*) Creation of neo-orifice at bladder mucosa. (*C, D*) Creation of submucosal tunnel with clamp to grasp tagged end of ureter. (*E*) Ureter pulled through tunnel and ureteral stent placed. (*F*) Anastomosis completed. Not shown: cystotomy repaired in standard fashion and extraperitoneal suction drain placed. If anastomotic site is not tension free, psoas hitch completed (see **Fig. 13**). (Illustration by Charlotte Holden.)

the ureteral orifice (**Fig. 10**). At the end of the tunnel, an oval segment of the bladder mucosa is removed to avoid obstruction of the neo-orifice. The ureter is passed through the tunnel and spatulated, and a tension-free anastomosis is made using fine absorbable suture. After placement of a ureteral catheter, the bladder is closed with fine absorbable suture through a double-layer technique, and an extraperitoneal suction drain is placed.[52]

To reduce tension on the ureteroneocystostomy anastomosis, a bladder (psoas) hitch or a possible bladder extension procedure (Boari flap) should be considered.[3] The psoas hitch is performed by creating an extraperitoneal cystotomy, then mobilizing the bladder toward the psoas muscle on the side of the planned repair. The

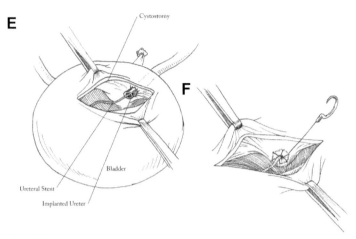

Fig. 9. (*continued*).

muscular wall of the bladder is sutured to the psoas muscle in a tension-free manner with several interrupted 0 or 2-0 delayed absorbable or nonabsorbable sutures (**Fig. 11**). The ureter is incorporated via tunneling, after which a stent is placed, the bladder is closed as previously described, and extraperitoneal suction drain is placed.[3,50,52] If bladder mobilization and a psoas hitch do not allow a satisfactory tension-free ureteral reanastomosis or reimplantation, then a Boari flap should be considered (**Fig. 12**). In this procedure, a rhombus with a 4-cm wide base and 3-cm wide top is demarcated on the anterior bladder wall, with intended base at the posterolateral bladder wall. Three sides are incised to create a wide rhombic flap, which is fixed to the psoas muscle. The ureter is reimplanted using the tunneling technique, a catheter is placed, and the remaining bladder flap is closed

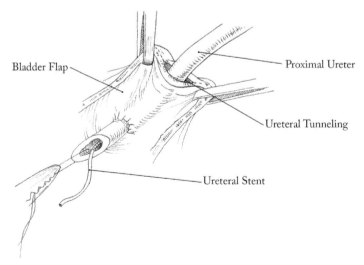

Fig. 10. Ureteral tunneling to minimize vesicoureteral reflux. (Illustration by Charlotte Holden.)

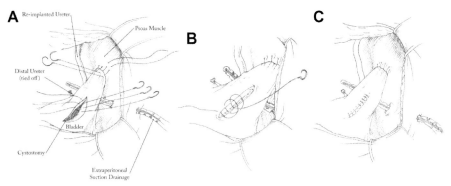

Fig. 11. (*A*) Bladder mobilized cephalad to relieve tension from anastomosis site and sutured to psoas muscle on ipsilateral side of repair. Extraperitoneal suction drain placed to prevent accumulation of fluids in the area and alert to an anastomotic leak. (*B*) Cystotomy closed in standard fashion. (*C*) Completed ureteroneocystostomy with bladder (psoas) hitch. (Illustration by Charlotte Holden.)

in a tubelike fashion by suturing together its lateral margins in a double-layer fashion.[3,52]

If a large portion of the ureter is damaged, rarely a transureteroureterostomy may be performed by joining the transected ureter to the contralateral ureter. Alternatively, an ileal-ureteroneocystostomy can be performed by using a segment of ileum as a bridge. Urinary diversion through cutaneous ureterostomy is a temporary method of urinary diversion to salvage renal function if definitive repair cannot be carried out during the primary procedure.[3,50]

Ureteral catheter placement is used in ureteral repair to promote ureteral healing, prevent urine extravasation, and to avoid anastomotic stenosis. Extraperitoneal suction drains must be placed in proximity to the anastomotic site to prevent fluid collection and detect anastomotic leakage promptly. Finally, if the ureter is reimplanted, indwelling bladder catheter must be maintained for 7 to 10 days, provided the daily drain output is low.[3,9,33,52]

Intraoperatively Recognized Bladder Injury

Intraoperative cystotomy repair and postoperative management are primarily determined by the location and size of the injury. Laparoscopic and vaginal approaches are used more often for repair (34.9% and 18.9%, respectively) with only 15% of bladder injuries requiring conversion to laparotomy.[17] If surgical management is indicated, nontrigonal bladder injuries are typically repaired after completion of the gynecologic procedure to guide dissection and prevent further iatrogenic injury.

Retroperitoneal cystotomy less than 2 mm, such as trocar perforation during sling placement (see **Fig. 5**), can be expectantly managed, granted that proper trocar placement is achieved on subsequent attempts.[53,54] Small nontrigonal defects (less than 1 cm) may be managed with bladder drainage for 1 week or repaired in a single- or double-layer closure with 3-0 absorbable suture followed by bladder drainage for 1 week. Nontrigonal injuries larger than 1 cm (**Fig. 13**) must be primarily suture repaired by a single- or double-layer closure followed by bladder drainage for 1 to 2 weeks. Nontrigonal injuries larger than 2 cm are typically repaired using a double-layer closure followed by bladder drainage for 1 to 2 weeks[9,50,53] (**Figs. 14** and **15**), although a small single-center retrospective review reported on single-layer closure of large

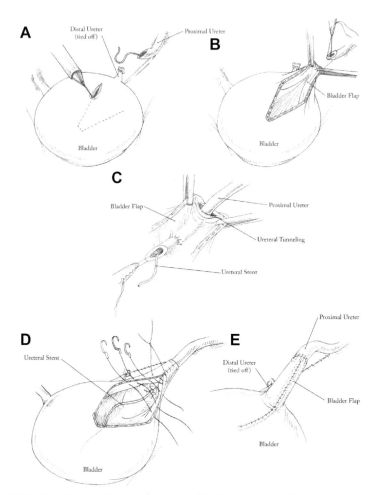

Fig. 12. (A) Bladder flap outlined and created. (B, C) Ureter reimplantation by submucosal tunneling technique. (D) Reanastomosis completed and ureteral stent placed. (E) Cystotomy closure completed. Not shown: psoas hitch performed to keep anastomotic site tension free. (Illustration by Charlotte Holden.)

cystotomies without major complications.[55] These repairs can be covered by a layer of peritoneum or an omental flap to separate the repair from the surrounding tissue, add bulk, and potentially provide blood supply.[3] Following closure of a bladder laceration, integrity of the repair should be assessed by filling the bladder with 300 mL of fluid. If leakage is observed, figure-of-8 sutures or additional layers of imbrication can be placed.[50,53]

Trigonal defects are more complex to repair, as this region contains the ureteral and urethral orifices, which must be evaluated before and following repair. Adequate exposure of this area can be difficult, and completion of any planned procedure is deferred until the bladder is evaluated and repaired by a specialist. The general principles for trigonal injury repair are similar to that of large nontrigonal injuries, including double-layer closure completed with absorbable suture, followed by bladder drainage for at least 10 to 14 days.[50]

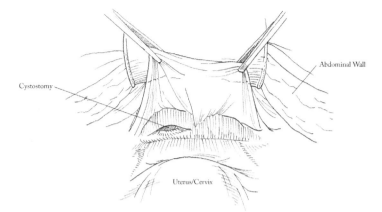

Fig. 13. Iatrogenic cystotomy during bladder dissection for abdominal hysterectomy. (Illustration by Charlotte Holden.)

Continuous bladder drainage for 5 to 14 days is performed following cystotomy repair or ureteroneocystostomy, with the duration of drainage determined by the extent of the injury and the patient's individual risk factors. Prophylactic antibiotic therapy for indwelling catheter maintenance is not routinely recommended.[56]

It is a common practice to assess repair integrity before removal of an indwelling bladder catheter. Routine cystography may not be necessary before catheter removal

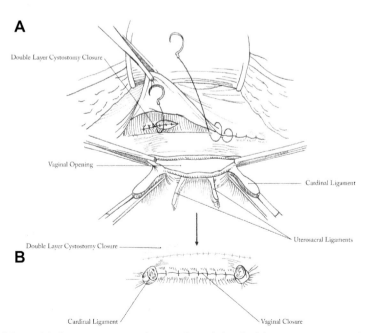

Fig. 14. (A) Double-layer cystotomy closure after abdominal hysterectomy completion. (B) Completed double-layer cystotomy closure and single-layer vaginal closure. (Illustration by Charlotte Holden.)

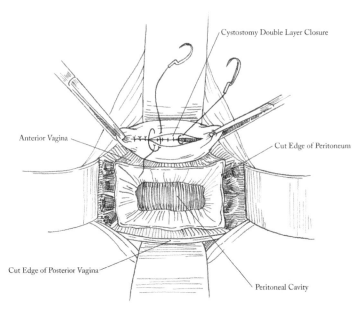

Fig. 15. Double-layer cystotomy closure after vaginal hysterectomy. (Illustration by Charlotte Holden.)

if the defect is small, and nontrigonal and prolonged drainage has occurred.[57] However, an analysis in 2016 found that almost 3% of voiding cystourethrogram (VCUG) studies evaluating LUT repairs were abnormal, directly influencing catheter management.[58] If a bladder injury was not primarily repaired, is large, complex (eg, involving the trigone or ureteral reimplantation), or has undergone short-term drainage, imaging should be performed before indwelling bladder catheter removal.[53,57,58]

Intraoperatively Recognized Urethral Injury

Urethral lacerations are repaired in a double-layer closure using 3-0 or 4-0 absorbable or delayed absorbable sutures over a transurethral catheter. The addition of a fat pad graft should be considered if additional tissue bulk is needed or the wound is poorly vascularized.[3,50] If injury is sustained during a synthetic mesh-based procedure, the procedure should be delayed until the urethra is healed to avoid future complications such as mesh erosion.[14,16] Patients may continue to experience irritative voiding symptoms for a prolonged period after repair.

Postoperatively Recognized Lower Urinary Tract Injury

There are no standard guidelines on the management of postoperatively identified iatrogenic ureteral transection and leakage. Although retrograde cystoscopic ureteral stenting is attempted in these cases, it is usually unsuccessful. In one study, if retrograde cystoscopic stenting failed, interventional radiologists proceeded with percutaneous nephrostomy (PCN) placement and subsequent antegrade ureteral stenting, demonstrating resolution of leakage in all patients without requiring surgical reintervention. PCN placement with antegrade ureteral stenting should be the preferred method of urinary diversion.[33,59] Postoperative ureteral strictures can be addressed with ureteral stenting or dilation procedures. Postoperative ureteral obstructions are typically secondary to suture ligation and can be managed with PCN placement until the suture absorbs.[9,33,60] If the aforementioned methods fail to resolve ureteral injury or restore normal urine flow, the surgical management procedures previously described should be used. A urinoma, if identified, can be managed with percutaneous drainage.

Management of postoperatively discovered cystotomies does not vary from intraoperative management. For defects less than 1 cm, indwelling bladder catheter should be placed for at least 7 days and removed after cystogram confirms appropriate healing. Larger injuries will require reoperation and bladder drainage for 7 to 14 days with a subsequent cystogram completed per surgeon preference. If suture material is found in the bladder after surgery, a transurethral resection is the method of choice for correction.[61]

Unrecognized iatrogenic LUT injuries found in the postoperative period can present as urogenital fistulae, urethral or bladder suture or mesh erosion, urethral diverticulum, or symptomatic outflow obstruction. These should be managed by a specialist trained in urologic pathology and management.[9,14] Although the management of these conditions is beyond the scope of this review, the general principles of management should be understood. Urethral or bladder mesh erosion repair requires meticulous operative technique and can be completed through vaginal or abdominal approaches. The general principles of repair include the complete excision of mesh, followed by 2-layer closure of the defect, bladder drainage for 7 to 14 days, and completion of VCUG before indwelling catheter removal.[62] Urogenital fistulae are generally managed first with bladder drainage, ureteral stenting, or urinary diversion before attempts at repair, as conservative techniques can lead to resolution of fistula or allow maturation of the tract and improve the chances of successful repair.[33] If a patient with urethrogenital fistula is asymptomatic and continent, surgery should be avoided.[50] If conservative management does not resolve a urogenital fistula, surgical repair is the next step. Vaginal or abdominal approaches can be used depending on the patient, fistula type, number of fistulas, and surgeon preference. General surgical principles of vesicovaginal fistulae (**Fig. 16**) repair include excision of the fistulous tract and tension-free, multilayer closure with delayed absorbable suture. Ureterovaginal fistulae (**Fig. 17**) are managed with ligation of ureter near the fistula and reimplantation.[9,22,23]

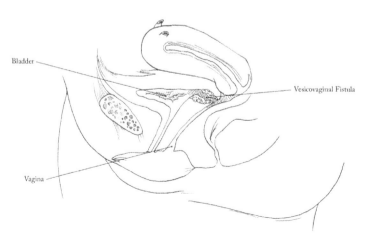

Bladder

Vesicovaginal Fistula

Vagina

Fig. 16. Vesicovaginal fistula. (Illustration by Charlotte Holden.)

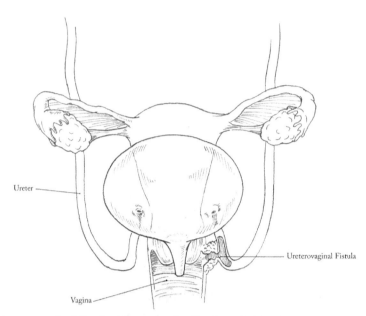

Fig. 17. Ureterovaginal fistula. (Illustration by Charlotte Holden.)

SUMMARY

LUT injuries are a recognized complication of gynecologic surgery, occurring as a consequence of the close proximity of the reproductive organs to the urologic organs. Considering the morbidity associated with LUT injury, prevention through knowledge of pelvic anatomy, high level of surgical skill, and understanding of patient risk factors are emphasized. In the setting of iatrogenic complications, the primary aim must be early intraoperative diagnosis and treatment. To combat delayed postoperative recognition of iatrogenic LUT injury, gynecologic surgeons must maintain an appropriate degree of suspicion for injuries by preserving familiarity with the types, locations, and mechanisms of injuries. Equally important, surgeons must be familiar with the wide range of patient symptoms and preferred diagnostic imaging to promptly diagnose LUT injury in the postoperative period. Finally, LUT injuries should be evaluated and repaired by a surgeon who is familiar with such procedures and the necessary postoperative management.

CLINICS CARE POINTS

- The authors recommend universal cystoscopy after all hysterectomies, with a goal of increasing intraoperative recognition of injuries and reducing the morbidity associated with delayed postoperative diagnosis.
- If there is high clinical suspicion of intraoperative ureteral injury, ureteral stent placement and retrograde imaging should be used to confirm ureteral integrity.
- Approach to LUT repair can be laparoscopic, vaginal, and abdominal, favoring minimally invasive approaches, but ultimately determined by surgeon preference.
- Cystotomy larger than 1 cm should generally be repaired in 2 layers, confirming that the repair is water-tight before completion, with bladder drainage for at least 7 days postoperatively.

- Routine prophylactic antibiotics are not indicated during bladder drainage after LUT injury repair.
- VCUG is recommended before indwelling bladder catheter removal if a bladder injury was not primarily repaired, is large, complex (eg, involving the trigone or ureteral reimplantation), or has undergone short-term drainage.
- In postoperatively identified ureteral transection injuries, PCN placement and subsequent antegrade ureteral stenting should be the approach of choice, as cystoscopic retrograde stenting is largely unsuccessful.

DISCLOSURE

The authors have nothing to disclose.

REFERENCES

1. Wallis CJD, Cheung DC, Garbens A, et al. Occurrence of and risk factors for urological intervention during benign hysterectomy: analysis of the national surgical quality improvement program database. Urology 2016;97:66–72.
2. Ozdemir E, Ozturk U, Celen S, et al. Urinary complications of gynecologic surgery: iatrogenic urinary tract system injuries in obstetrics and gynecology operations. Clin Exp Obstet Gynecol 2011;38:217–20.
3. Matthews CA, Gebhart JB. Avoiding and managing lower urinary tract injuries during pelvic surgery. In: Urogynecology and reconstructive pelvic surgery. Philadelphia: Elsevier Saunders; 2015. p. 431–42.
4. Stepp KJ, Walters MD. Anatomy of the lower urinary tract, pelvic floor, and rectum. In: Urogynecology and reconstructive pelvic surgery. Philadelphia: Elsevier Saunders; 2015. p. 19–31.
5. Rahn DD, Bleich AT, Wai CY, et al. Anatomic relationships of the distal third of the pelvic ureter, trigone, and urethra in unembalmed female cadavers. Am J Obstet Gynecol 2007;197:668e1–3.
6. Oelrich TM. The striated urogenital sphincter muscle in the female. Anatomical Rec 1983;205:223–32.
7. Buller JL, Thompson JR, Cundiff GW, et al. Uterosacral ligament: description of anatomic relationships to optimize surgical safety. Obstet Gynecol 2001;97:873–9.
8. Teeluckdharry B, Gilmour D, Flowerdew G. Urinary tract injury at benign gynecologic surgery and the role of cystoscopy: a systematic review and meta-analysis. Obstet Gynecol 2015;126:1161–9.
9. Blackwell RH, Kirshenbaum EJ, Shah AS, et al. Complications of recognized and unrecognized iatrogenic ureteral injury at time of hysterectomy: a population based analysis. J Urol 2018;199:1540–5.
10. Bai SW, Huh EH, Jung DJ, et al. Urinary tract injuries during pelvic surgery: incidence rates and predisposing factors. Int Urogynecol J Pelvic Floor Dysfunct 2006;17:360–4.
11. Ibeanu OA, Chesson RR, Echols KT, et al. Urinary tract injury during hysterectomy based on universal cystoscopy. Obstet Gynecol 2009;113:6–10.
12. Sharp HT, Adelman MR. Prevention, recognition, and management of urologic injuries during gynecologic surgery. Obstet Gynecol 2016;127:1085–96.
13. Fernbach SK, Feinstein KA, Spencer K, et al. Ureteral duplication and its complications. Radiographics 1997;17:109–27.

14. Morton HC, Hilton P. Urethral injury associated with minimally invasive mid-urethral sling procedures for the treatment of stress urinary incontinence: a case series and systematic literature search. BJOG 2009;116(8):1120–6. Available at: https://obgyn.onlinelibrary.wiley.com/journal/14710528. Accessed October 30, 2020.
15. Powers K, Lazarou G, Greston WM. Delayed urethral erosion after tension-free vaginal tape. Int Urogynecol J Pelvic Floor Dysfunct 2006;17:422.
16. Karram MM, Segal JL, Vassallo BJ, et al. Complications and untoward effects of the tension-free vaginal tape procedure. Obstet Gynecol 2003;101:929.
17. Wong JMK, Bortoletto P, Tolentino J, et al. Urinary tract injury in gynecologic laparoscopy for benign indication: a systematic review. Obstet Gynecol 2018;131:100.
18. Brummer TH, Jalkanen J, Fraser J, et al. FINHYST, a prospective study of 5279 hysterectomies: complications and their risk factors. Hum Reprod 2011;26:1741–51.
19. Tamussino KF, Hanzal E, Kölle D, et al, Austrian Urogynecology Working Group. Tension-free vaginal tape operation: results of the Austrian registry. Obstet Gynecol 2001;98:732–6.
20. Stav K, Dwyer PL, Rosamilia A, et al. Risk factors for trocar injury to the urinary bladder during midurethral sling procedures. J Urol 2009;182:174.
21. Packiam VT, Cohen AJ, Pariser JJ, et al. The impact of minimally invasive surgery on major iatrogenic ureteral injury and subsequent ureteral repair during hysterectomy: a national analysis of risk factors and outcomes. Urology 2016;98:183–8.
22. Bodner-Adler B, Hanzal E, Pablik E, et al. Management of vesicovaginal fistulas (VVFs) in women following benign gynaecologic surgery: a systematic review and meta-analysis. PLoS One 2017;12:e0171554.
23. Seth J, Kiosoglous A, Pakzad M, et al. Incidence, type and management of ureteric injury associated with vesicovaginal fistulas: report of a series from a specialized center. Int J Urol 2019;26:717–23.
24. Aarts JWM, Nieboer TE, Johnson N, et al. Surgical approach to hysterectomy for benign gynaecological disease. Cochrane Database Syst Rev 2015;(8):CD003677.
25. Dallas KB, Rogo-Gupta L, Elliott C. Urologic injury and fistula following hysterectomy for benign indications. Obstet Gynecol 2019;134:241–9.
26. Propst K, Harnegie MP, Ridgeway B. Evaluation of strategies to prevent urinary tract injury in minimally invasive gynecologic surgery: a systematic review. J Minim Invasive Gynecol 2021;28(3):684–91.e2.
27. Schimpf MO, Gottenger EE, Wagner JR. Universal ureteral stent placement at hysterectomy to identify ureteral injury: a decision analysis. Obstetrical Gynecol Surv 2008;63:699–700.
28. Lee Z, Kaplan J, Giusto L. Prevention of iatrogenic ureteral injuries during robotic gynecologic surgery: a review. Am J Obstet Gynecol 2016;214:566–71.
29. Phipps JH, Tyrrell NJ. Transilluminating ureteric stents for preventing operative ureteric damage. Br J Obstet Gynaecol 1992;99:81.
30. Siddighi S, Carr KR. Lighted stents facilitate robotic-assisted laparoscopic ureterovaginal fistula repair. Int Urogynecol J 2013;24:515–7.
31. Pedro RN, Kishore TA, Hinck BD, et al. Comparative analysis of lighted ureteral stents: lumination and tissue effects. J Endourol 2008;22:2555–8.
32. Hope-Ross M, Yannuzzi LA, Gragoudas ES. Adverse reactions due to indocyanine green. Ophthalmology 1994;101:529–33.

33. Brandes S, Coburn M, Armenakas N. Diagnosis and management of ureteric injury: an evidence-based analysis. BJU Int 2004;94:277–89.
34. Cadish LA, Ridgeway BM, Shepherd JP. Cystoscopy at the time of benign hysterectomy: a decision analysis. Am J Obstet Gynecol 2019;220. 369.e1-7.
35. Anand M, Casiano ER, Heisler CA, et al. Utility of intraoperative cystoscopy in detecting ureteral injury during vaginal hysterectomy. Female Pelvic Med Reconstr Surg 2015;21:70–6.
36. Nguyen MLT, Stevens E, LaFargue CJ, et al. Routine cystoscopy after robotic gynecologic oncology surgery. JSLS: J Soc Laparoendoscopic Surgeons 2014; 18:1–6.
37. Visco AG, Taber KH, Weidner AC, et al. Cost-effectiveness of universal cystoscopy to identify ureteral injury at hysterectomy. Obstet Gynecol 2001;97:685–92.
38. Delbo L, Gareau-Labelle AK, Langlais EL, et al. Sodium fluorescein for ureteral jet detection: a prospective observational study. J Soc Laparoendoscopic Surgeons 2018;22:1–5.
39. Espaillat-Rijo L, Siff L, Alas AN, et al. Intraoperative cystoscopic evaluation of ureteral patency. Obstet Gynecol 2016;128:1378–83.
40. Strom EM, Chaudhry ZQ, Guo MR, et al. Effectiveness of assessing ureteral patency using preoperative phenazopyridine. Female Pelvic Med Reconstr Surg 2019;25:289–93.
41. Patton S, Tanner JP, Prieto I, et al. Furosemide use and time to confirmation of ureteral patency during intraoperative cystoscopy. Obstet Gynecol 2019;133: 669–74.
42. Bitton-Tunitsky E, Huang WC. Radiologic studies of the lower urinary tract and pelvic floor. In: Urogynecology and reconstructive pelvic surgery. Philadelphia: Elsevier Saunders; 2015. p. 182–94.
43. Abboudi H, Ahmed K, Royle J, et al. Ureteric injury: a challenging condition to diagnose and manage. Nat Rev Urol 2013;10:108–15.
44. Siddighi S, Yune JJ, Kwon NB, et al. Perioperative serum creatinine changes and ureteral injury. Int Urol Nephrol 2017;49:1915–9.
45. Patel BN, Gayer G. Imaging of iatrogenic complications of the urinary tract. Radiologic Clin North America 2014;52:1101–16.
46. Esparaz AM, Pearl JA, Herts BR, et al. Iatrogenic urinary tract injuries: etiology, diagnosis, and management. Semin Interv Radiol 2015;32:195–208.
47. Bretschneider EC, Casas-Puig V, Sheyn D, et al. Delayed recognition of lower urinary tract injuries following hysterectomy for benign indications: a NSQIP-based study. Am J Obstet Gynecol 2019;221(2):132.e1–13. Available at: www.ncbi.nlm.nih.gov/pubmed/30926265. Accessed November 11, 2020.
48. El-Tabey NA, Ali-El-Dein B, Shaaban AA, et al. Urological trauma after gynecological and obstetric surgeries. Scand J Urol Nephrol 2006;40:225–31.
49. Keramida G, James JM, Prescott MC, et al. Pitfalls and limitations of radionuclide renal imaging in adults. Semin Nucl Med 2015;45:428–39.
50. Brubaker LT, Wilbanks GD. Urinary tract injuries in pelvic surgery. Surg Clin North America 1991;71:963–76.
51. De Cicco C, Dávalos ML, Van Cleynenbreugel B, et al. Iatrogenic ureteral lesions and repair: a review for gynecologists. J Minim Invasive Gynecol 2007;14: 428–35.
52. Stein R, Rubenwolf P, Ziesel C, et al. Psoas hitch and boari flap ureteroneocystostomy. BJU Int 2013;112:137–55.
53. Glaser LM, Milad MP. Bowel and bladder injury repair and follow-up after gynecologic Surgery. Obstet Gynecol 2019;133:313–22.

54. Richter HE, Albo ME, Zyczynski HM, et al. Retropubic versus transobturator mid-urethral slings for stress incontinence. N Engl J Med 2010;362:2066–76.
55. Chamsy D, King C, Lee T. The use of barbed suture for bladder and bowel repair. J Minimally Invasive Gynecol 2015;22:648–52.
56. Lo E, Nicolle L, Classen D, et al. Strategies to prevent catheter-associated urinary tract infections in acute care hospitals. Infect Control Hosp Epidemiol 2008;29: S41–50.
57. Inaba K, Okoye OT, Browder T, et al. Prospective evaluation of the utility of routine postoperative cystogram after traumatic bladder injury. J Trauma Acute Care Surg 2013;75:1019–23.
58. Bochenska K, Zyczynski HM. Utility of postoperative voiding cystourethrogram after lower urinary tract repair. Female Pelvic Med Reconstr Surg 2016;22: 369–72.
59. Trombatore C, Giordano G, San Lio VM. Interventional radiology in iatrogenic ureteral leaks: case series and literature review. La Radiologia Med 2017;122: 696–704.
60. Koukouras D, Petsas T, Liatsikos E, et al. Percutaneous minimally invasive management of iatrogenic ureteral injuries. J Endourol 2010;24:1921–7.
61. Küçükdurmaz F, Can S, Barut O. Endoscopic removal of intravesical polypropylene suture with plasmakinetic resection after abdominal hysterectomy. Int J Surg Case Rep 2014;5:1170–2.
62. Tijdink MM, Vierhout ME, Heesakkers JP, et al. Surgical management of mesh related complications after prior pelvic floor reconstructive surgery with mesh. Int Urogynecol J 2011;22:1395.

Female Pelvic Fistulae

Tasha Serna-Gallegos, MD, Peter C. Jeppson, MD*

KEYWORDS

- Pelvic fistula • Genitourinary fistula • Rectovaginal fistula • Vesicovaginal fistula
- Urethrovaginal fistula • Vesicouterine fistula

KEY POINTS

- Obstetric injury is the leading cause of pelvic fistulae worldwide; in developed nations, gynecologic surgery is the main cause of genitourinary fistulae.
- The diagnosis and evaluation of pelvic fistulae are accomplished with office-based procedures. Radiologic imaging may be required to optimize surgical planning.
- Pelvic fistulae are primarily treated with surgical intervention.
- A vaginal approach can be used for a variety of pelvic fistulae to decrease hospital stay, overall blood loss, operative time, and postoperative pain.
- The initial surgical repair has the highest chance of success. Success rates decrease with every subsequent attempt.

INTRODUCTION

Female pelvic fistulae have devastating effects on affected women around the world.[1,2] Pelvic fistulae that occur in developing countries are often the result of obstetric injuries and frequently result in women being abandoned by their husbands, leaving them without resources and alienated from their community. Fistulae have been present for millennia, with the first known historical report dating back to 2050 BC with a pelvic fistula identified on mummified Egyptian remains.[3] Pelvic fistula can be challenging to surgically repair. From a historic perspective, the first vaginal approach to fistula repair was described in the mid-1800s.[2] Many of the surgical principles initially reported for surgical fistula repair are still used today.[4]

Despite the impact fistula symptoms have on women worldwide, current literature guiding fistulae management is primarily based on observational data. Physicians therefore rely on expert opinion, such as that presented here, to guide their care of pelvic fistula. The purpose of this manuscript is to present a narrative review on the current management of pelvic fistula, including diagnosis, evaluation, conservative, and surgical treatment options.

Division of Female Pelvic Medicine & Reconstructive Surgery, Department of Obstetrics and Gynecology, MSC 10-5580, 1 University of New Mexico, Albuquerque, NM 87131-0001, USA
* Corresponding author.
E-mail address: pjeppson@salud.unm.edu

Obstet Gynecol Clin N Am 48 (2021) 557–570
https://doi.org/10.1016/j.ogc.2021.05.008
0889-8545/21/© 2021 Elsevier Inc. All rights reserved.

CAUSE AND EPIDEMIOLOGY OF FISTULAE

With the evolution of obstetric care, the cause of pelvic fistula has changed in developed nations but has remained unchanged in developing countries. In developed nations, gynecologic surgery is the leading cause of vesicovaginal fistulae (VVF), and obstetric trauma is the leading cause of rectovaginal fistulae (RVF).[2,4,5] The incidence of VVF after a benign hysterectomy ranges from 0.1% to 0.3%.[2,5] This further varies by route of surgery, with laparoscopy having the highest risk of VVF formation, followed by open abdominal and then vaginal approaches.[1] Other risk factors for development of a genitourinary fistula at the time of pelvic surgery include prior pelvic surgery, endometriosis, prior cesarean section, prior pelvic radiation, concurrent prolapse or antiincontinence procedure, diabetes mellitus, and pelvic inflammatory disease.[1,4]

In developing countries, the leading cause of both VVFs and RVFs is obstetric trauma, which affects 3.5 million women in sub-Saharan Africa and South Asia.[2,4] Because many women in these regions have limited access to hospitals, and these statistics are often extrapolated from hospital data, this likely represents an underestimation of women affected by pelvic fistulae. Obstetric injuries may occur with protracted or obstructed labor as a result of tissue ischemia and may also result from iatrogenic injury at the time of cesarean section. In developed countries, obstetric fistulae are rare but are more commonly reported following forceps-assisted deliveries, midline episiotomies, peripartum hysterectomy, or wound dehiscence of a perineal laceration.[4,6]

RVF are relatively more common in developed countries and can be caused by inflammatory bowel disease (IBD), infectious diseases, anorectal surgery, malignancy, radiation therapy, or congenital anomalies.[7] Crohn disease, a type of IBD, is the second most common cause of RVF. Interestingly, up to 10% of women with Crohn disease will develop an RVF during their disease course.[4,8] Infections, such as diverticulitis, lymphogranuloma venereum, or tuberculosis, can create inflammation and injury leading to a colovesical or a rectovaginal fistula.[2,9]

Vesicouterine, ureterovaginal, and urethrovaginal fistulae are rare entities. Vesicouterine fistulae comprise about 1% to 4% of all genitourinary fistulae, with most caused by surgery, either obstetric or gynecologic.[2,10] Similarly, ureterovaginal fistulae are most commonly caused by ureteral injury at the time of gynecologic surgery. In a systematic review published in 2015, the incidence of ureteral and bladder injury at the time of gynecologic surgery ranges from 0.03% to 1.5% and 0.2% to 1.8%, respectively.[3] Urethrovaginal fistulae have become more prominent with the increase in midurethral sling placement and are also a known complication of urethral diverticulum repair.[2,11] Specifically, the risk of a urethrovaginal fistula following surgical repair of a diverticulum ranges from 1.8% to 6%.[12]

DIAGNOSIS AND EVALUATION OF FISTULAE

Diagnosing a pelvic fistula requires a high level of suspicion, detailed history, and thorough pelvic examination. Additional procedures or imaging studies can aid in diagnosis and surgical planning. It is rare to have an iatrogenic fistula without any inciting event or predisposing risk factor, making a patient's medical history the first key step to diagnosis.

Clinical Presentation

Patients with genitourinary fistulae commonly present complaining of continuous urinary incontinence or watery vaginal discharge. Patients often report exacerbation of leakage when changing positions, particularly when going from supine to a sitting or standing position. As fistulae can be of variable size, the amount and frequency of leakage may vary from continuous to intermittent and in some cases mimic stress urinary incontinence. Patients also often complain of incontinent dermatitis from vulvovaginal irritation from persistent urinary leakage. Similarly, patients with RVF report leakage of gas or stool per vagina, but if the fistula is small, they may simply report a malodorous vaginal discharge.

Physical Examination

A physical examination should start with examination of the external female genitalia, which can show evidence of skin breakdown secondary to irritation from urine or feculent material, as seen in **Fig. 1**. A speculum examination will allow visualization of the vaginal walls to evaluate for scarring or puckering. A transparent plastic speculum can be particularly helpful in this regard. Large fistulae are more easily visible; however, a thorough evaluation is still important, as more than one fistula may be present. The examination should also specifically evaluate for abnormal discharge, fluid collections, or stool. Posthysterectomy genitourinary fistulae tend to be near the vaginal cuff, whereas RVF tend to be near the perineum.[4,6] In rare cases it may be helpful to send a sample of the watery vaginal discharge, as urine can be identified by creatinine or urea concentration. A bimanual examination is important to help determine the size and location of the fistula(e) but also to assess pelvic scar tissue, particularly in proximity of the fistula, as this will affect both the plan for and anticipated success of a surgical repair. A digital rectal examination, as shown in **Fig. 2**, should be done to localize an RVF and to assess the integrity of the anal sphincter complex; however, this is not particularly sensitive or specific.[2]

Office Procedures

There are a variety of office-based procedures that are frequently used to help identify the location of pelvic fistulae, which are described in detail in **Table 1**. With many options available, the workup should be individualized for each patient.

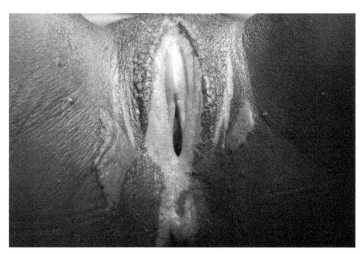

Fig. 1. Vulvar incontinence dermatitis and vitiligo secondary to a chronic vesicovaginal fistula.

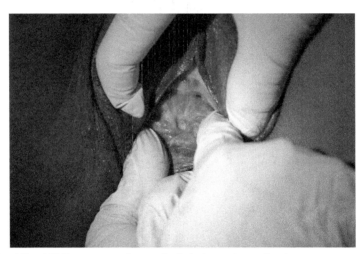

Fig. 2. A midlevel RVF seen on a thorough digital rectal examination.

Imaging Options

Although imaging is not necessary to diagnose pelvic fistulae, it can be helpful with complex fistulae and for surgical planning. MRI has become the imaging modality of choice to evaluate RVF, as computed tomography (CT) and ultrasound are less accurate.[13,14] For example, MRI is often superior to CT imaging, as it can help differentiate between active fistulae and fibrotic fistulae.[15] Endoanal ultrasound is inferior to clinical assessment for detection of fistulae but can evaluate the integrity of the anal sphincter complex.[15,16] MRI provides the most accurate and comprehensive imaging assessment of RVF, making it superior to other options.[4,14,15]

Selection of radiologic imaging is determined by clinical findings. In the setting of urinary tract fistulae, both the upper and lower urinary tract should be evaluated. Ureteral compromise has been reported in up to 12% of VVF.[4] Genitourinary fistulae may lead to ureteral strictures that can lead to obstruction or reflux with resultant hydronephrosis.[2] Retrograde pyelography, voiding cystourethrography, and CT urography are all common options chosen for evaluation.[2,4] Retrograde pyelography can visualize the distal ureters, whereas CT urography is better at visualizing the kidneys and upper ureters. Retrograde pyelography is a good option for patients with systemic contrast allergy or renal disease prohibiting intravenous contrast. A cystometrogram is performed by retrograde filling the bladder with radiopaque contrast under fluoroscopy to evaluate for bladder contour, vesicoureteral reflux, and fistulous communication. A voiding cystourethrogram can help identify small fistulous tracts in the bladder or urethra by adding a pressure-flow gradient during micturition.

CONSERVATIVE MANAGEMENT OF FISTULAE

RVF may heal spontaneously on rare occasions,[4] but conservative management is more likely to be directed at genitourinary fistulae. The mainstay of conservative treatment of VVFs is continuous bladder drainage such as use of a Foley catheter for 4 to 6 weeks. In a retrospective multicenter study with a total of 226 patients with VVF, 60 were initially managed conservatively with a Foley and 11.7% had spontaneous resolution.[17] A separate retrospective study found that prolonged Foley drainage only had a success rate of 1.9% when treating VVFs. They also noted that smaller fistulae,

Table 1
Office-based procedures to detect pelvic fistulae

Procedure	Fistula Detected	Technique/Findings
Tampon test	Vesicovaginal, rectovaginal	Dilute methylene blue is instilled into the bladder or rectum, then a tampon is placed into the vagina. The tampon is removed after 10–15 min and examined for the presence and location of any blue staining. This is often the first procedure done to evaluate a vesicovaginal fistula because it is cost-effective, easy to perform, and well tolerated by patients. The sensitivity and specificity of this test remain unknown.[6] Methylene blue should not be given to patients with a known hypersensitivity to it, and although rare, methemoglobinemia is a potential serious systemic side effect.
Double tampon test	Ureterovaginal, vesicovaginal	Phenazopyridine is taken orally and diluted methylene blue is instilled into the bladder, then a tampon is placed in the vagina. After 20 min, the tampon is removed and examined for the presence and location of blue or orange staining. Blue staining indicates a vesicovaginal fistula, whereas orange staining indicates a ureterovaginal fistula.
Bladder backfill test	Vesicovaginal	Dilute methylene blue or sterile milk is instilled into the bladder, whereas the posterior blade of a speculum is used to visualize any fluid leakage from the anterior vaginal wall/overlying bladder.
Trattner catheter double-balloon test	Urethrovaginal	The inner balloon lying against the urethrovesical junction and the outer balloon abutting the urethral meatus are inflated. Methylene blue or sterile milk is instilled into the catheter, which fills the urethral cavity between the 2 balloons. The posterior blade of a speculum is used to visualize any fluid leakage from the anterior vaginal wall/overlying urethra.
Cystourethroscopy	Vesicovaginal, urethrovaginal	A rigid 70° diagnostic cystoscope or flexible cystoscope is used to perform a full 360° evaluation of the bladder and the urethra evaluating for any visible fistulous tracts. It aids in identifying the location and size of the fistulous tract as well as its proximity to the trigone or ureteral orifices, which can be helpful in surgical planning. This can also allow for evaluation of ureteral involvement by the fistula or ureteral obstruction, which is better known before surgery.
Poppy seed test	Colovesical	Patients consume 50 g of poppy seeds in yogurt and monitor their urine for the next. If poppy seeds are present in their urine, a colovesical fistula is diagnosed. It does not provide information about the precise location of a fistula but it is a cheap test (~ $5.37/patient), with a sensitivity ranging from 94% to 100% and a specificity of nearly 100%.[12]

particularly less than 4 mm, were more likely to respond to conservative management.[18] It is reasonable to attempt a trial of continuous bladder drainage for 4 to 6 weeks in fistulae less than 1 cm, with success rates ranging from 12% to 80%.[4] There have also been case reports of spontaneous fistula closure secondary to pessary erosion following pessary removal.[19] Other types of nonsurgical management of genitourinary fistulae include electrocautery, cystoscopic laser ablation, or injection of fibrin or collage glue into the fistulous tract. Briefly, electrocautery and cystoscopic laser ablation deepithelialize the fistulous tract, allowing it to heal with prolonged continuous bladder drainage.[2,4] Fibrin and collage glue are injected into the fistulous tract after deepithelialization to promote closure. Many VVFs are given a trial of conservative management to allow for thorough tissue healing, making it more amenable to a successful surgical repair.

Ureterovaginal fistulae can be managed nonsurgically by placing an indwelling ureteral stent in the affected ureter for 6 to 8 weeks. A double-J stent is preferred to decrease the risk of stent migration out of the renal pelvis and can be done in either an antegrade or retrograde fashion. A retrospective study of 20 patients found that this endoscopic approach was successful in 64% of patients with ureterovaginal fistulae.[20] If the fistula resolves with ureteral stenting, the stent can be removed after 6 weeks. Some recommend serial CT urograms at 3-month intervals to evaluate for ureteral stricture formation.[2,4] If the fistula does not respond to conservative management, a plan for surgical intervention should be made. Nonsurgical treatments, for all types of genitourinary fistulae, should be used for patients who are poor surgical candidates; have very small, uncomplicated fistulae; or are strongly opposed to surgical interventions.

OPTIMIZING SURGICAL MANAGEMENT OF FISTULAE

Most pelvic of fistulae will require surgical intervention. It is also well established that the initial repair has the highest chance of success.[2,4,17] Being cognizant of factors that may optimize surgical repair including perioperative management and timing of surgical intervention can improve successful repair.

Timing of Surgical Repair

A controversial topic for fistula repair is timing of surgery. Optimal tissue integrity most amenable to surgical repair includes minimal inflammation, maximal pliability, and tissue mobilization with absent tissue necrosis. With these tissue characteristics, surgeons optimize their ability to secure a tension-free and watertight fistula closure. For some patients, this will occur within 72 hours of injury diagnosis, but for most of the patients with fistula, this will take 3 to 12 months to occur depending on the cause, location, and size of the fistula. Genitourinary injuries detected within 72 hours of surgery have an excellent chance of resolution if surgical repair is performed immediately.[21,22] In developed nations, this is not uncommon; however, in developing nations, patients present months to years after the original injury.[1,6] When the timing of surgical repair does not fall into this immediate or delayed diagnosis time frame, the decision becomes more difficult. Traditionally, for genitourinary fistulae, a 3- to 6-month waiting period has been discussed to maximize tissue integrity.[2,4,6,23] During this waiting period, some suggest monthly pelvic examinations so that surgery can proceed once tissue integrity is deemed adequate. Two studies done by Waaldijk showed a successful closure of greater than 90% of fistulas that were closed within 2 months of onset.[4,21,22] For RVFs, literature suggests a shorter standard waiting time from 8 to 12 weeks after injury. Obstetric third- and fourth-degree injuries should be repaired immediately, but nonobstetrical RVF do normally require a waiting period to allow optimization of medical conditions that may have contributed to fistula formation. Other factors such as prior radiation or active IBD may require additional time to allow the fistulous tract to mature before surgical repair. Timing of surgical repair is variable, and this decision should be highly individualized for each patient.

Perioperative Considerations

Thorough preoperative counseling is important to set realistic expectations when describing chances of a successful surgical repair including potential complications, risk of failure and need for repeat surgical repair, and the recovery period. Risk factors for failure include significant vaginal scarring, large fistula size, infection, and prior pelvic radiation. Preoperatively, barrier creams or ointments, in addition to routine perineal hygiene, are used to prevent skin breakdown or perineal dermatitis from urine or feculent material.[24] Preoperative antibiotic prophylaxis is universally recommended for urogynecologic procedures, including fistula repair, by the American College of Obstetricians and Gynecologists.[25] Following surgery, the need for continuous postoperative bladder drainage for 1 to 2 weeks cannot be overemphasized and dates back to at least 1852.[2,4,26] Before catheter removal, a cystometrogram should be performed to confirm resolution; if the findings suggest a persistent fistula, continued postoperative catheter use may ultimately result in successful closure. There is no literature to support the use of antibiotics for the duration of catheter placement following fistula repair, so the decision whether to use antibiotic prophylaxis in this setting rests with the surgeon.

SURGICAL TECHNIQUES FOR FISTULA REPAIR

The keys to a successful repair are represented in **Fig. 3** and include a tension-free, watertight, and well-vascularized fistula closure. Intraoperatively, adequate mobilization can help obtain a tension-free closure. The fistulous tract can be partially or completely resected. A partial resection leaves more durable tissue for reapproximation, whereas complete resection may result in greater vascularization by removing the scarred fistulous tract.[2] For very large fistulas, surgeons may opt to leave the fistulous tract in place in order to maximize the amount of tissue available for closure. Advancements in laparoscopic and robotic surgery allow for many minimally invasive surgical options; however, it is important to remember that many pelvic fistulae are amenable to a vaginal approach.[27] Vaginal surgery provides many advantages including shorter hospital stay, decreased intraoperative blood loss, decreased operative time, and less pain.[4,27] This section focuses on key pearls to the surgical management of the major types of pelvic fistulae.

Vaginal Approach to Vesicovaginal Fistula Repair

Current literature quotes success rates of 80% to 98%, with the first attempt at VVF repair through a vaginal approach.[2,4,28,29] These success rates drop exponentially with each subsequent attempt. One of the largest case series on genitourinary fistulae, including 303 patients, reported a 98% success rate for a VVF repair on first attempt, using a vaginal approach.[29]

Visualization is the first step to repair. Stay sutures can be placed to increase exposure, and a pediatric Foley catheter can be placed through the fistulous tract to bring the fistula into the surgical field. If the fistula tract is too small for a catheter, lacrimal duct dilators or vascular catheters can be used to cannulate the fistulous tract and aid in dissection and closure. Depending on the location of the VVF in relation to the

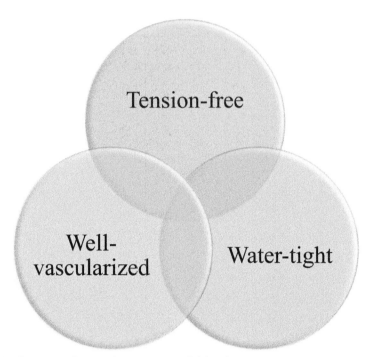

Fig. 3. The key surgical principles to a successful fistula repair.

bladder trigone and the ureteral orifices, intraoperative ureteral stents may be helpful for orientation and safety during repair.

The Latzko technique is used for simple VVF repairs and does not typically excise the fistula tract. It is best used for apical VVF repairs posthysterectomy. With this procedure, an elliptical incision is made around the fistula mobilizing 2 to 3 cm of vaginal epithelium around the fistula tract. The fistula is closed followed by imbricating the fibromuscular connective tissue over the tract in 1 or 2 layers. The vaginal epithelium is then closed with interrupted or mattress sutures. This technique is simple, efficacious, and requires minimal operating time with success rates greater than 90%.[2,4,17,30]

Larger fistulae may require more extensive dissection, and adequate closure may require a vaginal flap. Starting with an inverted "U" incision adjacent to the fistula, the vaginal epithelium is mobilized to allow for nonoverlapping suture lines, and the flap can help provide a tension-free closure of the underlying adventitia. Too much dissection compromises vascularity, but too little dissection can place undue tension on the surgical site, either of which can weaken the repair. The bladder wall should be closed in 2 layers with 3-0 vicryl in an interrupted or running fashion. If the fistula involves the trigone, the surgeon should consider whether a vertical or transverse closure would be better with regard to the position of the fistula relative the location of the ureters. Ideally, the first layer should result in a watertight closure with additional layers added for insurance. The remaining vesicovaginal fibromuscular connective tissue is then closed in 2 to 3 additional layers and the addition of a flap interposition could be considered for additional healthy vascular supply and/or to help fill significant dead space.[2,4] A complete discussion on pelvic flaps is beyond the scope of this manuscript but rectus, gracilis, Martius, or omental J-flap can be used. If a bladder backfill demonstrates the repair is watertight, a terminal cystoscopy may not be necessary and has the potential to place unwanted stress on the repair. A catheter should be left in place for 1 to 2 weeks, allowing for continuous bladder draining and minimal tension on the repair.

Urethrovaginal Fistula Repair

A layered urethrovaginal fistula repair has success rates greater than 90%.[31] They are approached very similarly to the described technique for VVF repairs discussed earlier. Very distal urethrovaginal fistulae may or may not be symptomatic depending on the location, but proximal urethrovaginal fistulae pose a challenging repair. Fistulae located in or near the urethrovesical junction may compromise the intrinsic sphincter mechanism of the urethra with resultant stress urinary incontinence (SUI) even if the fistula is successfully closed. Placing buttress sutures through the periurethral tissue may aid with both the fistula repair and improve symptoms of SUI, but a concomitant or staged antiincontinence procedure, such as an autologous fascial sling, could be considered. For a urethrovaginal fistula repair, a catheter is first placed through the urethra into the bladder. As described with VVF repair, a circumferential or "U" incision can be made around or adjacent to the urethrovaginal fistula. A scalpel, Metzenbaum, or tenotomy scissors can be used to sharply dissect the vaginal epithelium off of the underlying fibromuscular tissue. Adequate dissection can extend to the descending pubic rami and/or into the retropubic space, as needed to allow for tension free closure. The edges of the urethra are reapproximated with 2-0 or 3-0 absorbable sutures in an interrupted fashion followed by 2 to 3 additional layers of imbricating vaginal fibromuscular tissue and ultimately the vaginal epithelium. Depending on the extent of the dissection, an interposed flap can be used here as well. An indwelling Foley catheter is left in place for continuous bladder drainage for 1 to 2 weeks. In the setting of a urethrovaginal fistula, a synthetic mesh midurethral sling should not be placed at the time of fistula repair. Because SUI may be an issue for patients following urethrovaginal fistula is repaired, it may be reasonable to consider placing a concurrent pubovaginal sling during the fistula repair,[32] whereas others would wait to address SUI as a staged, secondary procedure.

Ureterovaginal Fistula Repair

Ureterovaginal fistulae can be repaired vaginally but are most commonly approached abdominally via laparotomy or laparoscopy (traditional or robot-assisted). Success rates for a traditional open ureterovaginal fistula repair are reported as ~90% in observational studies.[33,34] Once intraperitoneal access is obtained, the bowel is retracted into the upper abdomen using Trendelenburg and/or packing. The ureter is identified at the pelvic brim, and retroperitoneal access is obtained. The ureter is then mobilized to the level of the fistula, with care taken not to disrupt the periureteral tissue so as to not compromise ureteral blood flow. Once the fistula tract is released and the diseased ureter excised, the vagina is closed in 1 or 2 layers with absorbable sutures and a ureteroneocystostomy is performed at a site away from the prior fistula for the highest chances of a successful repair.[4,33] A ureteroneocystostomy involves transecting and then spatulating the ureter proximal to the fistula. The bladder dome is then incised and the ureter tunneled through and anchored to the bladder mucosa. The ureteral adventitia is also sutured to the overlying bladder peritoneum for added support. To avoid undue tension on the ureteroneocystostomy, either a psoas hitch or a Boari-Ockerblad flap can be performed.[4] Ureteral stents should be left in place for 4 to 6 weeks, and continuous bladder drainage with a Foley catheter should be maintained for 1 to 2 weeks to promote bladder recovery and prevent ureteral stricture formation.

Vesicouterine Fistula Repair

Vesicouterine fistula repairs are commonly performed through an abdominal approach using surgical techniques that can also be applied to an abdominal VVF repair. These types of fistulae are frequently seen after obstetric injury following a cesarean section. Once intraperitoneal access is obtained, the bladder is dissected off of the uterus to level of the fistula where the fistula tract is then resected. Once the bladder and uterus are free from each other, each is closed in 1 to 2 layers in a perpendicular fashion as to avoid overlapping suture lines. To further separate these 2 otherwise abutting repairs, an omental, peritoneal, or sigmoid epiploic flap can be interposed and anchored with absorbable sutures between the bladder and uterus.[2,33] The most definitive treatment of a vesicouterine fistula is a hysterectomy at the time of repair if childbearing is complete.[6]

Rectovaginal Fistulae Repair

RVF repair approach depends on the location of the injury. **Fig. 4** demonstrates a very distal RVF likely as seen with a chronic fourth degree obstetric laceration as well as a mid-level RVF with a probe delineating the fistulous tract. High rectovaginal or colovaginal fistulae are best suited for an abdominal approach, whereas midlevel and distal RVF can be repaired via a transvaginal, perineal, or transrectal approach. RVF repairs have a lower probability of success than genitourinary fistulae.[2] In a retrospective cohort study, success rates at 1 year postoperatively ranged from 35.2% to 95% with the average success of transvaginal and transanal repairs being 55.6%.[35] Most of the RVF that gynecologists see are those related to an obstetric injury seen in the postpartum time period.[4,35] With a fistula at the mid to distal vagina and an intact perineal body, a transverse or vertical incision encircling the fistula tract or a "U" incision in the vagina or the perineum can be used to gain access to the fistula tract. Either an upright or an inverted "U" perineal incision can be used when a sphincteroplasty is planned as part of the repair. One nonrandomized comparative cohort study compared a traditional inverted "U" perineal incision with an upright "U" posterior fourchette incision and found the latter approach decreased postoperative wound complications while maintaining a similar functional outcome.[36] A vaginal repair is performed as follows: the vagina is dissected off of the anterior rectal wall. This dissection is continued laterally around the fistulous tract to allow for a tension-free repair. The fistula tract is excised or used as part of the rectal closure. The rectal muscularis and submucosa are then imbricated over the rectal mucosa. An additional 2 to 3 layers of interrupted 2-0 or 3-0 absorbable sutures are used to provide additional support between the rectum and posterior vaginal wall. Flaps, such as a sphincteroplasty or Martius, could be used if needed. Finally, the vaginal epithelium is closed. For low RVF with a damaged perineal body and separated anal sphincter, an episioproctotomy is done, by first making an incision between the vagina and rectum. Once this is mobilized, the repair proceeds similarly to a fourth-degree obstetric laceration repair. which includes reapproximating the rectal mucosa, then the internal anal sphincter is imbricated over the rectal mucosa. The external anal sphincter is closed by either an end-to-end or an overlapping technique based on surgeon preference, as there are no data to favor one over the other.[37] The perineal body is reconstructed by bringing together the bulbocavernosus muscles, then the transverse perineal muscles after which the vaginal epithelium is reapproximated.

A diverting colostomy can be considered but is commonly reserved for recurrent fistula repairs.[38] It is also important to be able to distinguish a normally nonpainful RVF from its painful relative, the fistula-in-ano. A fistula-in-ano is a result of infected anal

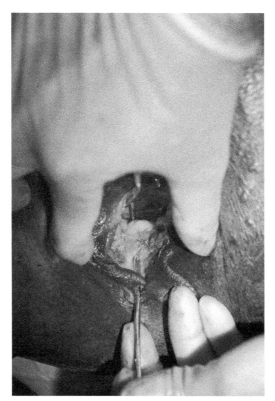

Fig. 4. A patient with both a distal RVF involving the anal sphincter complex and a midlevel RVF approximately proximal to the hymen.

glands that rupture through the rectum and vagina, leading to a high chance of failure with typical RVF repair.[39] Postoperative care has evolved for RVF surgery and based on colorectal data, there is no need for a low-residual diet, delayed feeding, or postoperative antibiotics.[2,40]

SUMMARY

Pelvic fistulae remain challenging for both patients and surgeons. Successful repair is most likely to result if an accurate diagnosis is obtained and appropriate surgical repair planned. Success rates for initial surgical repair of genitourinary fistulae are typically greater than 90%, whereas rectovaginal fistula repairs are approximately 55%. Regardless of the fistula type, ensuring a tension-free, "watertight", well-vascularized closure is the cornerstone to successful fistula repairs. Literature guiding pelvic fistula care is predominantly based on observational data and expert opinion.

CLINICS CARE POINTS

- Current literature guiding clinical care for pelvic fistulae management is based on observational data with very limited level I evidence.

- A trial of continuous bladder drainage for 4 to 6 weeks can be used in pelvic fistulae less than 1 cm, with success rates ranging from 12% to 80%.[4]
- Timing of surgical repair is variable but should be deferred until tissue integrity is maximized.
- Most of the pelvic fistulae are best repaired vaginally with success rates for initial surgical repair of genitourinary fistulae greater than 90%, whereas rectovaginal fistula repairs are ~55%.

DISCLOSURE

The authors have nothing to disclose.

REFERENCES

1. Mellano EM, Tarnay CM. Management of genitourinary fistula. Curr Opin Obstet Gynecol 2014;26(5):415–23.
2. Rogers RG, Jeppson PC. Current Diagnosis and Management of Pelvic Fistulae in Women. Obstet Gynecol 2016;128(3):635–50.
3. Polan ML, Sleemi A, Bedane MM, et al. Obstetric Fistula. In: Debas HT, Donkor P, Gawande A, et al, editors. Essential surgery: disease control priorities, vol. 1, 3rd edition. Washington (DC): The International Bank for Reconstruction and Development / The World Bank © 2015 International Bank for Reconstruction and Development / The World Bank.; 2015. p. 1–4.
4. Walters MD, Karram MM. Urogynecology and reconstructive pelvic surgery. 4th edition. Philadelphia: Elsevier Saunders; 2015.
5. Dallas KB, Rogo-Gupta L, Elliott CS. Urologic Injury and Fistula After Hysterectomy for Benign Indications. Obstet Gynecol 2019;134(2):241–9.
6. Wong MJ, Wong K, Rezvan A, et al. Urogenital fistula. *Female pelvic medicine.* Reconstr Surg 2012;18(2):71–8 [quiz: 78].
7. Simpson AN, Garbens A, Dossa F, et al. A Cost-Utility Analysis of Nonsurgical Treatments for Stress Urinary Incontinence in Women. Female Pelvic Med Reconstr Surg 2019;25(1):49–55.
8. El-Gazzaz G, Hull T, Mignanelli E, et al. Analysis of function and predictors of failure in women undergoing repair of Crohn's related rectovaginal fistula. J Gastrointest Surg 2010;14(5):824–9.
9. Melchior S, Cudovic D, Jones J, et al. Diagnosis and surgical management of colovesical fistulas due to sigmoid diverticulitis. J Urol 2009;182(3):978–82.
10. Rajamaheswari N, Chhikara AB. Vesicouterine fistulae: our experience of 17 cases and literature review. Int Urogynecol J 2013;24(2):275–9.
11. Blaivas JG, Mekel G. Management of urinary fistulas due to midurethral sling surgery. J Urol 2014;192(4):1137–42.
12. Antosh DD, Gutman RE. Diagnosis and management of female urethral diverticulum. Female Pelvic Med Reconstr Surg 2011;17(6):264–71.
13. VanBuren WM, Lightner AL, Kim ST, et al. Imaging and Surgical Management of Anorectal Vaginal Fistulas. Radiographics 2018;38(5):1385–401.
14. Dwarkasing S, Hussain SM, Hop WC, et al. Anovaginal fistulas: evaluation with endoanal MR imaging. Radiology 2004;231(1):123–8.
15. Dwarkasing S, Hussain SM, Krestin GP. Magnetic resonance imaging of perianal fistulas. Semin Ultrasound CT MR 2005;26(4):247–58.

16. Choen S, Burnett S, Bartram CI, et al. Comparison between anal endosonography and digital examination in the evaluation of anal fistulae. Br J Surg 1991; 78(4):445–7.
17. Oakley SH, Brown HW, Greer JA, et al. Management of vesicovaginal fistulae: a multicenter analysis from the Fellows' Pelvic Research Network. Female Pelvic Med Reconstr Surg 2014;20(1):7–13.
18. Kumar A, Goyal NK, Das SK, et al. Our experience with genitourinary fistulae. Urol Int 2009;82(4):404–10.
19. Arias BE, Ridgeway B, Barber MD. Complications of neglected vaginal pessaries: case presentation and literature review. Int Urogynecol J Pelvic Floor Dysfunct 2008;19(8):1173–8.
20. Al-Otaibi KM. Ureterovaginal fistulas: The role of endoscopy and a percutaneous approach. Urol Ann 2012;4(2):102–5.
21. Waaldijk K. The immediate surgical management of fresh obstetric fistulas with catheter and/or early closure. Int J Gynaecol Obstet 1994;45(1):11–6.
22. Waaldijk K. The immediate management of fresh obstetric fistulas. Am J Obstet Gynecol 2004;191(3):795–9.
23. Hadley HR. Vesicovaginal fistula. Curr Urol Rep 2002;3(5):401–7.
24. Gray M. Optimal management of incontinence-associated dermatitis in the elderly. Am J Clin Dermatol 2010;11(3):201–10.
25. ACOG practice bulletin No. 104: antibiotic prophylaxis for gynecologic procedures. Obstet Gynecol 2009;113(5):1180–9.
26. Shittu OS, Ojengbede OA, Wara LH. A review of postoperative care for obstetric fistulas in Nigeria. Int J Gynaecol Obstet 2007;99(Suppl 1):S79–84.
27. Frajzyngier V, Ruminjo J, Asiimwe F, et al. Factors influencing choice of surgical route of repair of genitourinary fistula, and the influence of route of repair on surgical outcomes: findings from a prospective cohort study. BJOG 2012;119(11): 1344–53.
28. Lee D, Zimmern P. Vaginal approach to vesicovaginal fistula. Urol Clin North Am 2019;46(1):123–33.
29. Lee RA, Symmonds RE, Williams TJ. Current status of genitourinary fistula. Obstet Gynecol 1988;72(3 Pt 1):313–9.
30. Margolis T, Mercer LJ. Vesicovaginal fistula. Obstet Gynecol Surv 1994;49(12): 840–7.
31. Clifton MM, Goldman HB. Urethrovaginal fistula closure. Int Urogynecol J 2017; 28(1):157–8.
32. Leng WW, Amundsen CL, McGuire EJ. Management of female genitourinary fistulas: transvesical or transvaginal approach? J Urol 1998;160(6 Pt 1):1995–9.
33. Shaw J, Tunitsky-Bitton E, Barber MD, et al. Ureterovaginal fistula: a case series. Int Urogynecol J 2014;25(5):615–21.
34. Symmonds RE. Ureteral injuries associated with gynecologic surgery: prevention and management. Clin Obstet Gynecol 1976;19(3):623–44.
35. Byrnes JN, Schmitt JJ, Faustich BM, et al. Outcomes of rectovaginal fistula repair. Female Pelvic Med Reconstr Surg 2017;23(2):124–30.
36. Tan M, O'Hanlon DM, Cassidy M, et al. Advantages of a posterior fourchette incision in anal sphincter repair. Dis colon rectum 2001;44(11):1624–9.
37. Farrell SA. Overlapping compared with end-to-end repair of third and fourth degree obstetric anal sphincter tears. Curr Opin Obstet Gynecol 2011;23(5): 386–90.
38. Fu J, Liang Z, Zhu Y, et al. Surgical repair of rectovaginal fistulas: predictors of fistula closure. Int Urogynecol J 2019;30(10):1659–65.

39. Delancey JO, Berger MB. Surgical approaches to postobstetrical perineal body defects (rectovaginal fistula and chronic third and fourth-degree lacerations). Clin Obstet Gynecol 2010;53(1):134–44.

40. Andersen HK, Lewis SJ, Thomas S. Early enteral nutrition within 24h of colorectal surgery versus later commencement of feeding for postoperative complications. Cochrane database Syst Rev 2006;(4):Cd004080.

Recognition and Management of Pelvic Floor Disorders in Pregnancy and the Postpartum Period

Annetta M. Madsen, MD[a],*, Lisa C. Hickman, MD[b],
Katie Propst, MD[c]

KEYWORDS

- Postpartum pelvic floor • Pregnancy pelvic floor • Obstetric anal sphincter injury
- Obstetric laceration • Pelvic floor disorders

KEY POINTS

- Start early. Women should be educated on their pelvic floor, normal changes, and pelvic floor disorders that can occur in pregnancy and postpartum.
- Screen often. Providers should make an effort to screen for pelvic floor symptoms in pregnancy and postpartum, as early recognition and management could improve quality of life during this critical time in a woman's life.
- Avoid overnormalization. Connect pregnant and postpartum women experiencing pelvic floor disorder symptoms with education, support, early treatment, and referral to subspecialty care, as needed.

INTRODUCTION

Although women have experienced pregnancy and childbirth since the beginning of humankind, there remains a lack in basic knowledge of its effect on the pelvis.[1,2] Women report dismissive reactions by health care providers, personal lack of knowledge, and feelings of embarrassment and shame that keep them from accessing care that could significantly improve their quality of life.[3] The American College of Obstetricians and Gynecologists recently acknowledged insufficiencies in postpartum care, including pelvic health.[4] However, no consensus on the standard of care for pelvic health in pregnancy or postpartum exists. Diagnosis and management of postpartum

[a] Division of Female Pelvic Medicine & Reconstructive Surgery, Department of Obstetrics & Gynecology, Mayo Clinic, 200 First Street SW, Rochester, MN 55905, USA; [b] Division of Female Pelvic Medicine & Reconstructive Surgery, Department of Obstetrics & Gynecology, The Ohio State University Wexner Medical Center, 395 West 12th Avenue, Room 504, Columbus, OH 43210, USA; [c] Urogynecology & Reconstructive Pelvic Surgery, OB/Gyn and Women's Health Institute, Cleveland Clinic, 9500 Euclid Avenue, Desk A-81, Cleveland, OH 44195, USA
* Corresponding author.
E-mail address: Madsen.Annetta@mayo.edu

Obstet Gynecol Clin N Am 48 (2021) 571–584
https://doi.org/10.1016/j.ogc.2021.05.009
0889-8545/21/© 2021 Elsevier Inc. All rights reserved.

pelvic floor disorders (PFDs) were extensively reviewed in a recent article by Meekins and Siddiqui.[5] This article builds on that knowledge to recommend a broader clinical approach to education, recognition, and care for women with PFDs and perineal lacerations in pregnancy and postpartum.

DISCUSSION
Start Early: Education, Awareness, and Promotion of Pelvic Health

General knowledge of PFDs, including the effects of pregnancy and childbirth, is lacking for women of all ages.[1,6–8] Women report a desire for more information, but antenatal education about PFDs is scant. Utilizing a team of nurses and physical therapists could help to initiate pelvic health education early in pregnancy, maintain awareness through the continuum of care, and promote early identification of PFDs.[9,10] During pregnancy and early postpartum, it can be difficult to determine if symptoms are transient normal changes or indicative of a PFD. Educating women on what is normal, not normal, and what can be done to optimize pelvic health can start the conversation at the onset of pregnancy care and lead to earlier recognition of a disorder (**Table 1**).

Outcomes research on prenatal pelvic floor education programs is limited but has shown some improvement in symptoms with no change in mode of delivery.[11] Therefore, a belief that more knowledge would lead to fear and increased cesarean section rates is not supported by the literature. Education on the risks of pelvic floor injury and PFDs should be considered an important aspect of informed consent for delivery, especially during discussions about operative vaginal delivery and episiotomy.

Education: normal physiologic changes to the pelvis and related symptoms

The physiologic changes of pregnancy are vast, affecting nearly every organ system, in an effort to accommodate the gravid uterus and support the growing fetus, as well as prepare the body for the events necessary for parturition. Changes related to the pelvis and urinary tract during pregnancy are outlined in **Fig. 1**.[12,13] As the bony pelvis progressively widens and tilts anteriorly to prepare for vaginal delivery, women are also predisposed to low back and pelvic girdle pain that can persist postpartum.[12] Physical examination studies show that women with relaxation in anterior, apical, and genital hiatus Pelvic Organ Prolapse Quantification (POP-Q) measurements in the third trimester were significantly more likely to have an uncomplicated spontaneous vaginal delivery that included no operative assistance or obstetric anal sphincter injury.[14] Thus, changes to the pelvic floor muscles, vagina, and pelvic floor support serve an important role in mitigating the risk of neuromuscular injury during childbirth. However, it is not surprising that increased pressure from the gravid uterus

Table 1		
Normal transient symptoms versus a pelvic floor disorder		
Symptom	**Normal Symptoms**	**Pelvic Floor Disorder Symptoms**
Urinary	Frequency, urgency, nocturia	Incontinence or other urinary symptoms affecting quality of life
Bowel	Slower transit	Constipation, straining, incomplete emptying, incontinence
Vaginal	Changes in vaginal caliber and vaginal support	Pelvic organ prolapse

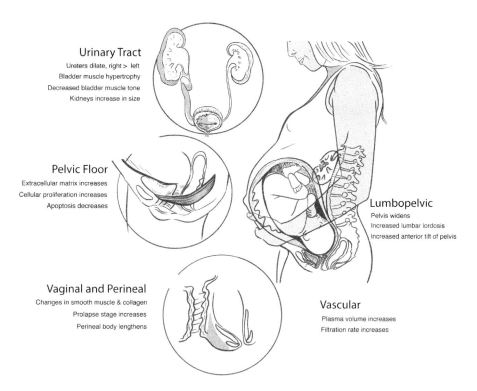

Urinary Tract
Ureters dilate, right > left
Bladder muscle hypertrophy
Decreased bladder muscle tone
Kidneys increase in size

Pelvic Floor
Extracellular matrix increases
Cellular proliferation increases
Apoptosis decreases

Lumbopelvic
Pelvis widens
Increased lumbar lordosis
Increased anterior tilt of pelvis

Vaginal and Perineal
Changes in smooth muscle & collagen
Prolapse stage increases
Perineal body lengthens

Vascular
Plasma volume increases
Filtration rate increases

Fig. 1. Changes to the pelvis and urinary tract in pregnancy. (*Courtesy of* Polina Sawyer, MD, University of Texas Southwestern).

in addition to these changes can impose early, transient symptoms of defects in pelvic floor support.[15]

Defining normal pelvic floor support after vaginal or cesarean delivery is complex and an area of ongoing research.[16,17] Studies demonstrate increases in the levator hiatus and bladder neck mobility and relaxation in all POP-Q measurements, most commonly the anterior wall.[18] These changes are more notable after vaginal compared with cesarean delivery, but tend to improve during the first 6 postpartum months, with little change between 6 months and 1 year.[18,19] The only change independently associated with the later development of symptomatic pelvic organ prolapse is an enlarged genital hiatus.[19]

The urinary system undergoes significant changes in pregnancy, starting as early as the first trimester.[12,13] Despite an increase in functional bladder volume, an increase in urine production caused by increased plasma volume and glomerular filtration rate causes women in pregnancy to experience urinary frequency and nocturia, which are the most common lower urinary tract symptoms in pregnancy.[12,13] Both estrogen and progesterone can exert a negative impact on urethral pressure, which when combined with chronically increased intra-abdominal pressure from the gravid uterus and decreased pelvic floor muscle tone, likely exacerbate stress-related urinary incontinence.[13] Taken together, these changes can explain the prevalent urinary tract symptoms women experience in pregnancy. Postpartum, urinary frequency and urgency may persist for 3 to 4 months.[20] Although postpartum incontinence can improve with time, it should not be considered normal.

Awareness: Pelvic floor disorder recognition, risks, and impact in pregnancy, postpartum, and beyond

In contrast to transient physiologic changes that can be normal in pregnancy, PFDs are persistent conditions that negatively impact quality of life and include urinary incontinence, anal incontinence, and pelvic organ prolapse. These symptoms can start in pregnancy and persist postpartum or develop after delivery.

PFDs starting in pregnancy are relatively common. In a cohort of pregnant women in the third trimester who were assessed using the validated Pelvic Floor Distress Inventory, 29.0% reported prolapse symptom distress; 41.8% reported urinary symptom distress, and 24.2% reported colorectal symptom distress.[21] Colorectal symptoms specific to fecal incontinence are rare, occurring in 3.9% of women at 12 weeks of gestation.[22] During delivery, obstetric perineal lacerations are the most commonly identified form of pelvic trauma and classified by degree, summarized in **Table 2**.[23] Up to 79% of women experience an obstetric laceration at the time of vaginal delivery, and most these are first- or second-degree lacerations.[23] Severe perineal lacerations that injure the anal sphincter complex are called obstetric anal sphincter injuries (OASIs) and include third- and fourth-degree lacerations.[23] OASIs occur in up to 3.3% of vaginal deliveries and are independently associated with fecal incontinence at 12 months postpartum.[22]

Women can develop postpartum pelvic floor disorders without a clear perineal injury. The role of occult neuromuscular injury, especially to the levator ani, and the subsequent development of PFDs, is an area of ongoing research.[24] Currently, the main factors associated with developing a postpartum PFD are vaginal delivery and presence of OASI, described in **Table 3**.[16,19,25,26] Aging, increasing parity, vaginal birth, and especially operative vaginal birth, are all associated with development of PFDs later in life.[19] Additionally, 76% of women who experience urinary incontinence at 3 months postpartum reported urinary incontinence at 12 years, even if it initially resolved.[27] This indicates that women with postpartum urinary incontinence are a high-risk group of women who would benefit from screening because they have a high probability of experiencing incontinence in their lifetime.

Regardless of the long-term implications, the significant impact of PFD symptoms experienced during pregnancy and postpartum should not be underestimated. In a longitudinal study of over 600 women during pregnancy, urinary incontinence, fecal incontinence, and perineal pain increased between first and third trimesters, with third-trimester urinary incontinence associated with a significant decrease in quality of life.[28] During pregnancy, up to 52% of women report psychological strain attributed to at

Table 2 Perineal laceration classification	
Laceration Degree	**Description of Injury**
1st	Involves only perineal skin
2nd	Involves skin and muscles of the perineal body
3rd	Extends into anal sphincter complex 3a: <50% of external anal sphincter torn 3b: >50% of the external anal sphincter torn 3c: injury to the internal and external anal sphincters
4th	Extends through perineal body muscles, anal sphincter complex, and anal-rectal epithelium

Data from: ACOG Practice Bulletin No. 198: Prevention and Management of Obstetric Lacerations at Vaginal Delivery. Obstet Gynecol 2018;132(3).

Table 3 Proportion of women with postpartum pelvic floor disorders by delivery type			
Pelvic Floor Disorder	Postpartum Vaginal Delivery	Postpartum Vaginal Delivery + OASI[a]	Postpartum Cesarean Delivery
Urinary incontinence	35% at 6 wks 31% at 6 mo	34% at 6 wks 33% at 6 mo	25% at 6 wks 22% at 6 mo
Fecal incontinence	11% at 6 wks 8% at 6 mo	26% at 6 wks 17% at 6 mo	10% at 6 wks 7% at 6 mo
Pelvic organ prolapse (Stage 2 on examination)	29% at 6–12 mo 7% at 5–10 y 14% at 20 y	38% at 6–12 mo	21% at 6–12 mo 6% at 20 y

[a] OASI: obstetric anal sphincter injury.
Data from Handa VL, Nygaard I, Kenton K, et al. Pelvic organ support among primiparous women in the first year after childbirth. Inter Urogynecol J 2009;20(12):1407-1411; Handa VL, Blomquist JL, Roem J, et al. Longitudinal study of quantitative changes in pelvic organ support among parous women. Am J Obstet Gynecol 2018;218(3):320; Borello-France D, Burgio KL, Richter HE, et al. Fecal and urinary incontinence in primiparous women. Obstet Gynecol 2006;108(4):863-872; Gyhagen M, Bullarbo M, Nielsen T, et al. Prevalence and risk factors for pelvic organ prolapse 20 years after childbirth: a national cohort study in singleton primiparae after vaginal or caesarean delivery. BJOG 2013;120(2):152-160.

least 1 domain of bladder, bowel, prolapse, or sexual dysfunction symptoms.[29] Urinary incontinence and pain have also been independently associated with postpartum depression.[30] Qualitative studies reveal a negative impact on partnership and sexual function, somatic and psychological effects, and trauma.[3] Even more concerning is patient report of feelings of isolation, embarrassment, and shame when their symptoms were dismissed by comments such as "it will get better" without further information or attention by their health care provider.[3] Health care providers must be equipped to provide resources, support, and care to women who have the courage to mention their pelvic floor symptoms in pregnancy and postpartum.

Promotion of pelvic health and prevention of pelvic floor disorders
No comprehensive evidence-based prevention strategies for PFDs or prediction models that clearly improve outcomes exist. A Cochrane review describing the effects of pelvic floor muscle exercises performed in pregnancy showed a lower incidence of new urinary symptoms in pregnancy, but no clear benefit in treatment of existing urinary incontinence or prevention and treatment of fecal incontinence.[31] Evidence for the benefits of physical therapy in treating all types of pelvic floor disorders in nonpregnant women is strong.[32] There are also significant gaps in knowledge of general exercise and pelvic floor disorders.[33] Evidence supports the recommendation that women be encouraged to exercise in pregnancy and postpartum for promotion of overall mental and physical well-being and to incorporate pelvic floor muscle exercise into their general exercise routine.[34] The best types of general exercise to perform, or avoid, in pregnancy for the promotion of pelvic health are unclear. National guidelines on prevention of pelvic floor injury also vary significantly, with no current international consensus.[35] Pregnancy and intrapartum measures of limiting pelvic floor trauma and OASI have limited supportive data and are described in **Table 4**.[23,36]

Screen Often: Recognition of Pelvic Floor Disorders in the Clinical Setting
Women with pre-existing or new-onset PFDs may benefit from early identification and support. Clinicians may miss these diagnoses due to lack of screening questions.[37]

Table 4
Risk factors and prevention of obstetric anal sphincter injury

Risk Factors	Odds Ratio (95% Confidence Interval)
Forceps-assisted delivery	5.50 (3.17–9.55)
Forceps-assisted delivery + midline episiotomy	
Fourth degree laceration	10.55 (10.29–10.81)
Third degree laceration	5.65 (5.55–5.75)
Vacuum-assisted delivery	3.98 (2.60–6.09)
Midline episiotomy	3.82 (1.96–7.42)
Primiparity	3.24 (2.20–4.76)
Occiput posterior position	3.09 (1.81–5.29)
Asian ethnicity	2.74 (1.31–5.72)
Labor induction	1.08 (1.02–1.14)
Epidural anesthesia	1.95 (1.66–2.32)
Birthweight >4000g[a]	2.10 (1.60–2.60)
Second stage of labor (>30 min)[a]	1.80 (1.40–2.30)
Prevention Strategies	*Relative Risk (95% CI)*
Perineal massage started at 34 weeks' gestation	0.91 (0.86–0.96)
Restricted (versus routine) use of mediolateral episiotomy	0.67 (0.49–0.91)
Perineal massage in second stage of labor (versus hands off)	0.52 (0.29–0.94)
Warm compresses on perineum during second stage of labor	0.48 (0.28–0.84)
Perineal protection during delivery	Inconsistent data
Birthing position	I data

[a] Data on risk for recurrent OASI from: van Bavel J, et al. Risk factors for the recurrence of obstetric anal sphincter injury and the role of a mediolateral episiotomy: an analysis of a national registry. BJOG 2020;127(8):951 to 56.
Data from: ACOG Practice Bulletin No. 198: Prevention and Management of Obstetric Lacerations at Vaginal Delivery. Obstet Gynecol 2018;132(3):e87-e102.

There are no known pregnancy-specific PFD screening tools, but the B[3] (Bulge, Bladder, Bowel) questionnaire is straight-forward and could be easily implemented into a typical review of systems (**Box 1**).[38]

Clinical evaluation and diagnosis of PFDs was previously reviewed, but the primary consideration is a woman's report of her symptoms.[5] Various symptom and quality of life questionnaires are available. Although none are specifically validated for pregnant or postpartum populations, these can be efficient, useful adjuncts to screen and evaluate women for pregnancy-related PFDs. The Pelvic Floor Distress Inventory (PFDI-20) and Pelvic Floor Impact Questionnaire (PFIQ) are commonly used, because they assess urinary, prolapse, and bowel symptoms.[39] The PFIQ is the only tool validated in a postpartum population and is especially useful, because all questions are asked in relation to before childbirth.[40] Five domains are used to assess sexual function, pelvic floor function, and pelvic organ support, but it does not include urinary or bowel symptoms.

Avoid Overnormalization: Addressing Pelvic Floor Concerns in Pregnancy and Postpartum

Pregnancy and postpartum can be a difficult time for new mothers as they adjust to the challenges of a new baby and significant changes to their body. Providers must

---

Box 1
B³ (bulge, bladder, bowel) screening tool for pelvic floor disorders

Bulge
  Do you have a sensation that there is a bulge in your vagina or that something is falling out of your vagina?

Bladder
  Do you experience bothersome leakage of urine?

Bowel
  In the past month, have you experienced accidental bowel leakage (liquid or solid stool)?

Data from: Barr SA, Crisp CC, White AB, Malik SA, Kenton K. FACE: Female Pelvic Medicine and Reconstructive Surgery Awareness Campaign: *Increasing Exposure*. Female Pelvic Med Reconstr Surg 2018;24(2):115-19.

---

walk a line to avoid overnormalization of PFDs while also providing reassurance about normal body changes. Although postpartum PFD management was extensively reviewed recently, the clinical approach to intervening in pregnancy and the postpartum period, addressing prior pelvic surgeries, and incorporating future childbearing goals into a woman's management plan are additional considerations for providing comprehensive care.[5]

Pregnancy in women with pre-existing pelvic floor disorders or prior pelvic surgery
Pregnant women with pre-existing PFDs are at risk of worsening symptoms with increasing gestation and childbirth. Evidence-based recommendations for these women is lacking. The authors recommend providing support through early optimization of conservative management strategies, team-based care with a physical therapist, and a proactive postpartum care plan to provide reassurance. Women who have undergone prior treatments or surgery for a PFD should be counseled on the potential impacts of subsequent pregnancy and delivery.[41]

Potential risks include:

1. Voiding dysfunction and urinary retention with a history of stress urinary incontinence surgery[41]
2. Pain or uterine constriction with increasing gestation with a history of mesh placement for pelvic organ prolapse[41]
3. Lead migration, need for revision, or decreased postpartum efficacy of a sacral neuromodulation device[41]

Despite these potential risks, current knowledge supports the safety of pregnancy and vaginal delivery following all types of PFD surgery.[41] Although there may be a risk of PFD recurrence, this does not appear to be affected by mode of delivery.[41]

The decision regarding delivery mode after OASI repair is especially complex. A recent meta-analysis reports overall risk of OASI of 5.7% in first pregnancy, with a risk of recurrent OASI increasing to 6.3% with a second pregnancy compared to 1.5% in women with no prior OASI.[42] Although prior OASI certainly increases the risk of subsequent OASI, the overall risk is low, and no evidence supports that mode of subsequent delivery is protective of long-term anal incontinence outcomes.[43] Among women with anal incontinence, cesarean section may prevent worsening of anal incontinence.[44] Providers should engage patients in a shared decision-making process, taking into consideration modifiable and nonmodifiable risk factors, current symptoms and prior wound complications, emotional trauma related to their prior birth experience, and the outcomes most important to each individual.[23] As risk for OASI is greatest in the setting of operative vaginal delivery and/or episiotomy, discussion of these potential interventions is an important part of the shared decision-making process.

Another special consideration is women with history of type 3 circumcision (female genital cutting), who are at increased risk of complex perineal lacerations and episiotomy during delivery. Comprehensive antenatal and postpartum care for women with circumcision is summarized by the World Health Organization and includes starting in preconception or early pregnancy with evaluation, counseling on risks, and

---

Box 2
Proposed clinical approach to new-onset pelvic floor symptoms in pregnancy and postpartum

1. Consider symptom time course.
   - Review normal changes in pregnancy and postpartum.
   - Provide reassurance that early symptoms can improve with time and care.

2. Do not overnormalize bothersome symptoms.
   - Although symptoms may improve, a significant proportion of women with postpartum PFDs will have persistent or recurrent symptoms.
   - A proactive, supportive, and reassuring approach is recommended.

3. Recommend early, low-risk interventions.
   - Self-directed pelvic floor muscle exercises can improve symptoms in women who are able to correctly perform them on clinical examination.
   - Kegel apps are available and can be a good adjunct to a home regimen.
   - Physical therapy is low-risk, although associated with a cost, and is likely to provide benefit. This is especially helpful for women who need additional support or are unable to contract pelvic floor muscles on clinical examination
   - Consider pessary management for improvement in prolapse or urinary symptoms, even if symptoms may be transient.
   - Vaginal estrogen therapy can benefit vaginal and urinary symptoms in breastfeeding women.

4. Outline a follow-up plan.
   - Recommend earlier postpartum follow-up (2 weeks) for women with complex perineal lacerations or PFD symptoms.
   - Consider referral to subspecialty female pelvic medicine and reconstructive surgery or postpartum perineal care clinic for
     ○ Severe perineal lacerations
     ○ Wound breakdown
     ○ Complex symptoms requiring close monitoring or surgical intervention
     ○ Women with significant concerns who need additional support
   - Define a follow-up timepoint to check on symptomatic improvement to decrease anxiety:
     ○ 3-month follow-up for women performing independent home exercises or attending physical therapy
     ○ Women with severe symptoms, complex lacerations, or poor wound healing need closer follow-up, possibly weekly, until improvement is seen

5. Provide reassurance that symptoms can improve with treatment.
   - Affirm that the patient has options for management and need not suffer until childbearing is complete.
   - Consider the patient's goals, in light of the risks and benefits of each management option, at any age.
   - Remember that PFD surgery does not always require hysterectomy, can improve quality of life and functioning, and is not an absolute contraindication for future childbearing in women who understand their risks.

shared decision-making on deinfibulation and mode of delivery.[45] Women with circumcision can also develop PFDs and may experience additional barriers to seeking care. Starting respectful pelvic health conversations early can improve communication, provide best care at the right time in pregnancy, limit misunderstanding and expectation mismatch at the time of delivery, and avoid underrecognition of PFDs in this group of women.

Table 5
Conservative interventions in pregnancy and postpartum

Pelvic Floor Condition	Initial Intervention
Stress urinary incontinence: Involuntary leakage of urine with coughing, laughing, sneezing, or activity	• Pelvic floor muscle exercises • Pelvic floor physical therapy ± biofeedback for women who lack ability to squeeze pelvic floor muscles or do not improve with pelvic floor muscle exercises • Incontinence pessary
Overactive bladder: Urinary urgency, frequency and/or nocturia in absence of infection. Urgency urinary incontinence: Involuntary leakage of urine associated with a sense of urgency	• Behavioral and dietary modification ○ Limitation of excessive fluid intake ○ Avoidance of irritants (ie, caffeine) ○ Timed voiding ○ Bladder calming techniques • Pelvic floor physical therapy ± biofeedback • Vaginal estrogen therapy in breastfeeding women • Judicious prescribing of anticholinergic medications (pregnancy category B; may reduce lactation)
Fecal incontinence (accidental bowel leakage): Involuntary loss of feces	• Behavioral and dietary modification ○ Avoidance of irritants (ie, lactose, caffeine) ○ Dietary fiber or fiber supplement • Pelvic floor physical therapy ± biofeedback • Occasional loperamide for loose stool (pregnancy category B; low level of breastmilk secretion)
Constipation: Although not a PFD, this can be a symptom of, or contribute to, pelvic floor dysfunction and can be caused by slow colonic transit and/or outlet obstruction	• Dietary fiber or fiber supplement • Adequate hydration • Osmotic laxatives (polyethylene glycol) or stool softeners (docusate sodium) • Pelvic floor physical therapy ± biofeedback
Pelvic organ prolapse: Symptomatic descent of one or more of the vaginal walls or uterus, typically to the level of the hymen or beyond	• Pelvic floor physical therapy ± biofeedback • Vaginal pessary ○ Need for pessary may decrease with increasing gestation and may be needed again postpartum
Vaginal pain and sexual dysfunction: Although not a PFD, this may be a symptom of underlying pelvic floor dysfunction	• Vaginal estrogen therapy in breastfeeding women • Pelvic floor physical therapy ± biofeedback

Data from: Meekins AR, Siddiqui NY. Diagnosis and management of postpartum pelvic floor disorders. Obstet Gynecol Clin North Am 2020;47(3):477-86.

Clinical approach to new-onset pelvic floor disorder symptoms in pregnancy and postpartum

Box 2 summarizes a proposed clinical approach to women who develop new symptoms in pregnancy and postpartum. The American College of Obstetrician Gynecologists recommends all patients have contact with an obstetric provider within the first 3 weeks following delivery.[4] For patients who experienced an OASI, follow-up within 2 weeks of delivery is recommended, given the increased prevalence of wound complications and bowel control issues.[46,47] Similar consideration for early

Table 6
Patient education resources on postpartum pelvic health and pelvic floor disorders

Resource	Website	Description
American Urogynecologic Society: Patient Fact Sheets	https://www.augs.org/patient-fact-sheets/	Printable fact sheets on pelvic floor disorders and treatment options, including one specifically addressing third and fourth degree perineal tears Information in English and Spanish
American Urogynecologic Society "Voices for PFD" Web site: Information for New Moms	https://www.voicesforpfd.org/new-mothers/new-moms/)	Covers basics on the pelvic floor and postpartum changes, patient stories, pregnancy-related pelvic floor symptoms, and additional patient resources both on the web and in print Information in English and Spanish
International Urogynecological Association: Your Pelvic Floor	https://www.yourpelvicfloor.org/leaflets/	Printable patient leaflets on pelvic floor disorders and treatments, including maternal pelvic floor trauma and third and fourth degree perineal tears Information in multiple languages
Royal College of Obstetricians & Gynecologists (RCOG)	https://www.rcog.org.uk/en/patients/tears?source=tearsPIL	Comprehensive Web site on perineal tears and episiotomies in childbirth, the pelvic floor, perineal breakdown. Also provides anticipatory guidance before and after delivery. *Information in English*
RCOG Patient Experience	https://www.rcog.org.uk/en/guidelines-research-services/audit-quality-improvement/oasi-care-bundle/oasi-videos/	Patient experience videos Information in English

follow-up should be given for patients with advanced obstetric injury not involving the anal sphincter complex or for women experiencing PFDs immediately postpartum. At this point of contact, in addition to a comprehensive history and physical examination, the patient can be screened for difficulties with bladder or bowel control, breast-feeding, pain, and postpartum mood disorders. Further follow-up, either via an in-person visit with the obstetric provider or a subspecialist referral, can be arranged if needed.[48]

The authors recommend providing support and conservative management of PFDs during pregnancy and up to 6 months postpartum, as summarized in **Table 5**.[5] However, women with persistent postpartum PFDs should be offered the full spectrum of management options. Although it has been typically recommended to delay surgical management until childbearing is complete, given the growing literature on the safety of pregnancy after PFD surgery and increasing popularity of hysteropexy techniques, this decision is best made as a shared decision between a patient and surgeon through comprehensive counseling on the risks and benefits of all options. There is a growing number of subspecialty peripartum pelvic floor disorder clinics nationally and internationally.[48] These clinics are typically run by subspecialists in female pelvic medicine and reconstructive surgery and serve as an excellent resource for pregnant or postpartum women experiencing advanced obstetric lacerations or PFDs.

Patient education and support resources
Educational resources on pregnancy-related PFDs are available from major national and international organizations for patients and providers (**Table 6**). Although many women turn to social media and Web site searches to find relevant information and peer support postpartum, directing them to sites such as these ensures accurate and useful information is provided.

SUMMARY

Often considered a condition of aging women, PFDs will initially present during pregnancy and postpartum for a subset of individuals. These conditions can have a negative impact on quality of life during this important time and also increase a woman's lifetime risk of persistent or recurrent PFD symptoms. Whole-woman care should integrate pelvic health beginning early in pregnancy and continue postpartum. Routine screening for PFDs can be efficiently accomplished with a brief questionnaire and should be routinely performed throughout pregnancy and the postpartum period to reach women who may otherwise not seek care out of embarrassment and shame. Avoidance of overnormalization, validating patient concerns, and providing support, resources, treatment, and referrals for women with PFD symptoms could improve the peripartum experience and connect women at high risk for PFDs with early access to pelvic health care.

CLINICS CARE POINTS

- Normal physiologic changes in pregnancy and postpartum may result in urinary frequency, urgency, nocturia, changes in pelvic organ support, and slower bowel transit.

- PFDs, in contrast to normal changes, are persistent conditions affecting the bowel, bladder, and vaginal support that negatively affect quality of life and may lead to psychological stress, trauma, depression, and decreased sexual function in postpartum women.

- PFDs are more common with vaginal delivery compared with cesarean section, and anal incontinence is associated with vaginal delivery that involves an anal sphincter injury.

- A simple screening tool can be used to identify women with a PFD in pregnancy and postpartum.
- Conservative treatments for PFDs include behavioral and dietary changes, pelvic floor muscle exercises or physical therapy, and medications.
- Prior surgery for a PFD is not an absolute contraindication for pregnancy or vaginal delivery, and women of all ages should be comprehensively counseled on the risks and benefits of all PFD management options and delivery decisions.

DISCLOSURE

All authors have nothing to disclose.

REFERENCES

1. Geynisman-Tan JM, Taubel D, Asfaw TS. Is something missing from antenatal education? A survey of pregnant women's knowledge of pelvic floor disorders. Female Pelvic Med Reconstr Surg 2018;24(6):440–3.
2. Cooke CM, O'Sullivan OE, O'Reilly BA. Urogynaecology providers' attitudes towards postnatal pelvic floor dysfunction. Int Urogynecol J 2018;29(5):751–66.
3. Skinner EM, Barnett B, Dietz HP. Psychological consequences of pelvic floor trauma following vaginal birth: a qualitative study from two Australian tertiary maternity units. Arch Womens Ment Health 2018;21(3):341–51.
4. McKinney J, Keyser L, Clinton S, et al. ACOG Committee Opinion No. 736: optimizing postpartum care. Obstet Gynecol 2018;132(3):784–5.
5. Meekins AR, Siddiqui NY. Diagnosis and management of postpartum pelvic floor disorders. Obstet Gynecol Clin North Am 2020;47(3):477–86.
6. Parden AM, Griffin RL, Hoover K, et al. Prevalence, awareness, and understanding of pelvic floor disorders in adolescent and young women. Female Pelvic Med Reconstr Surg 2016;22(5):346–54.
7. Neels H, Tjalma WAA, Wyndaele J-J, et al. Knowledge of the pelvic floor in menopausal women and in peripartum women. J Phys Ther Sci 2016;28(11):3020–9.
8. McKay ER, Lundsberg LS, Miller DT, et al. Knowledge of pelvic floor disorders in obstetrics. Female Pelvic Med Reconstr Surg 2019;25(6):419–25.
9. Li T, Wang J, Chen X, et al. Obstetric nurses' knowledge, attitudes, and professional support related to actual care practices about urinary incontinence. Female Pelvic Med Reconstr Surg 2020;27(2):e377–84.
10. Dufour S, Hondronicols A, Flanigan K. Enhancing pelvic health: optimizing the services provided by primary health care teams in Ontario by integrating physiotherapists. Physiother Can 2019;71(2):168–75.
11. Hyakutake MT, Han V, Baerg L, et al. Pregnancy-associated pelvic floor health knowledge and reduction of symptoms: the PREPARED randomized controlled trial. J Obstet Gynaecol Can 2018;40(4):418–25.
12. Cunningham FG, Leveno KJ, Bloom SL, et al, editors. Maternal physiology. Wiliams obstetrics. 25th edition. New York: McGraw-Hill Education; 2018.
13. Gregory WT, Sibai BM. Obstetrics and Pelvic Floor Disorders. In: Walters MD, Karram MM, editors. Urogynecology and reconstructive pelvic surgery. 4th edition. Philadelphia: WB Saunders; 2015. p. 224–37.
14. Oliphant SS, Nygaard IE, Zong W, et al. Maternal adaptations in preparation for parturition predict uncomplicated spontaneous delivery outcome. Am J Obstet Gynecol 2014;211(6):630.e1–7.

15. O'Boyle AL, O'Boyle JD, Ricks RE, et al. The natural history of pelvic organ support in pregnancy. Int Urogynecol J Pelvic Floor Dysfunct 2003;14(1):46–9.
16. Handa VL, Nygaard I, Kenton K, et al. Pelvic organ support among primiparous women in the first year after childbirth. Inter Urogynecol J 2009;20(12):1407–11.
17. Handa VL, Blomquist JL, Roem J, et al. Longitudinal study of quantitative changes in pelvic organ support among parous women. Am J Obstet Gynecol 2018;218(3):320.
18. Van Geelen H, Ostergard D, Sand P. A review of the impact of pregnancy and childbirth on pelvic floor function as assessed by objective measurement techniques. Inter Urogynecol J 2018;29(3):327–38.
19. Handa VL, Blomquist JL, Knoepp LR, et al. Pelvic floor disorders 5–10 years after vaginal or cesarean childbirth. Obstet Gynecol 2011;118(4):777–84.
20. Chaliha C, Stanton SL. Urological problems in pregnancy. BJU Int 2002;89(5):469–76.
21. Yohay D, Weintraub AY, Mauer-Perry N, et al. Prevalence and trends of pelvic floor disorders in late pregnancy and after delivery in a cohort of Israeli women using the PFDI-20. Eur J Obstet Gynecol Reprod Biol 2016;200:35–9.
22. van Brummen HJ, Bruinse HW, van de Pol G, et al. Defecatory symptoms during and after the first pregnancy: prevalences and associated factors. Int Urogynecol J Pelvic Floor Dysfunct 2006;17(3):224–30.
23. ACOG Practice Bulletin No. 198. Prevention and management of obstetric lacerations at vaginal delivery. Obstet Gynecol 2018;132(3):e87–102.
24. Handa VL, Blomquist JL, Roem J, et al. Pelvic floor disorders after obstetric avulsion of the levator ani muscle. Female Pelvic Med Reconstr Surg 2019;25(1):3–7.
25. Borello-France D, Burgio KL, Richter HE, et al. Fecal and urinary incontinence in primiparous women. Obstet Gynecol 2006;108(4):863–72.
26. Gyhagen M, Bullarbo M, Nielsen T, et al. Prevalence and risk factors for pelvic organ prolapse 20 years after childbirth: a national cohort study in singleton primiparae after vaginal or caesarean delivery. BJOG 2013;120(2):152–60.
27. MacArthur C, Wilson D, Herbison P, et al. Urinary incontinence persisting after childbirth: extent, delivery history, and effects in a 12-year longitudinal cohort study. BJOG 2016;123(6):1022–9.
28. Rogers RG, Ninivaggio C, Gallagher K, et al. Pelvic floor symptoms and quality of life changes during first pregnancy: a prospective cohort study. Int Urogynecol J 2017;28(11):1701–7.
29. Bodner-Adler B, Kimberger O, Laml T, et al. Prevalence and risk factors for pelvic floor disorders during early and late pregnancy in a cohort of Austrian women. Arch Gynecol Obstet 2019;300(5):1325–30.
30. Swenson CW, Deporre JA, Haefner JK, et al. Postpartum depression screening and pelvic floor symptoms among women referred to a specialty postpartum perineal clinic. Am J Obstet Gynecol 2018;218(3):335.
31. Woodley SJ, Boyle R, Cody JD, et al. Pelvic floor muscle training for prevention and treatment of urinary and faecal incontinence in antenatal and postnatal women. Cochrane Database Syst Rev 2020;5(5):CD007471.
32. Wallace SL, Miller LD, Mishra K. Pelvic floor physical therapy in the treatment of pelvic floor dysfunction in women. Curr Opin Obstet Gynecol 2019;31(6):485–93.
33. Nygaard IE, Shaw JM. Physical activity and the pelvic floor. Am J Obstet Gynecol 2016;214(2):164–71.
34. Bø K, Artal R, Barakat R, et al. Exercise and pregnancy in recreational and elite athletes: 2016/2017 evidence summary from the IOC expert group meeting,

Lausanne. Part 5. Recommendations for health professionals and active women. Br J Sports Med 2018;52(17):1080–5.

35. Roper JC, Amber N, Wan OYK, et al. Review of available national guidelines for obstetric anal sphincter injury. Int Urogynecol J 2020;31(11):2247–59.

36. van Bavel J, Ravelli A, Abu-Hanna A, et al. Risk factors for the recurrence of obstetrical anal sphincter injury and the role of a mediolateral episiotomy: an analysis of a national registry. BJOG 2020;127(8):951–6.

37. Brown S, Gartland D, Perlen S, et al. Consultation about urinary and faecal incontinence in the year after childbirth: a cohort study. BJOG 2015;122(7):954–62.

38. Barr SA, Crisp CC, White AB, et al. FACE: female pelvic medicine and reconstructive surgery awareness campaign: increasing exposure. Female Pelvic Med Reconstr Surg 2018;24(2):115–9.

39. Barber MD, Walters MD, Bump RC. Short forms of two condition-specific quality-of-life questionnaires for women with pelvic floor disorders (PFDI-20 and PFIQ-7). Am J Obstet Gynecol 2005;193(1):103–13.

40. Thibault-Gagnon S, Yusuf S, Langer S, et al. Do women notice the impact of childbirth-related levator trauma on pelvic floor and sexual function? Results of an observational ultrasound study. Int Urogynecol J 2014;25(10):1389–98.

41. Wieslander CK, Weinstein MM, Handa VL, et al. Pregnancy in women with prior treatments for pelvic floor disorders. Female Pelvic Med Reconstr Surg 2020; 26(5):299–305.

42. Jha S, Parker V. Risk factors for recurrent obstetric anal sphincter injury (rOASI): a systematic review and meta-analysis. Int Urogynecol J 2016;27(6):849–57.

43. Webb SS, Yates D, Manresa M, et al. Impact of subsequent birth and delivery mode for women with previous OASIS: systematic review and meta-analysis. Int Urogynecol J 2017;28(4):507–14.

44. Jangö H, Langhoff-Roos J, Rosthøj S, et al. Mode of delivery after obstetric anal sphincter injury and the risk of long-term anal incontinence. Am J Obstet Gynecol 2016;214(6):733.

45. Pallitto C, Stein K. Care of girls & women living with female genital mutliation: a clinical handbook. In: World Health Organization. Sexual and reproductive health. 2018. Available at: https://apps.who.int/iris/bitstream/handle/10665/272429/9789241513913-eng.pdf?ua=19789241513913-eng.pdf?ua51. Accessed November 28, 2020.

46. Lewicky-Gaupp C, Leader-Cramer A, Johnson LL, et al. Wound complications after obstetric anal sphincter injuries. Obstet Gynecol 2015;125(5):1088–93.

47. Jibrel F, Cox CK, Fairchild PS, et al. Indications for surgical intervention in a postpartum pelvic floor specialty clinic. Int Urogynecol J 2020;31(11):2233–6.

48. Hickman LC, Propst K, Swenson CW, et al. Subspecialty care for peripartum pelvic floor disorders. Am J Obstet Gynecol 2020;223(5):709–14.

Painful Bladder Syndrome/Interstitial Cystitis and High Tone Pelvic Floor Dysfunction

Catherine Chandler Moody, MD[a], Tola B. Fashokun, MD[b],*

KEYWORDS

- Interstitial cystitis • Painful bladder syndrome • High tone pelvic floor dysfunction
- Chronic pelvic pain • Pelvic floor physical therapy

KEY POINTS

- Painful bladder syndrome/interstitial cystitis (PBS/IC) is a condition that consists of a constellation of symptoms and the diagnosis is based on exclusion, in which other possible conditions have been eliminated.
- Clinicians should suspect PBS/IC in patients who present with symptoms of recurrent urinary tract infection and are found to have negative cultures.
- Treatment should be systematic and stepwise, with conservative options exhausted before moving to more invasive treatments.
- High tone pelvic floor dysfunction often coexists with PBS/IC and is characterized by hypertonicity of the pelvic floor muscles resulting in their inability to appropriately relax, contract, or function in a coordinated manner.

INTRODUCTION

Painful bladder syndrome/interstitial cystitis (PBS/IC) is a complex condition that may be challenging to accurately characterize and manage effectively. Even the nomenclature itself has been disputed and reclassified over the years: the etymology of "cystitis" implies a process of inflammation that may or may not be histologically present in the bladder. Several societies have attempted to propose terminology and guidelines that can adequately characterize this condition, which is primarily diagnosed by symptoms more consistent with a syndrome than with an end-organ disease. Accepted and often preferred alternatives to the historically used term interstitial cystitis now include painful bladder syndrome (PBS), bladder pain syndrome, and hypersensitive bladder syndrome.[1–3] The term "interstitial cystitis" (IC)

[a] Department of Obstetrics and Gynecology, Sinai Hospital of Baltimore, 2401 West Belvedere Avenue, Mower Building Suite 209, Baltimore, MD 21215, USA; [b] Female Pelvic Medicine and Reconstructive Surgery Faculty, Institute of Female Pelvic Medicine at Sinai Hospital of Baltimore, Sinai Hospital of Baltimore, 2401 West Belvedere Avenue, Mower Building Suite 209, Baltimore, MD 21215, USA
* Corresponding author.
E-mail address: tfashoku@lifebridgehealth.org

Obstet Gynecol Clin N Am 48 (2021) 585–597
https://doi.org/10.1016/j.ogc.2021.05.010
0889-8545/21/© 2021 Elsevier Inc. All rights reserved.

has remained a primary diagnostic term despite revised, more accurate nomenclature, partially due to limitations of billing and coding, with insurance companies often reluctant to cover treatments when they are billed under newer terminology. Confounding the clinical picture is that IC frequently coexists with other chronic pain syndromes, including endometriosis, irritable bowel syndrome, and high tone pelvic floor dysfunction (HTPFD).[2,3]

HTPFD is a chronic pelvic pain condition characterized by involuntary contracted pelvic floor muscles that are tight, shortened, and tender to palpation, and may have palpable myofascial nodules or trigger points.[4,5] This hypertonicity renders the pelvic floor muscles unable to appropriately relax, contract, or function in a coordinated manner.[5] The prevalence of HTPFD in the general population is unknown. It frequently coexists with other chronic pelvic pain conditions (PBS/IC, endometriosis, vulvodynia). In one study, 87% of women with PBS/IC and pelvic pain had levator spasms noted on examination. HTPFD also exacerbates the symptomatology of women with PBS/IC causing more severe and debilitating symptoms.[5–9]

This article reviews the existing literature on the evaluation and management of women with PBS/IC and HTPFD.

BACKGROUND

PBS/IC symptoms were described in the 1830s by a Philadelphia surgeon named Joseph Parrish as "tic douloureux of the bladder."[10] The term "interstitial cystitis" was introduced in the 1870s by physician Alexander Skene,[11] who described this inflammatory condition of the bladder wall in his text *Diseases of the Bladder and Urethra in Women.* Following the invention of the cystoscope in the early 1900s, Dr Guy Hunner described bleeding, ulcerated lesions in the female bladder that are pathognomonic for but found in less than 10% of patients with IC.[12] As the study and understanding of the syndrome has evolved, a shift in focus from cystoscopic and histologic features that may be nonspecific or only present in a subset of patients, to symptom-based diagnosis has occurred.

Multiple theories exist regarding the etiology of IC, including autoimmune, mast cell–mediated, and infectious pathways. The glycosaminoglycan (GAG) layer of the bladder protects against bacterial adherence and irritation from urine.[13] Disruption of this layer exposes the epithelium to noxious stimuli, and bladder wall damage precipitates an inflammatory cascade that can become pathologically upregulated. Histologic sampling of bladders of patients with IC may demonstrate infiltration by mast cells,[14] which release histamine, serotonin, cytokines, and neuropeptides, and may similarly upregulate pain.[14] The infectious hypothesis posits that there is a yet undiscovered pathogen responsible. Other cell factors suggested to play a role in the development of IC include defective Tamm-Horsfall proteins, overexpression of E-cadherin mediated by anti-proliferative factor, altered cytokeratin profile, and enhanced expression of interleukin-6.[15]

Epidemiologic estimates of the prevalence of IC vary in large part because of varying definitions and guidelines for diagnosis. IC is more common in women than men (5:1 ratio) and is diagnosed most commonly in the second to fifth decades of life.[16,17] The 2011 RAND Interstitial Cystitis Epidemiology Study estimated that 3.3 to 7.9 million adult US women have IC, a chronic disease without curative treatment.[17]

Proposed theories for the development of HTPFD include neuroplasticity, neural convergence with centralized pain phenomenon, neuromuscular trauma, metabolic changes at the cellular level, and even learned or acquired behaviors.[18] HTPFD has been linked to prior pelvic surgery, vaginal trauma, sexual abuse, and anxiety.[18]

Sustained muscle contraction may result from a persistent perceived threat or an overreaction of the general defense reaction as a mechanism of involuntary pelvic floor muscle activity.[19,20] HTPFD may originate from behaviors learned during early childhood or adulthood. A common misperception that tight pelvic floor muscles are optimal may prompt women to "overperform" pelvic floor strengthening exercises (eg, Kegels), which may increase spasms and pain.

CLINICAL PRESENTATION AND EVALUATION OF PAINFUL BLADDER SYNDROME/ INTERSTITIAL CYSTITIS AND HIGH TONE PELVIC FLOOR DYSFUNCTION

The diagnosis of IC is based primarily on symptoms: urinary frequency; pelvic or suprapubic pain, pressure or discomfort associated with bladder filling; and relief following voiding; in the absence of urinary tract infection.[17] IC sufferers experience both daytime (>7) and nighttime (>2) urinary frequency, and often report a history of culture-negative recurrent "urinary tract infection."[17,21] This is most likely due to the episodic exacerbation of symptoms or "flares" that can occur without any identified cause but have been associated with dietary irritants, emotional stressors, and physical activity, including sexual intercourse.[21]

Organic causes of symptoms that may mimic IC include urethral diverticulum, chemical cystitis, bladder or ureteral calculi, genital herpes, and malignancy.[21] Symptom chronicity is important, with varying guidelines specifying duration of symptoms required for diagnosis ranging from 6 weeks to 6 months.[22] Validated questionnaires such as the O'Leary-Sant symptom and Problem Index questionnaire and Pelvic Pain and Urinary Urgency Frequency Patient Symptom Scale may be used to objectively characterize the nature and degree of bother of symptoms.[22,23]

Women with HTPFD may present with pain and/or a variety of nonspecific symptoms of heaviness, pressure, and bowel or bladder dysfunction. Symptoms may be continuous or waxing and waning, with or without precipitating factors. Symptoms may develop insidiously, even beginning in childhood with bowel or bladder issues, or abruptly after pelvic surgery or trauma.[18] Any woman with chronic pelvic pain is at risk for HTPFD. Women with HTPFD may report pain in the pelvis, bladder, urethra, vagina, vulva, rectum, lower back, abdomen, buttocks, or thighs. Pain may be localized or generalized. It may occur with prolonged sitting or standing, walking, intercourse, orgasm, or tampon insertion; resting or lying down may improve symptoms. Many women report vaginal pain symptoms only after sex. Pain may be described as aching, spasms, soreness, pressure, like a "headache in the vagina" or "being kicked in the vaginal area." Urinary symptoms may include urinary frequency, urgency, urinary retention, and voiding dysfunction. Bowel symptoms may include fecal incontinence, diarrhea, constipation, and painful defecation.[18–20] HTPFD can produce both local and referred pain and is categorized as both a somatic muscular and sensory abnormality with contraction or tightness of the muscle resulting in impaired function and reproducible tenderness with palpation of the pelvic floor muscles. Its etiology is likely multifactorial and remains poorly understood. Dysfunction in the muscles of the hip girdle, thighs, low back, and abdominal wall can also contribute to pelvic pain via neurophysiological changes and referred somatic pain.

It is often difficult to distinguish the primary symptoms of PBS/IC from HTPFD because the symptoms often overlap (**Table 1**). This may be due to neural "cross talk" among pelvic muscles and viscera that share common innervation pathways.[20] HTPFD should be suspected in patients with PBS/IC who symptoms have been refractory or in the absence of any bladder findings.

Table 1
Painful Bladder Syndrome/Interstitial Cystitis (PBS/IC) and High Tone Pelvic Floor Dysfunction (HTPFD) Symptoms

PBS/IC Symptoms	HTPFD Symptoms
Bladder pain/suprapubic pain	Low back pain/tail bone pain
Urethral pain/dysuria	Hip and groin pain
Urinary urgency/frequency/nocturia	Dyspareunia
Pressure or discomfort worse with bladder filling	Constipation, voiding, and defecatory dysfunction

Although self-reported symptoms form the cornerstone of diagnosis for both PBS/IC and HTPFD, physical assessment is required to exclude other pathology. A thorough pelvic examination should be performed. Physical examination should begin with general observation of the patient's posture and stance. Patients with HTPFD may prefer to stand due to exacerbation of symptoms with sitting. Muscles outside the pelvis (abdominal wall, upper and lower back, hip girdle, and thighs) should be examined first to identify referred pain or trigger points. Trigger points are pathognomonic for HTPFD and are described as hyper-irritable areas within a taut band of muscle that are painful on compression, contraction, or stretching of the affected and surrounding muscle.[24]

Pelvic examination begins with a visual inspection of the perineum at rest and when patients are asked to contract their pelvic floor musculature, assessing symmetry, coordination, and movement. Palpation of the pelvic floor muscles with a single digit, applying consistent, gentle but firm pressure, identifies resting tone, trigger points, and pain along the levator ani, piriformis, and obturator internus muscles. With a single digit still in the vagina, the patient is instructed to perform a pelvic floor muscle contraction (Kegel) to evaluate strength and coordination. In patients with severe anxiety or concerns about worsening pain, we recommend deferring pelvic examination to a later visit. For these patients it may be more beneficial to establish trust, set shared goals, and review possible treatment options at the initial visit, rather than increasing anxiety by performing internal examination.[24]

The potassium sensitivity test is no longer recommended because it is neither sensitive nor specific.[25,26] The author has used a "lidocaine challenge" test in patients undergoing initial evaluation for PBS/IC in which the source of the pain is unclear: 10 mL of viscous 2% lidocaine (xylocaine) is placed directly in the urethra and bladder. Improvement or resolution of symptoms suggests that the origin of the pain is bladder and not due to pelvic floor dysfunction.

All patients should have a urinalysis with microscopy and urine culture performed. Microscopic hematuria should prompt guideline-informed workup to exclude malignancy (usually computed tomography urography and cystoscopy). Urine culture should be performed regardless of findings on urinalysis because treatment may improve symptoms even in those with normal urinalysis. Testing for mycoplasma and ureaplasma requires special culture media and should be considered when symptoms persist despite negative standard culture.[27,28]

Clinical circumstances may warrant other diagnostic procedures. Urodynamic testing in patients with PBS/IC may reveal decreased compliance, low volume at normal desire to void, low volume urgency, and low capacity, in addition to bladder pain.[29] Cystoscopy may reveal characteristic findings of IC, including glomerulations (**Fig. 1**) and Hunner lesions, and can exclude alternative causes of symptoms (eg, malignancy, stones). Normal cystoscopy does not preclude IC, and the presence of

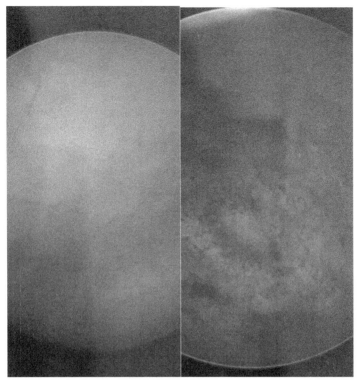

Fig. 1. Bladder urothelium pre and post hydrodistension (cytoscopic image of posterior bladder in same patient pre and post hydrodistension). Glomerulations and hemorrhages note.

glomerulations following hydrodistension may suggest the diagnosis but can also occur in patients without IC.[30,31] Cystoscopy should be considered as part of the initial evaluation of women with unexplained hematuria and culture-confirmed recurrent urinary tract infections.

THERAPEUTIC OPTIONS (PAINFUL BLADDER SYNDROME/INTERSTITIAL CYSTITIS)

Guidelines for the treatment of PBS/IC recommend a stepwise approach, starting with low-risk treatments and escalating to more invasive options.[32] First-line treatments involve self-care strategies, including general stress and pain management, patient education, and behavioral modification. Nonsteroidal anti-inflammatory drugs (NSAIDs), acetaminophen, and short courses of bladder analgesics such as phenazopyridine are suggested. The use of narcotics is not routinely recommended but may be warranted in patients with severe and persistent pain.

Behavioral modifications include changing voiding and eating patterns. Bladder training involves extending the interval between voids through urge suppression and distraction.[33,34] Avoidance of foods and beverages that trigger symptoms, such as caffeine, alcohol, and acidic and spicy foods, may also be helpful. Patients may use baking soda, potassium citrate, or calcium glycerophosphate to alkalinize the urine.

Second-line treatments include manual physical therapy, oral therapies, and intravesical therapies. Oral therapies include tricyclic antidepressants (amitriptyline), antihistamines (hydroxyzine, cimetidine), and pentosan polysulfate (PPS), or Elmiron.

Amitriptyline, gabapentin, and pregabalin are modulators of neuropathic pain. In a randomized controlled trial, 63% of patients with IC who received amitriptyline reported clinically significant improvement versus 4% of placebo group.[35] PPS, theorized to repair the GAG layer and reduce its permeability, is the only Food and Drug Administration (FDA)-approved oral medication to treat IC.[36] The efficacy of PPS compared with placebo is unclear because trials have shown mixed results.[36] It takes 3 to 6 months to improve symptoms, and recent data link PPS to rare ophthalmologic complications. A previously unidentified pigmentary maculopathy characterized by difficulty reading and prolonged dark adaptation was diagnosed and linked to patients with documented chronic PPS exposure.[37] The incidence appears to be rare, with 0.6% of 1604 patients at 7-year follow-up identified with a new diagnosis of atypical maculopathy outcome in a recent retrospective, matched cohort study.[38] All patients considering PPS therapy should be counseled about this potential side effect and routine eye examinations are recommended for those patients using it chronically.

Intravesical therapy entails instillation of medication into the bladder via catheter. This is usually an office-based procedure that can be performed once as a "rescue instillation" to manage severe and refractory symptoms due to an acute flare or as an ongoing therapy; performed as a weekly procedure over an indeterminate number of weeks required to reduce PBS/IC symptoms. Many patients are often able to perform home installations after education and if intravesical medication is readily available. The solution is held (dwell time) for varying periods of time, from a few seconds to 30 minutes before being drained or voided.

Commonly used intravesical treatments are dimethyl sulfoxide (DMSO), heparin, and lidocaine. DMSO is the only FDA-approved intravesical therapy for PBS/IC. It is an organosulfur compound with a multifactorial method of action that includes reduction of inflammation, detrusor relaxation, dissolve collagen, in addition to acting as an analgesic. In one placebo-controlled trial, 53% of patients receiving intravesical DMSO exhibited an improvement in symptoms as compared with 18% receiving placebo.[39]

Intravesical heparin functions similarly to oral PPS, by restoring the GAG layer. Lidocaine is a topical anesthetic but also has anti-inflammatory properties; provides temporary relief (rarely longer than 2 weeks).[40] Many practitioners combine the aforementioned medications to create a "bladder cocktail" for intravesical therapy based on anecdotal evidence that multiple medications are more effective than a single agent. Sodium bicarbonate has also been added for alkalinization and steroids for anti-inflammatory properties. A common instillation schedule is weekly for 6 to 8 weeks. If symptoms improve, the interval of time between instillations is increased gradually from weekly to every 2 weeks, 3 weeks, 1 month, and then discontinued. There is no evidence to recommend a specific type of intravesical therapy or standard duration of treatment.

Third-line therapies include cystoscopy under anesthesia with hydrodistension and fulguration of Hunner lesions if found. Hydrodistension involves filling the bladder to a low pressure (60–80 cm H_2O) for a short time (<10 minutes). The bladder volume is then drained, allowing the clinician to assess bladder capacity, and repeat cystoscopy may reveal glomerulations. Hydrodistension may provide therapeutic pain relief for up to 6 months.[41,42] The mechanism by which hydrodistension provides relief is unclear, but it has been proposed that hydrodistension results in breakdown and subsequent reconstruction of damaged nerve pathways.[43] Although generally believed to have minimal morbidity, there have been case reports of significant bladder necrosis following the procedure.[44] Fulguration of the bladder involves using high-frequency energy via electrocautery or laser and is performed after hydrodistension when the Hunner lesions are more visible and to minimize the risk of bladder rupture. The purpose of this procedure is to promote healing of these areas; results have shown greater than 50% improvement in pain in more than 90% of patients, in addition to significant improvement in refractory urgency and frequency symptoms. Low-dose steroids (Triamcinolone 40 mg/dL diluted in 10 mL) when injected into Hunner lesions have also been shown to be an effective therapy with low morbidity.[45]

Fourth-line treatments include intradetrusor onabotulinum toxin A injection and neuromodulation.[46] Onabotulinum toxin A may work by preventing apoptosis of urothelial cells during the inflammatory cascade, preventing urothelial damage and increasing in bladder capacity.[47] Sacral nerve stimulation involves placement of a lead wire and implantable pulse generator that stimulate the pelvic and pudendal nerves. This therapy is effective and FDA approved for the treatment of urinary urgency and frequency, which occur in many patients with IC, but is not FDA approved for the indication of IC specifically.[32]

Final therapeutic options for IC include oral Cyclosporine A (CyA) and surgery. CyA is used for immunomodulation in transplant recipients and those with autoimmune disorders. Theorized to suppress bladder inflammation, 75% of patients with IC who received CyA experienced clinically significant improvement, compared with 19% of those who received PPS, in a randomized trial.[48] Side effects of CyA include nephrotoxicity, hypertension, neurotoxicity, metabolic abnormalities, infections, and increased risk of malignancy.[49] Finally, urinary diversion or substitution cystoplasty should be considered only when all other treatment options have been exhausted.

Ongoing research focuses on IC biomarkers, understanding cellular changes that underlie the development of the disease, and development of novel treatments. Implantable lidocaine eluding devices have promising initial results.[50] Chondroitin sulfate and/or hyaluronic acid may be beneficial as an intravesical instillation, functioning similarly to heparin as a GAG replenisher.[51,52]

THERAPEUTIC OPTIONS (HIGH TONE PELVIC FLOOR DYSFUNCTION)

A multidisciplinary approach including clinicians, pelvic floor physical therapy (PFPT), and, when warranted, pain psychologists, can lead to significant symptomatic improvement in patients with HTPFD. PFPT is the mainstay of treatment and should be considered first line, with adjunct therapies initiated to help facilitate PFPT or if symptoms are refractory despite appropriate PFPT. Ideally, PFPT is provided by a physical therapist with training and experience treating women with HTPFD. Patients should be counseled that PFPT often includes internal examination and should be reassured that it is performed in a private room rather than a shared therapy space, because it differs from other types of physical therapy.

The use of manual therapy with specific pelvic floor muscle massage was first described in 1930 by Dr George Thiele. "Thiele's Massage" involves massaging the pelvic floor muscles with firm pressure applied by an index finger in the rectum or vagina.[53–55] Myofascial massage reduces pain in 59% of women, versus global muscle massage, which reduces pain in only 26%.

PFPT for the management of HTPFD may also include biofeedback, electrical stimulation, dilator use, and dry needling. Providers should encourage patients to continue therapy outside of scheduled sessions with their therapist with a home exercise program. The optimal duration for PFPT for HTPFD has not been established. Because HTPFD is chronic and may wax and wane, many patients continue PFPT for months to years. Providers may need to advocate for patients when insurance restrictions prohibit therapy continuation; especially in patients with a positive response to therapy.

Adjunct medication can improve treatment of HTPFD. Several studies have evaluated intravaginal Diazepam suppositories with conflicting results.[55] Low-dose muscle relaxers have been used in several different formulations, including oral, vaginal, or rectal suppositories to treat HTPFD. Additional medication therapies include NSAIDs, neuromodulators, and topical lidocaine cream, all of which are considered adjunctive treatment not to be used in isolation.

Trigger point injections may be beneficial in patients whose symptoms persist after treatment with PFPT. Injections may be performed with steroids, lidocaine, or onabotulinum toxin A. Trigger point injections may be performed in the office or operating room under sedation if preferable for both the patient and provider. Trigger points should be identified before any sedation or muscle relaxant is given to ensure the correct muscles are identified before injection. First, digital muscle palpation is used to locate tender and contracted points along major pelvic floor muscles that required injection. A 20-gauge pudendal block needle with a trumpet guide is advanced to the target site piercing through the vaginal mucosa to the intended muscle groups and injecting 1 to 3 mL at each injection site. Targeted muscles include the coccygeus, iliococcygeus, pubococcygeus, puborectalis, obturator, and pyriformis muscles. Injection locations are individualized to findings on physical examination and patient-reported tenderness at each site. Intravaginal pressure should be applied for a few minutes as required for hemostasis. Patients are usually monitored in the

Table 2
Botulinum trigger point injection for the treatment of high tone pelvic floor dysfunction

Study	Number of Participants (n)	Botulinum Toxin (Units)	Outcome
Morrissey et al,[57] 2015	21	Up to 300	EMG-guided Botox injection into PFM 61.9% of subjects reported improvement on GRA at 4 wk and 80.9% at 8, 12, and 24 wk post injection. Dyspareunia VAS score significantly improved at 12 and 24 wk. AE: worsening of preexisting conditions: constipation (28.6%), stress urinary incontinence (4.8%), fecal incontinence (4.8%), and new onset stress urinary incontinence (4.8%).
Adelowo et al,[58] 2013	29	100–300	79.3% reported improvement in pain, compared to 20.7% reported no improvement. Median pain with levator palpation was significantly lower post injection (P<.0001). 51.7% elected to have a second Botox injection; median time to the second injection was 4.0 mo AE: 10.3 de novo urinary retention; (6.9%) fecal incontinence, (10.3%) constipation and/or rectal pain; all AEs resolved spontaneously.
Dessie et al (2019)[59]	59	200	Double-blind, randomized, placebo-controlled trial No significant differences in participant-reported pain on palpation for any muscle group Participants in the intervention group reported greater declines in overall pelvic pain on the VAS compared with the placebo these differences were not statistically significant (both P = .16) AE: 10.1% reporting de novo constipation in both placebo and intervention group. urinary incontinence in the intervention group (22%) and urinary tract infection (9%) in the placebo group.

Abbreviations: AE, adverse events; EMG, electromyography; GRA, global response assessment; VAS, visual analogue scale.

office for at least 20 to 30 minutes post injection for any bleeding or side effects. Clinical outcomes for women with HTPFD are variable (**Table 2**). The most common side effects after trigger point injection are pain at the injection site, urinary retention, urinary and/or fecal incontinence, constipation, and hematoma. Fortunately, the overall occurrence for these complications is low and resolved spontaneously.

Onabotulinumtoxin A (Botox; Allergan Inc., Irvine, CA) causes reversible flaccid paralysis and has been shown to decrease pain associated with hypertonic muscles.[56] Because this is an off-label non–FDA-approved use for this medication, insurance restrictions exist; the out-of-pocket expense limits its use for many patients. Before injecting Botox for HTPFD, clinicians should confirm that patients do not have active infection and have not received Botox injections in the past 12 weeks due to potential for developing "neutralizing" antibodies. Although the ideal dosing and interval timing for administration of Botox has not been established for patients with HTPFD, using the lowest effective dose with a gap of 3 to 4 months between injections is supported from several studies.

SUMMARY

PBS/IC is a complex disease that can be challenging for both patients and clinicians. PBS/IC should be suspected in patients who present with symptoms of recurrent urinary tract infection with negative cultures. Clinicians should exclude alternate urinary pathology and perform a pelvic examination to identify any other etiologies for chronic pelvic pain. Treatment should be systematic and stepwise, whenever possible, exhausting conservative options first. Behavioral and diet modifications should be emphasized, and clinicians should have a low threshold to refer patients to a pelvic floor physical therapist. Different patients may have different triggers for IC flares and treatments that work for one patient may not work for another; therefore, treatment should be individualized and often multimodal for optimal results. Increased awareness has prompted advances in research and management of PBS/IC but it remains a syndrome without curative treatment.

HTPFD is an underdiagnosed condition that commonly occurs with chronic pelvic pain conditions including PBS/IC. Providers should have a high degree of suspicion for HTPFD in women presenting with pelvic pain, bladder or bowel dysfunction, and/or sexual dysfunction. Effective treatments often require a multidisciplinary approach to achieve the best clinical outcomes.

CLINICS CARE POINTS

- A thorough history and physical exam is of paramount importance to the diagnosis of Painful bladder syndrome/interstitial cystitis (PBS/IC) because there is no definitive test for this condition; diagnosis is based on the exclusion of other conditions with similar presenting symptoms.

- It may be difficult to distinguish the primary symptoms of PBS/IC from high tone pelvic floor dysfunction (HTPFD) because the symptoms often overlap. HTPFD should be suspected in patients with PBS/IC who symptoms have been refractory or in the absence of any bladder findings

- Clinical guidelines exist to aid in the treatment of women with PBS/IC but clinicians should individualized therapy based on patient's symptoms and treatment goals to optimize outcomes.

DISCLOSURE

The authors have nothing to disclose.

REFERENCES

1. Doggweiler R, Whitmore KE, Meijlink JM, et al. A standard for terminology in chronic pelvic pain syndromes: a report from the chronic pelvic pain working group of the international continence society. Neurourol Urodyn 2017;36(4): 984–1008.
2. Homma Y, Ueda T, Tomoe H, et al. Clinical guidelines for interstitial cystitis and hypersensitive bladder updated in 2015. Int J Urol 2016;23(7):542–9.
3. Van de Merwe JP, Nordling J, Bouchelouche P, et al. Diagnostic criteria, classification, and nomenclature for painful bladder syndrome/interstitial cystitis: an ESSIC proposal. Eur Urol 2008;53:60–7.
4. Rogers RG, Pauls RN, Thaker R, et al. An International Urogynecological Association (IUGA)/International Continence Society (ICS) joint report on the terminology for the assessment of sexual health of women with pelvic floor dysfunction. Neurourol Urodyn 2018;37(4):1.
5. Bassaly R, Tidwell N, Bertolino S, et al. Myofascial pain and pelvic floor dysfunction in patients with interstitial cystitis. Int Urogynecol J 2011;22:413–8.
6. Peters KM, Carrico DJ, Kalinowski SE, et al. Prevalence of pelvic floor dysfunction in patients with interstitial cystitis. Urology 2007;70:16–8, 220-1240.
7. Meister MR, Sutcliffe S, Badu A, et al. Pelvic floor myofascial pain severity and pelvic floor disorder symptom bother: is there a correlation? Am J Obstet Gynecol 2019;221(3):235.e1-15.
8. Tu FF, As-Sanie S, Steege JF. Prevalence of pelvic musculoskeletal disorders in a female chronic pelvic pain clinic. J Reprod Med 2006;51(3):185–9.
9. Brookoff D. Genitourinary pain syndromes: interstitial cystitis, chronic prostatitis, pelvic floor dysfunction, and related disorders. In: Smith H, editor. Current therapy in pain. Philadelphia: W. B. Saunders; 2009. p. 205–15. Q20.
10. Parrish J. Tic douloureux of the urinary bladder. Practical observations on strangulated hermia and some of the diseases of the urinary organs. Philadelphia: Key and Biddle; 1836. p. 309–13.
11. Skene AJC. Diseases of the bladder and urethra in women. New York: William Wood; 1887.
12. Teichman JM. Hunner's lesions. Can Urol Assoc J 2009;3(6):478.
13. Adams K, Denman MA. Bladder pain syndrome: a review. Female Pelvic Med Reconstr Surg 2011;17(6):279–89.
14. Gamper M, Regauer S, Welter J, et al. Are mast cells still good biomarkers for bladder pain syndrome/interstitial cystitis? J Urol 2015;193(6):1994–2000.
15. Parsons CL, Stein P, Zupkas P, et al. Defective Tamm-Horsfall protein in patients with interstitial cystitis. J Urol 2007;178(6):2665–70.
16. Berry SH, Elliott MN, Suttorp M, et al. Prevalence of symptoms of bladder pain syndrome/interstitial cystitis among adult females in the United States. J Urol 2011;186(2):540–4.
17. Bogart LM, Berry SH, Clemens JQ. Symptoms of interstitial cystitis, painful bladder syndrome and similar diseases in women. J Urol 2007;177(2):450–6.
18. Butrick CW. Pathophysiology of pelvic floor hypertonic disorders. Obstet Gynecol Clin North Am 2009;36(3):699–705.

19. Kutch JJ, Ichesco E, Hampson JP, et al. Brain signature and functional impact of centralized pain; a multidisciplinary approach to the study of chronic pelvic pain (MAPP) network study. Pain 2017;158:1979–91.
20. Rudick CN, Chen MC, Mongiu AK, et al. Organ cross talk modulates pelvic pain. Am J Physiol Regul Integr Comp Physiol 2007;293(3):R1191–8.
21. Hurst RE, Moldwin RM, Mulholland SG. Bladder defense molecules, urothelial differentiation, urinary biomarkers, and interstitial cystitis. Urology 2007;69(4 Suppl): 17–23.
22. O'Leary MP, Sant GR, Fowler FJ, et al. The interstitial cystitis symptom index and problem index. Urology 1997;49(suppl 5A):58–63.
23. Parsons CL, Dell J, Stanford EJ, et al. Increased prevalence of interstitial cystitis: previously unrecognized urologic and gynecologic cases identified using a new symptom questionnaire and intravesical potassium sensitivity. Urology 2002; 60(4):573–8.
24. Meister MR, Sutcliffe S, Ghetti C, et al. Development of a standardized, reproducible screening examination for assessment of pelvic floor myofascial pain. Am J Obstet Gynecol 2019;220(3):255.e1-9.
25. Jiang YH, Jhang JF, Kuo HC. Revisiting the role of potassium sensitivity testing and cystoscopic hydrodistention for the diagnosis of interstitial cystitis. PLoS One 2016;11(3):e0151692.
26. Parsons CL, Greenberger M, Gabal L, et al. The role of urinary potassium in the pathogenesis and diagnosis of interstitial cystitis. J Urol 1998;159(6):1862–7 [published correction appears in J Urol 2014;191(6);1936. Dosage error in article text].
27. Garner CM, Hubbold LM, Chakraborti PR. Mycoplasma detection in cell cultures: a comparison of four methods. Br J Biomed Sci 2000;57(4):295–301.
28. Potts JM, Ward AM, Rackley RR. Association of chronic urinary symptoms in women and Ureaplasma urealyticum. Urology 2000;55(4):486–9.
29. Kim SH, Kim TB, Kim SW, et al. Urodynamic findings of the painful bladder syndrome/interstitial cystitis: a comparison with idiopathic overactive bladder. J Urol 2009;181(6):2550–4.
30. Haylen BT, de Ridder D, Freeman RM, et al. An International Urogynecological Association (IUGA)/International Continence Society (ICS) joint report on the terminology for female pelvic floor dysfunction. Int Urogynecol J 2010;21:5–26.
31. Hanno PM. Interstitial Cystis-epidemiology, diagnostic criteria, clinical markers. Rev Urol 2002;4(Suppl 1):S3–8.
32. Hanno PM, Burks DA, Clemens JQ, et al. Interstitial cystitis guidelines panel of the American Urological Association Education and Research, Inc. AUA guideline for the diagnosis and treatment of interstitial cystitis/bladder pain syndrome. J Urol 2011;185(6):2162–70.
33. Colaco M, Evans R. Current guidelines in the management of interstitial cystitis. Transl Androl Urol 2015;4(6):677–83.
34. Atchley MD, Shah NM, Whitmore KE. Complementary and alternative medical therapies for interstitial cystitis: an update from the United States. Trans Androl Urol 2015;4(6):662–7.
35. van Ophoven A, Pokupic S, Heinecke A, et al. A prospective, randomized, placebo controlled, double-blind study of amitriptyline for the treatment of interstitial cystitis. J Urol 2004;172(2):533–6.
36. Nickel JC, Herschorn S, Whitmore KE, et al. Pentosan polysulfate sodium treatment for treatment of interstitial cystitis/bladder pain syndrome: insights from a randomized, double-blind, placebo-controlled study. J Urol 2015;193(3):857–62.

37. Pearce WA, Chen R, Jain N. Pigmentary maculopathy associated with chronic exposure to pentosan polysulfate sodium. Ophthalmology 2018;125(11): 1793–802.
38. Jain N, Li AL, Yu Y, et al. Association of macular disease with long-term use of pentosan polysulfate sodium: findings from a US cohort. Br J Ophthalmol 2020; 104:1093–7.
39. Perez-Marrero R, Emerson LE, Feltis JT. A controlled study of dimethyl sulfoxide in interstitial cystitis. J Urol 1988;140:36–9.
40. Henry RA, Morales A, Cahill CM. Beyond a simple anesthetic effect: lidocaine in the diagnosis and treatment of interstitial cystitis/bladder pain syndrome. Urology 2015;85(5):1025–33.
41. Hsieh CH, Chang WC, Huang MC, et al. Hydrodistension plus bladder training versus hydrodistension for the treatment of interstitial cystitis. Taiwan J Obstet Gynecol 2012;51(4):591–5.
42. Aihara K, Hirayama A, Tanaka N, et al. Hydrodistension under local anesthesia for patients with suspected painful bladder syndrome/interstitial cystitis: safety, diagnostic potential and therapeutic efficacy. Int J Urol 2009;16(12):947–52.
43. Niimi A, Nomiya A, Yamada Y, et al. Hydrodistension with or without fulguration of hunner lesions for interstitial cystitis: long term outcomes and prognostic predictors. Neurourol Urodyn 2016;35(8):965–9.
44. Zabihi N, Allee T, Maher MG, et al. Bladder necrosis following hydrodistension in patients with interstitial cystitis. J Urol 2007;177(1):149–52.
45. Funaro MG, King AN, Stern JNH, et al. Endoscopic injection of low dose triamcinolone: a simple, minimally invasive, and effective therapy for interstitial cystitis with hunner lesions. Urology 2018;118:25–9.
46. Smith CP, Radziszewski P, Borkowski A, et al. Botulinum toxin a has antinociceptive effects in treating interstitial cystitis. Urology 2004;64(5):871–5 [discussion: 875].
47. Shie JH, Liu HT, Wang YS, et al. Immunohistochemical evidence suggests repeated intravesical application of botulinum toxin A injections may improve treatment efficacy of interstitial cystitis/bladder pain syndrome. BJU Int 2013; 111(4):638–46.
48. Sairanen J, Tammela TL, Leppilahti M, et al. Cyclosporine A and pentosan polysulfate sodium for the treatment of interstitial cystitis: a randomized comparitive study. J Urol 2005;174(6):2235–8.
49. Crescenze IM, Tucky B, Li J, et al. Efficacy, side effects, and monitoring of oral cyclosporine in interstitial cystitis-bladder pain syndrome. Urology 2017;107: 49–54.
50. Nickel JC, Jain P, Shore N, et al. Continuous intravesical lidocaine treatment for interstitial cystitis/bladder pain syndrome: safety and efficacy of a new drug delivery device. Sci Transl Med 2012;4(143):143ra100.
51. Downey A, Hennessy DB, Curry D, et al. Intravesical chondroitin sulphate for interstitial cystitis/painful bladder syndrome. Ulster Med J 2015;84(3):161–3.
52. Pyo J-S, Cho WJ. Systematic review and meta-analysis of intravesical hyaluronic acid and hyaluronic acid/chondroitin sulfate instillation for interstitial cystitis/painful bladder syndrome. Cell Physiol Biochem 2016;39:1618–25.
53. Oyama IA, Rejba A, Lukban JC, et al. Modified Thiele massage as therapeutic intervention for female patients with interstitial cystitis and high-tone pelvic floor dysfunction. Urology 2004;64:862–5.
54. FitzGerald MP, Payne CK, Lukacz ES, et al, Interstitial Cystitis Collaborative Research Network. Randomized multicenter clinical trial of myofascial physical

therapy in women with interstitial cystitis/painful bladder syndrome and pelvic floor tenderness. J Urol 2012;187(6):2113–8.

55. Stone RH, Abousaud M, Abousaud A, et al. A systematic review of intravaginal diazepam for the treatment of pelvic floor hypertonic disorder. J Clin Pharmacol 2020;60(Suppl 2):S110–20.

56. Bhide AA, Puccini F, Khullar V, et al. Botulinum neurotoxin type A injection of the pelvic floor muscle in pain due to spasticity: a review of the current literature. Int Urogynecol J 2013;24(9):1429–34.

57. Morrissey D, El-Khawand D, Ginzburg N, et al. Botulinum Toxin A Injections into pelvic floor muscles under electromyographic guidance for women with refractory high-tone pelvic floor dysfunction: a 6-month prospective pilot study. Female Pelvic Med Reconstr Surg 2015;21(5):277–82.

58. Adelowo A, Hacker MR, Shapiro A, et al. Botulinum toxin type A (BOTOX) for refractory myofascial pelvic pain. Female Pelvic Med Reconstr Surg 2013;19(5): 288–92.

59. Dessie SG, Von Bargen E, Hacker MR, et al. A randomized, double-blind, placebo-controlled trial of onabotulinumtoxin A trigger point injections for myofascial pelvic pain. Am J Obstet Gynecol 2019;221(5):517.e1-9.

Urethral Masses

Emily C. Serrell, MD, Sarah E. McAchran, MD, FACS*

KEYWORDS

- Urethral mass • Periurethral mass • Urethral carcinoma • Urethral diverticulum

KEY POINTS

- Urethral and periurethral masses are rare and include both benign and malignant entities.
- Patients may present with a variety of symptoms, including palpable mass with or without pain, urinary symptoms, or bleeding.
- In most cases, clinicians may diagnose the lesion on physical examination. Imaging, particularly ultrasound and MRI, may be helpful for evaluation, diagnosis, and surgical planning.

URETHRAL AND PERIURETHRAL MASSES

Urethral or periurethral masses in women are rare and may be difficult to differentiate (**Table 1**). Given the scarcity, the overall incidence of these lesions is difficult to quantitate. Although malignancy is rare, differentiating between benign and malignant lesions is essential for management and surveillance. A series of women with urinary symptoms found to have periurethral masses reported 88.0% were diverticula, 7.0% vaginal cyst, 5.0% leiomyoma, 2.5% squamous cell carcinoma, 2.5% ectopic ureter, and 1.0% granuloma.[1] A multidisciplinary approach with urology and gynecology may be beneficial for patient care.

Anatomy of the Female Urethra

Anatomy and support of the female urethra and pelvis are complex (**Fig. 1**). The female urethra is 3 to 4 cm long and 6 mm in diameter. The urethra is suspended beneath the pubic bone by pubourethral ligaments (posterior) and suspensory ligaments of the clitoris (anterior). It begins at the bladder neck, courses through the distal third of the vagina under the anterior vaginal wall, and terminates at the external urethral orifice. The urethral meatus is anterior to the vaginal opening and 2 cm posterior to the glans clitoris.

The innermost urethral layer is an epithelial layer lining the lumen, spongy submucosa with vascular layers, and then mucosa. This is surrounded by 2 smooth muscle

Department of Urology, University of Wisconsin SMPH, 1685 Highland Avenue, Madison, WI 53705, USA
* Corresponding author.
E-mail address: mcachran@urology.wisc.edu

Obstet Gynecol Clin N Am 48 (2021) 599–616
https://doi.org/10.1016/j.ogc.2021.05.011
0889-8545/21/© 2021 Elsevier Inc. All rights reserved.

obgyn.theclinics.com

Table 1
Urethral and periurethral masses in women

Congenital	Acquired	Benign	Malignant
Ectopic ureter	Urethral diverticulum	Hemangioma	Primary urethral carcinoma
Duplicated ureter	Urethral fistula	Leiomyoma	Leiomyosarcoma
Duct cyst	Duct cyst	Endometrioma	Melanoma
Hypospadias, epispadias	Urethral prolapse or caruncle	Condyloma	Lymphoma
Sarcoma botryoides	Pelvic organ prolapse	Granuloma	Other
Ureterocele	Hemangioma	Adenoma	
	Stone		
	Coaptite		

layers (inner longitudinal, outer circular) and, most exteriorly, a skeletal muscle layer. The internal sphincter is a complex landmark where detrusor smooth muscle joins the longitudinal mucosal tissue: the sphincter is innervated by the autonomic sympathetic nervous system via the hypogastric nerve (L1-L4) and thus involuntary control. The external sphincter is located distal to the bladder neck and is composed of striated skeletal muscle layers with longitudinal fibers. Stimulation is provided by the somatic nervous system via the pudendal nerve (S2-S4 nerve roots) to voluntarily compress or relax depending on the timing of micturition. At the middle third of the urethra, the sphincter forms a U-shape with circular fibers thicker ventrally; this is the location of the highest closing pressure and an important continence mechanism.[2]

The types of cells in urethral mucosa depend on embryologic development. The bladder trigone transitions to transitional cells (derived from mesonephric duct). More distally, the urethra transitions to pseudostratified and squamous epithelium

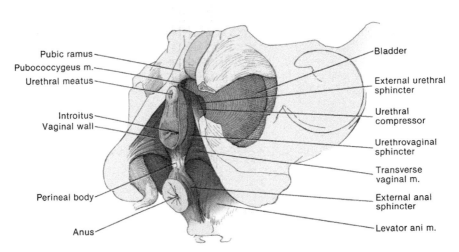

Fig. 1. Urethral anatomy. (*From:* MacLennan F, Hinman's Atlas of UroSurgical Anatomy, ed. 2, 2012, p 303; with permission.)

that is derived from the urogenital sinus, which also gives rise to the distal two-thirds of the vagina and vestibule.[3]

The female urethra can be divided into the posterior (proximal two-thirds) and anterior (distal one-third), the latter of which can be excised without disrupting continence. This also determines lymphatic drainage, as the anterior urethra drains to the superficial and inguinal lymph nodes and the posterior drains to the iliac and obturator lymph nodes. Arterial inflow to the urethra is primarily provided by the vaginal artery, although the proximal urethra has blood supply from the adjacent bladder through the inferior vesical and internal pudendal arteries. Venous drainage occurs via the inferior, middle, and superior vesical veins as well as the clitoral plexus.

Periurethral glands in the submucosal layer are prominent distally and drain into the distal urethra. The paraurethral Skene's glands are located in the vestibule of the vulva on either side of the urethral meatus and act to lubricate the urethral opening.

Workup of a Urethral Mass

Urethral masses are generally diagnosed through history and physical examination. This should include obstetric history, history of personal or familial malignancy, and prior pelvic surgery. Although no clear guidelines for workup of a urethral or periurethral mass exist, it is our practice to obtain a urinalysis and culture. For suspicious lesions, clinicians may obtain voided cytology or biopsy for pathology.

Radiographic imaging may include ultrasound, computed tomography (CT), MRI, contrast cystogram or urethrogram, voiding cystourethrography (VCUG), or cystourethroscopy. For suspected malignancy, a CT or bone scan may be helpful in assessing for the presence of locally advanced or metastatic disease.

Ultrasound may be performed via transvaginal, transperineal, or transurethral approach and is helpful in differentiating between solid and cystic masses. Although the diagnostic accuracy of ultrasound is operator-dependent, advantages include absence of radiation, cost-effectiveness, and ability to evaluate the urethra during activity. MRI has the highest sensitivity of all imaging modalities for urethral pathology and preoperative planning. Disadvantages include higher cost and more limited access. On MRI (**Fig. 2**), the normal urethra has a targetlike appearance due to alternating signal intensity that correlates to the urethral layers: hypointense outer

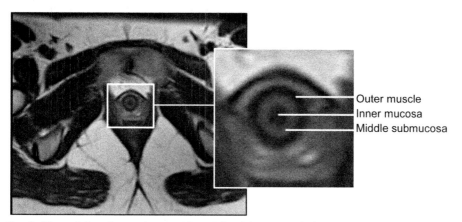

Outer muscle
Inner mucosa
Middle submucosa

Fig. 2. Normal female urethra on T2-weighted image with hypointense outer muscular layer, hyperintense middle submucosal layer, and hypointense inner mucosal layer.

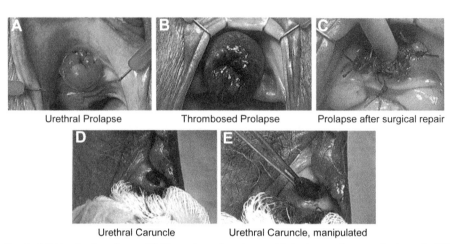

Fig. 3. (A) Urethral prolapse. (B) Thrombosed prolapse. (C) Prolapse after surgical repair. (D) Urethral caruncle. (E) Urethral caruncle, manipulated.

smooth and striated muscle fibers, hyperintense submucosa, hypointense mucosal layer, and hyperintense urine in the lumen of the urethra.

Benign Urethral Masses

Urethral prolapse and caruncle

Urethral prolapse is a herniation of the urethral mucosa at the meatus. This occurs in a bimodal distribution of premenarchal girls or postmenopausal women and may be more common in African American female individuals.[4] The mucosa appears beefy red and circumferentially encompasses the meatus in a donut shape (**Fig. 3**A–C). Conversely, urethral caruncles are small, single-quadrant mucosal prolapses seen more commonly in postmenopausal women. The mucosa is beefy red but appears at only a small area of the meatus (**Fig. 3**D, E). Risk factors for acquired prolapse include low estrogen and chronically increased intra-abdominal pressure.[5] Patients may present with vaginal bleeding, hematuria, pain at the meatus (particularly with thrombosis), dysuria, or sloughing of tissue. Asymptomatic patients may be managed with reassurance and education. Mild to moderate symptoms may be addressed with supportive care such as Sitz baths and topical estrogen. If this is not effective, prolapse may be reduced or excised.[6] Surgical excision of the prolapse in 4 quadrants (for total prolapse) or involved quadrants (for caruncle) has excellent success with low complications or recurrence.[5,7]

Urethral diverticula

Urethral diverticula (**Fig. 4**A) are outpouchings of the urethra, contiguous with the lumen, caused by a congenital or acquired defect in periurethral fascia. Anatomic variances include extension of the diverticulum to contralateral side of urethra (saddlebag) or circumferentially around the urethra. Diverticula are thought to originate from inflammation of the periurethral glands in the submucosal spongy layer of the urethra. Glands that become infected may become obstructed and form an abscess that ruptures and drains into the urethral lumen. Cycles of reinfection contribute to growth and maturation of the diverticula. More than 90% of ostia (diverticula neck) are located at the posterolateral mid or distal urethra.[8]

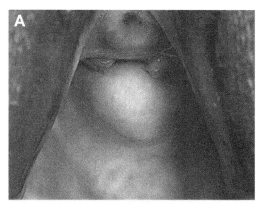

Urethral Diverticulum

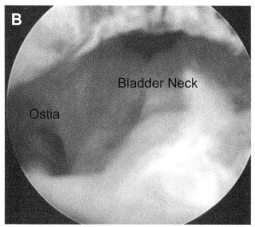

Urethral Diverticulum during cystoscopy

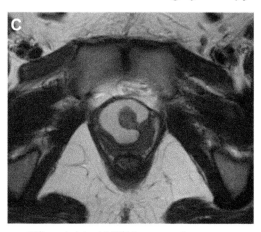

T2 weighted MRI image of near-
circumferential diverticulum. The fluid filled
diverticulum appears hyperintense.

Fig. 4. (*A*) Urethral diverticulum. (*B*) Urethral diverticulum during cystoscopy. (*C*) T2-weighted MRI image of near-circumferential diverticulum. The fluid-filled diverticulum appears hyperintense.

The prevalence of urethral diverticula has been reported as 1% to 10%, with higher rates in women with lower urinary tract symptoms,[9,10] in their fifth decade of life, and without a clear ethnic preponderance.[11] Presenting symptoms of urethra diverticulum may include the "3Ds" (dyspareunia, dysuria, postvoid dribbling), although contemporary series demonstrate this triad occurs in only 5% of patients.[12] Instead, patients present with a variety of symptoms, including painless mass of the anterior vaginal wall, stress incontinence, dyspareunia, recurrent infections, urethral bleeding, or, less commonly, lower urinary tract symptoms (frequency, urgency, dysuria).[11,12] Fewer than 10% will have diverticular calculi.[11]

Physical examination should include a careful vaginal examination (**Fig. 4**). Although not widely used, the L/N/S/C3 classification system may be used to document the location, number, size, and anatomic configuration, urethral communication, and continence status.[13] Diverticula appear as anterior vaginal wall masses that may or may not express fluid from the meatus on palpation. Laboratory tests should include urinalysis and culture. The diverticula may be directly visualized via cystourethroscopy (see **Fig. 4**B). Preoperative imaging may include double-balloon positive-pressure urethrography (balloons obstruct the bladder neck and urethral meatus, and contrast is instilled into the urethra, collecting in the diverticulum), VCUG, CT urogram (for upper tract evaluation), ultrasound (diverticula appear anechoic/hypoechoic), or MRI. In our practice, we use MRI, as it is not only highly specific but also aids in surgical planning: diverticula appear as areas of decreased intensity on T1 and high intensity on T2 (see **Fig. 4**C). Images should be interpreted cautiously, as one case series reports a 24.4% discrepancy between MRI and surgical findings.[14] In addition, transurethral bulking agents may be mistaken for diverticula if radiologists are not made aware of such implants before interpretation of imaging (**Fig. 5**).[15]

Pathology is benign in 97% of cases and most are composed of benign squamous or columnar epithelial cells.[16] However, rare cases of diverticular malignancy have been reported.[17,18] Most commonly these are adenocarcinoma, followed by urothelial and squamous cell carcinoma.[11,18] Given the thin layer of muscle around the urethra, diverticular cancer is advanced at diagnosis; more than 80% are T2 and above at presentation.[11]

Asymptomatic urethral diverticula may be managed conservatively with patient education regarding risk of symptoms or possible malignancy. To reduce the risk of infection, women may take prophylactic antibiotics or proximally to distally digitally strip the urethra to express retained urine. Based on patient preference, symptomatic patients may elect for surgery. Transvaginal marsupialization includes incision, drainage, and eversion of cyst wall with approximation to vestibular skin with absorbable suture; this allows drainage into the vagina. This is a quick procedure with low recurrence rates, but is associated with a risk of dyspareunia or stress incontinence if the sphincter mechanism is damaged.[19] Diverticulectomy requires excision of the entire diverticular sac, watertight closure of the urethra, and a multilayered closure of the surrounding deep and superficial tissue. For patients with diverticula associated with preoperative stress urinary incontinence, providers may offer simultaneous or staged anti-incontinence procedure,[20] although most providers would not use mesh in the repair. Conversely, for patients who are not incontinent preoperatively, there is a low but significant 33% risk of de novo incontinence that may require future intervention.[21] Overall, a recent systemic review failed to identify superiority for a specific surgical approach, and so providers should approach each case on an individual basis.[22]

Benign lesions

Rare cases of sarcoidosis and amyloidosis have presented with isolated urethral masses.[23] Extrapelvic endometriosis may rarely involve the urinary tract and most

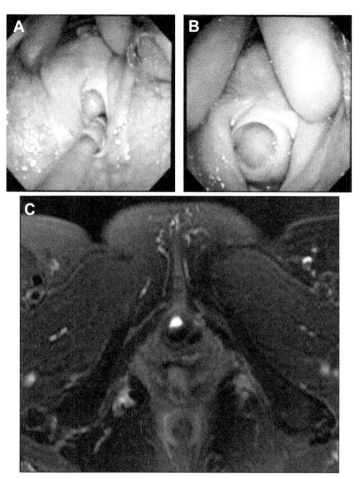

Fig. 5. Coaptite injection presenting as urethral mass. (*A, B*) A gross image demonstrating the bulking agent extending into and protruding from the urethral meatus. (*C*) On this T2 fat-saturated image, the bulking agent appears hypointense, in contradistinction to a fluid-filled urethral diverticulum that appears hyperintense.

commonly involves the bladder.[24] Periurethral endometriomas occur most commonly in patients with prior gynecologic surgery but may occur spontaneously. Consider this diagnosis for patients with dysuria and monthly gross hematuria.[25,26]

Leiomyoma are benign smooth muscle tumors of the genitourinary system (**Fig. 6**A). Periurethral and urethral leiomyoma are rare and occur most commonly in premenopausal women. They enlarge during pregnancy and regress in the postpartum or postmenopausal period, suggesting a hormonal relationship.[27,28] Leiomyoma of the urethra present as fixed masses of the anterior wall of the proximal urethra that may protrude from the meatus, whereas paraurethral leiomyoma are mobile lesions of the anterior vaginal wall that do not involve the urethral mucosa. Patients may be asymptomatic or present with complaint of palpable mass, dysuria, frequency, hesitancy, gross hematuria, and very rarely urinary retention or recurrent urinary tract infection.[29,30] Evaluation may be aided by voiding cystourethrogram demonstrating

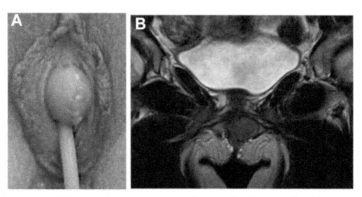

Fig. 6. Leiomyoma. (*A*) Gross image demonstrating protruding urethral leiomyoma Photo courtesy of Dr. Lee Ponsky, Cleveland, Ohio. (*B*) On this T2-weighted coronal MRI, a leiomyoma is seen displacing the urethra to the right. Note well-demarcated borders and low signal intensity.

filling defect, cystoscopy, or ultrasound demonstrating a smooth and homogenous solid mass. MRI demonstrates a solid mass with well-demarcated borders, moderate signal intensity in T1-weighted images, and low signal intensity on T2-weighted images (**Fig. 6**B).[31] Asymptomatic patients may be monitored, although clinicians may consider biopsy for counseling. Surgical excision may be performed through a transvaginal, transurethral, or abdominal approach with overall good outcomes,[27,29] although patients should be counseled on the risk of de novo stress urinary incontinence based on the location of the lesion.[29]

Hemangioma are vascular tumors but do not communicate with surrounding vessels. They are bluish, sessile lesions that present at any age with a mass, painless bleeding, or gross hematuria.[32,33] Asymptomatic lesions may be monitored, with the risk being missed diagnosis, slow growth over time, or thrombosis with associated pain.[33,34] Endoscopic treatment with electrocoagulation, laser fulguration, or ablation has been described for small lesions in men, but it is unclear if this approach may be used in women.[35] Because hemangioma may extend more deeply than they appear, MRI may be valuable for planning resection. Incomplete resection results in a recurrent mass.[36,37] Recurrent and extensive hemangioma in women are best managed with wide local excision.[32,38]

A variety of genital stromal tumors may develop from subepithelial stromal or mesenchymal cells that extend from the cervix to vulva and present as periurethral masses.[39] These are described in small series or case reports and, in general, are well managed with excision and have low recurrence rates. Fibroepithelial stromal polyp (also known as mesodermal stromal polyp, cellular pseudosarcomatous fibroepithelial stromal polyp, pseudosarcoma botryoides) is a benign, vaginal polypoid growth or growths found in young women of childbearing age. Less commonly they occur in postmenopausal women taking estrogen and infants, possibly due to maternal hormones.[40,41] Superficial myofibroblastoma (**Fig. 7**) is a benign, solid, nodular, or polypoid mass that occurs in the cervix, vagina, or vulva of middle-aged and postmenopausal women.[39,42] Cellular angiofibroma is a benign, solid, fibrous mass arising from the vulvovaginal or inguinal regions in middle-aged women.[43,44] Angiomyofibroblastoma is a benign, small, well-circumscribed rubbery mass of the vulva and vagina that may occur in women of any age and appears similar to a Bartholin gland cyst.[45]

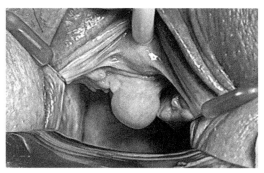

Fig. 7. Benign stromal neoplasm, myofibroblastoma.

Unlike other benign mesenchymal masses, aggressive angiomyxoma are locally aggressive and may invade the pelvis, perineum, and retroperitoneum. They occur in young and middle-aged women and present as a large, cystic mass with fingerlike projections into the adjacent soft tissue.[46,47] They are likely hormone dependent, and so preoperatively patients may benefit from gonadotropin-releasing hormone analogues to reduce operative morbidity.[48] The lack of capsule and invasive nature makes full resection difficult; there are consequently high rates of local recurrence, usually in the first 5 years.[39,47]

Infectious lesions
Inflammatory and infectious processes may present with urethral lesions. *Escherichia coli* malakoplakia,[49] tuberculosis granulomas,[50] or fungal lesions[51] have been rarely reported. Condyloma acuminata caused by human papillomavirus, the most common sexually transmitted disease, may result in multiple small, papillary growths. These occur most commonly in the genitalia and rectum but may also occur in or on the urethra.[52,53] Cases of circumferential, pan-urethral polyps have been described in men, and rare cases of female obstruction have been caused by lesions at the urethral meatus.[53–55] Topical therapies for vulvovaginal lesions include imiquimod, podophyllotoxin, polyphenon E, and cidofovir. Destructive options including trichloroacetic acid, cryotherapy, electrocoagulation, or laser vaporization are associated with higher rates of recurrence, scarring, and urethral stenosis or stricture. Local excision of vaginal or urethral polyps is the most effective definitive therapy.[53,56]

Periurethral gland masses
Bartholin, Skene, and Gartner duct cysts may present as cystic lesions or abscesses that abut but do not communicate with the urethra. The Bartholin gland is the female analogue to the male bulbourethral gland. They are pea-sized glands that secrete mucus that is discharged from ducts at the 4 and 8 o'clock positions on either side of the vaginal introitus. Bartholin gland cysts occur in approximately 2% of women, most commonly of reproductive age.[57] Bartholin abscess is more common in women with cysts but may occur spontaneously.[58] Although there are rare case reports of malignancy arising from the Bartholin gland, asymptomatic simple cysts may be observed.[59] Historically, patients with infected cysts were managed with antibiotics and drainage,[58] but this is associated with a high rate of recurrence. Similar efficacy and low recurrence rates (10%) have been reported with marsupialization and fistulization with placement of a Word catheter (bulb-tipped catheter that is placed into the cyst cavity and inflated with saline) to maintain a drainage tract.[60] Silver nitrate

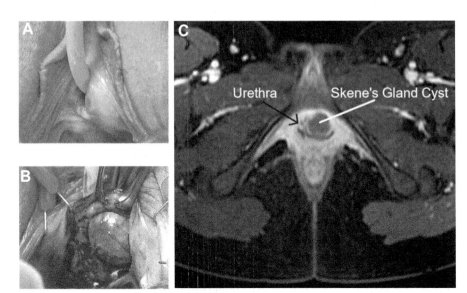

Fig. 8. Skene duct cyst. (*A*) Gross image of a Skene duct cyst presenting as paramedian mass displacing urethra. (*B*) Skene duct cyst unroofed during surgery, demonstrating the separation between vaginal/urethral mucosa and cyst capsule. (*C*) T1-weighted image with hypointense, fluid-filled cyst displacing the urethra to the right. Note that diverticula have a horseshoe appearance that encompasses and does not displace the urethra.

application or CO2 laser ablation are other minimally invasive approaches that may have the benefit of lower scar formation.[61,62] If office-based treatments have failed and a cyst recurs, patients may require surgical excision.[57]

The Skene glands are the female homologue to the male prostate. They are located laterally within the urethral meatus and secrete lubricating fluid. The Skene duct may develop a cyst due to inflammation, infection, or possibly degeneration of embryonic remnants of the paraurethral glands (**Fig. 8**).[63,64] Cysts may present as asymptomatic, bulging interlabial masses that displace the urethral meatus in premenarchal or middle-aged women.[63,65,66] Cysts of the Skene and Bartholin glands are difficult to differentiate: Skene gland cysts occur midline and anterior to the urethra, and Bartholin gland cysts occur off of midline and posterior to the urethra. Cysts may be monitored, as most resolve spontaneously.[67] More definitive management includes aspiration, incision and drainage, marsupialization, or excision.[64–66]

Gartner duct cysts are embryonic remnants. During normal development, the distal mesonephric duct is resorbed; however, if it persists, it may present as a paraovarian cyst between the layers of the broad ligament or as a Gartner duct cyst in the anterolateral vaginal wall. This may be associated with congenital vesicovaginal fistula or ectopic ureter, the latter of which may be associated with abnormalities in the ipsilateral kidney.[68] These patients present with urinary symptoms, history of chronic stress urinary incontinence (since childhood), and recurrent urinary tract infection.[69,70] Gartner duct cysts present as an ureterocele or a palpable anterior vaginal mass along the mid-urethra, but they will not involve or distort the urethra (**Fig. 9**). Imaging of the pelvis and abdomen should be obtained; abdominal imaging is necessary to evaluate for renal and ureteral abnormality.[70] VCUG should be considered if planning ureteral reimplantation, which may require extensive reconstruction.[69,71] One cautionary report

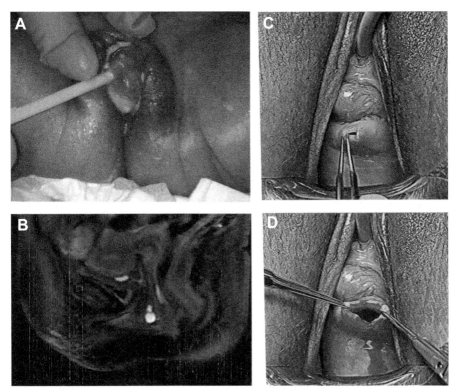

Fig. 9. Gartner duct cyst. (*A*) Gross image of congenital cyst in a newborn (Courtesy of Dr Walid Farhat). (*B*) T2 sagittal MRI with hyperintense appearance of dual-compartment, fluid-filled cyst that does not communicate with the urethra. (*C, D*) Gross image of intraoperative dissection of the Gartner duct cyst.

describes excision of a presumed diverticulum (in fact an ectopic ureterocele) and resulted in ureterovaginal fistula.[71] Excision of Gartner duct cysts may require excision of fistulous tracts, excision of cysts, and layered closure with grafts.

Urethral malignancies
Primary urethral cancer is rare. Traditional teaching is that urethral carcinoma preferentially affects women,[72] but this has been refuted by multiple international population analyses; these indicate that urothelial carcinoma is more common in older individuals, men, and possibly African American individuals.[73–75] Risk factors include chronic inflammation, recurrent infection,[76] sexually transmitted infection (particularly human papillomavirus),[77] and urethral diverticula.[17,18] Synthetic mesh has not been shown to increase risk of urethral carcinoma.[78]

Patients may present with palpable mass (**Fig. 10**), hematuria, dysuria, bloody discharge, infection, or obstruction. Physical examination should include bimanual examination, speculum examination, and palpation of inguinal lymph nodes. Clinicians should consider evaluation of voiding symptoms with VCUG or retrograde urethrogram. Urine cytology should be interpreted cautiously given varying sensitivity of 77% in women with squamous cell but only 50% with transitional cell carcinoma.[72] Cystoscopy should be performed to identify extent of urethral or bladder involvement.[79] Transvaginal biopsy or transurethral resection should be performed for

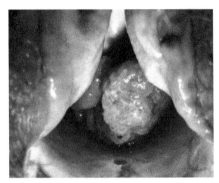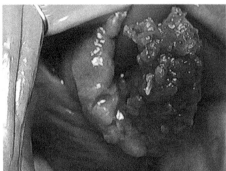

Fig. 10. This patient presented with vaginal bleeding and a palpable mass, as pictured in the left image. The right image was taken during examination under anesthesia. The mass was noted to be composed of papillary, friable lesions. This was resected and diagnosed as high-grade urothelial carcinoma with lamina propria invasion.

pathologic diagnosis. Imaging should include abdominal and chest imaging to evaluate for local, regional, and metastatic disease. Guidelines recommend staging with MRI of the pelvis with and without contrast and chest radiograph or CT.[80,81] MRI has high sensitivity in evaluation of urethral tumors, which appear hypointense on T1-weighted images and hyperintense on T2 images.[82]

Urothelial carcinoma is classified according to the eighth edition of the tumor, node, metastasis (TNM) classification.[83] In this classification, depth of invasion is qualified as Tis carcinoma in situ, T1 invading subepithelial connective tissue, T2 invading periurethral muscle, T3 invading anterior vagina or bladder neck, and T4 invading bladder or adjacent organs. Notably, urethral diverticula herniate between muscle fibers and so cannot be staged as T2.[84] Urothelial carcinoma is graded by the 2016 World Health Organization grading system: well, moderately, and poorly differentiated.[84]

It remains unclear if there is a difference in histologic variant of urethral malignancy based on gender. Men have a higher incidence of urothelial carcinoma, and some studies demonstrate a predominance of urothelial carcinoma in both men and women.[74,75,85] However, other studies report a higher incidence in women of adenocarcinoma (47%) as compared with squamous cell carcinoma (24%), and urothelial carcinoma (25%).[72,73] Adenocarcinoma may present more commonly as locally advanced disease, but it is unclear if there is a difference in cancer-free survival between histologic variants.[73,85,86] Overall, prognosis is worse in older individuals.[86] Overall and cancer-free survival depend primarily on stage at presentation, with a 5-year survival rate between 43% and 50%[75,86] (67% in stage 0 to 2, 53% in stage 3, and 17% in stage 4).[85] African American individuals tend to present with more advanced stage disease and thus have worse outcomes.[86]

Treatment of localized Ta-T2 urethral carcinoma most commonly includes urethrectomy with concurrent cystectomy, partial urethrectomy, or chemoradiotherapy. Radical urethrectomy includes resection of a cylinder of urethral and periurethral soft tissue: from the meatus to the pubic symphysis and bladder neck, posteriorly including the anterior vaginal wall, and laterally to the bulbocavernosus muscles.[87] Carefully selected patients with distal malignancy may be treated with endoscopic resection or partial urethrectomy with or without chemoradiotherapy, although a 2-cm margin is technically difficult to achieve without impacting sphincter patency and continence.[80,81] Partial urethrectomy is associated with a high rate of urethral recurrence (22% for primary urethral cancer, 60% for melanoma).[87,88] Most evidence regarding primary treatment with radiotherapy is older, although outcomes appear to be similar to surgical series. However, there is selection bias in the reported series as well as high rates of complication (up to 50% stenosis, fistula, or cystitis with bleeding), although the addition of brachytherapy to external beam therapy may reduce morbidity.[89–91] Radiotherapy is rarely used alone and is instead used as part of a multimodal approach for primary chemoradiation, locally advanced disease, or recurrent cancer.[80,81,92]

Patients with locally advanced T3-T4 or metastatic disease require multimodal therapy with a combination of chemotherapy, radiotherapy, with or without consolidative surgery (eg, pelvic exenteration).[80,81] Notably, locally advanced squamous cell carcinoma of the urethra has been shown to respond well to local radiotherapy with concurrent chemotherapy.[93] For patients with locally advanced disease considering extirpative surgery, neoadjuvant cisplatin-based therapy should be considered.[94] Multimodal therapy confers a survival benefit. Unfortunately, most patients do not receive chemotherapy or radiotherapy before surgery.[95]

Rare malignant tumors

Rare cases have been reported of urethral masses diagnosed as lymphoma,[96] neuroendocrine small cell carcinoma,[97] sarcoma,[98] or paraganglioma.[99] Melanoma may present as a dark brown or black mass with irregular border on an older woman with lower urinary tract symptoms.[88] A review of 73 articles describing 112 women with primary urethral melanoma managed with urethrectomy or pelvic exenteration found no superiority among treatments. Survival is poor, with a 5-year survival of 10%.[100] This may be due to inadequate resection and subsequent recurrence, as it has been suggested surgeons aim for a 2.5-cm margin.[88,100]

SUMMARY

Urethral and periurethral masses in women are rare. Most may be diagnosed on physical examination, although imaging with ultrasound and MRI may aid in diagnosis and management. Most benign-appearing urethral masses may be observed. Surgical management is generally effective and may be pursued based on patient preference. Care must be taken to avoid the sphincter mechanism in order to preserve continence. Primary urethral carcinoma is rare and optimal treatment modality may vary depending on the stage at presentation. However, cancer-free survival is poor, so clinicians should have a high suspicion when evaluating a urethral mass.

CLINICS CARE POINTS

- Urethral and periurethral masses are rare, and the incidence is likely underreported. Most are benign.

- On MRI T2-weighted imaging, the normal female urethra will appear targetlike with a hypointense outer muscular layer, hyperintense middle submucosal layer, and hypointense inner mucosal layer.

- Many urethral masses may be effectively managed with surgery. The distal one-third of the female urethra may be excised without disrupting continence. More proximal resection may disrupt the sphincter and thus the patient's continence mechanism. Patients electing surgical management should be counseled about the risk of de novo stress urinary incontinence.

- Workup of suspected urethral malignancy should include MRI of the pelvis, diagnostic cystoscopy, transvaginal biopsy or transurethral resection, and chest radiograph or CT scan.

- MRI has high sensitivity in evaluation of urethral malignancy, which appears hypointense on T1-weighted and hyperintense on T2-weighted images.
- For urethral malignancy in women, overall and cancer-free survival depends primarily on stage at presentation, with a 5-year survival rate between 43% and 50%. Outcomes are worse in older and African American women.

DISCLOSURE

The authors have nothing to disclose.

REFERENCES

1. Blaivas JG, Flisser AJ, Bleustein CB, et al. Periurethral masses: etiology and diagnosis in a large series of women. Obstet Gynecol 2004;103:842.
2. Herschorn S. Female pelvic floor anatomy: the pelvic floor, supporting structures, and pelvic organs. Rev Urol 2004;(6 Suppl 5):S2.
3. Carlile A, Davies I, Faragher E, et al. The epithelium in the female urethra: a quantitative study. J Urol 1987;138:775.
4. Nussbaum AR, Lebowitz RL. Interlabial masses in little girls: review and imaging recommendations. AJR Am J Roentgenol 1983;141:65.
5. Hillyer S, Mooppan U, Kim H, et al. Diagnosis and treatment of urethral prolapse in children: experience with 34 cases. Urology 2009;73:1008.
6. Holbrook C, Misra D. Surgical management of urethral prolapse in girls: 13 years' experience. BJU Int 2012;110:132.
7. Hall ME, Oyesanya T, Cameron AP. Results of surgical excision of urethral prolapse in symptomatic patients. Neurourol Urodyn 2017;36:2049.
8. Mackinnon M, Pratt JH, Pool TL. Diverticulum of the female urethra. Surg Clin North Am 1959;39:953.
9. EJ B. Die Pathologie der weiblichen urethra und des parurethrium 1959.
10. Lorenzo AJ, Zimmern P, Lemack GE, et al. Endorectal coil magnetic resonance imaging for diagnosis of urethral and periurethral pathologic findings in women. Urology 2003;61:1129.
11. O'Connor E, Iatropoulou D, Hashimoto S, et al. Urethral diverticulum carcinoma in females-a case series and review of the English and Japanese literature. Transl Androl Urol 2018;7:703.
12. Baradaran N, Chiles LR, Freilich DA, et al. Female urethral diverticula in the contemporary era: is the classic triad of the "3Ds" still relevant? Urology 2016; 94:53.
13. Leach GE, Sirls LT, Ganabathi K, et al. A proposed classification system for female urethral diverticula. Neurourol Urodyn 1993;12:523.
14. Chung DE, Purohit RS, Girshman J, et al. Urethral diverticula in women: discrepancies between magnetic resonance imaging and surgical findings. Int Braz J Urol 2010;36:504.
15. Chulroek T, Wangcharoenrung D, Cattapan K, et al. Can magnetic resonance imaging differentiate among transurethral bulking agent, urethral diverticulum, and periurethral cyst? Abdom Radiol (Ny) 2019;44:2852.
16. Tsivian M, Tsivian A, Shreiber L, et al. Female urethral diverticulum: a pathological insight. Int Urogynecol J Pelvic Floor Dysfunct 2009;20:957.
17. Cameron AP. Urethral diverticulum in the female: a meta-analysis of modern series. Minerva Ginecol 2016;68:186.

18. Thomas AA, Rackley RR, Lee U, et al. Urethral diverticula in 90 female patients: a study with emphasis on neoplastic alterations. J Urol 2008;180:2463.
19. Roehrborn CG. Long term follow-up study of the marsupialization technique for urethral diverticula in women. Surg Gynecol Obstet 1988;167:191.
20. Greiman A, Rittenberg L, Freilich D, et al. Outcomes of treatment of stress urinary incontinence associated with female urethral diverticula: a selective approach. Neurourol Urodyn 2018;37:478.
21. Lee UJ, Goldman H, Moore C, et al. Rate of de novo stress urinary incontinence after urethal diverticulum repair. Urology 2008;71:849.
22. Bodner-Adler B, Halpern K, Hanzal E. Surgical management of urethral diverticula in women: a systematic review. Int Urogynecol J 2015;27:993.
23. Ho KL, Hayden MT. Sarcoidosis of urethra simulating carcinoma. Urology 1979; 13:197.
24. Comiter C. Endometriosis of the urinary tract. The Urol Clin North America 2002; 29:625.
25. Wu YC, Liang CC, Soong YK. Suburethral endometrioma. A case report. J Reprod Med 2003;48:204.
26. Chowdhry AA, Miller FH, Hammer RA. Endometriosis presenting as a urethral diverticulum: a case report. J Reprod Med 2004;49:321.
27. Migliari R, Buffardi A, Mosso L. Female paraurethral leiomyoma: treatment and long-term follow-up. Int Urogynecol J 2015;26:1821.
28. Fry M, Wheeler JS Jr, Mata JA, et al. Leiomyoma of the female urethra. J Urol 1988;140:613.
29. Cornella JL, Larson TR, Lee RA, et al. Leiomyoma of the female urethra and bladder: report of twenty-three patients and review of the literature. Am J Obstet Gynecol 1997;176:1278.
30. Özel B, Ballard C. Urethral and paraurethral leiomyomas in the female patient. Int Urogynecol J 2006;17:93.
31. Ikeda R, Suga K, Suzuki K. MRI appearance of a leiomyoma of the female urethra. Clin Radiol 2001;56:76.
32. Parshad S, Yadav SP, Arora B. Urethral hemangioma. An unusual cause of hematuria. Urol Int 2001;66:43.
33. Jahn H, Nissen HM. Haemangioma of the urinary tract: review of the literature. Br J Urol 1991;68(113).
34. Tabibian L, Ginsberg DA. Thrombosed urethral hemangioma. J Urol 1942;170: 2003.
35. Khaitan A, Hemal AK. Urethral hemangioma: laser treatment. Int Urol Nephrol 2000;32:285.
36. Uchida K, Fukuta F, Ando M, et al. Female urethral hemangioma. J Urol 2001; 166:1008.
37. Hayashi T, Igarashi K, Sekine H. Urethral hemangioma: case report. J Urol 1997; 158:539.
38. Rao AR, Motiwala H. Urethral hemangioma. Urology 2005;65:1000.
39. Schoolmeester JK, Fritchie KJ. Genital soft tissue tumors. J Cutan Pathol 2015; 42:441.
40. Nucci MR, Young RH, Fletcher CD. Cellular pseudosarcomatous fibroepithelial stromal polyps of the lower female genital tract: an underrecognized lesion often misdiagnosed as sarcoma. Am J Surg Pathol 2000;24:231.
41. Norris HJ, Taylor HB. Polyps of the vagina. A benign lesion resembling sarcoma botryoides. Cancer 1966;19:227.

42. Laskin WB, Fetsch JF, Tavassoli FA. Superficial cervicovaginal myofibroblastoma: fourteen cases of a distinctive mesenchymal tumor arising from the specialized subepithelial stroma of the lower female genital tract. Hum Pathol 2001;32:715.
43. Nucci MR, Granter SR, Fletcher CD. Cellular angiofibroma: a benign neoplasm distinct from angiomyofibroblastoma and spindle cell lipoma. Am J Surg Pathol 1997;21:636.
44. Iwasa Y, Fletcher CD. Cellular angiofibroma: clinicopathologic and immunohistochemical analysis of 51 cases. Am J Surg Pathol 2004;28:1426.
45. Nielsen GP, Rosenberg AE, Young RH, et al. Angiomyofibroblastoma of the vulva and vagina. Mod Pathol 1996;9:284.
46. Fetsch JF, Laskin WB, Lefkowitz M, et al. Aggressive angiomyxoma: a clinicopathologic study of 29 female patients. Cancer 1996;78:79.
47. Haldar K, Martinek IE, Kehoe S. Aggressive angiomyxoma: a case series and literature review. Eur J Surg Oncol 2010;36:335.
48. McCluggage WG, Jamieson T, Dobbs SP, et al. Aggressive angiomyxoma of the vulva: dramatic response to gonadotropin-releasing hormone agonist therapy. Gynecol Oncol 2006;100:623.
49. Sloane BB, Ernesto Figueroa T, Ferguson D, et al. Malacoplakia of the urethra. The J Urol 1988;139:1300.
50. Indudhara R, Vaidyanathan S, Radotra BD. Urethral Tuberculosis. Urol Int 1992;48:436.
51. Pal DK, Moulik D, Chowdhury MK. Genitourinary rhinosporidiosis. Indian J Urol 2008;24:419.
52. Scheurer ME, Tortolero-Luna G, Adler-Storthz K. Human papillomavirus infection: biology, epidemiology, and prevention. Int J Gynecol Cancer 2005;15:727.
53. Cinar O, Suat Bolat M, Akdeniz E, et al. A rare cause of acute urinary retention in women: meatal condyloma accuminata, a case report. Pan Afr Med J 2016;24:87.
54. Chae JY, Bae JH, Yoon CY, et al. Female urethral condyloma causing bladder outlet obstruction. Int Neurourol J 2014;18:42.
55. Timm B, Connor T, Liodakis P, et al. Pan-urethral condylomata acuminata - A primary treatment recommendation based on our experience. Urol Case Rep 2020;31:101149.
56. Fathi R, Tsoukas MM. Genital warts and other HPV infections: established and novel therapies. Clin Dermatol 2014;32:299.
57. Pundir J, Auld BJ. A review of the management of diseases of the Bartholin's gland. J Obstet Gynaecol 2008;28:161.
58. Cheetham DR. Bartholin's cyst: marsupialization or aspiration? Am J Obstet Gynecol 1985;152:569.
59. Lee MY, Dalpiaz A, Schwamb R, et al. Clinical pathology of Bartholin's glands: a review of the literature. Curr Urol 2015;8:22.
60. Kroese JA, van der Velde M, Morssink LP, et al. Word catheter and marsupialisation in women with a cyst or abscess of the Bartholin gland (WoMan-trial): a randomised clinical trial. BJOG 2017;124:243.
61. Ozdegirmenci O, Kayikcioglu F, Haberal A. Prospective randomized study of marsupialization versus silver nitrate application in the management of Bartholin gland cysts and abscesses. J Minim Invas Gynecol 2009;16:149.
62. Frega A, Schimberni M, Ralli E, et al. Complication and recurrence rate in laser CO2 versus traditional surgery in the treatment of Bartholin's gland cyst. Arch Gynecol Obstet 2016;294:303.

63. Moralıoğlu S, Bosnalı O, Celayir AC, et al. Paraurethral Skene's duct cyst in a newborn. Urol Ann 2013;5:204.
64. Shah SR, Biggs GY, Rosenblum N, et al. Surgical management of Skene's gland abscess/infection: a contemporary series. Int Urogynecol J 2012;23:159.
65. Centonze A, Salerno D, Capillo S, et al. Skene gland cyst in post puberal girl. J Pediatr Surg Case Rep 2019;42:9.
66. Lee NH, Kim SY. Skene's duct cysts in female newborns. J Pediatr Surg 1992; 27:15.
67. Wright JE. Paraurethral (Skene's duct) cysts in the newborn resolve spontaneously. Pediatr Surg Int 1996;11:191.
68. Gotoh T, Koyanagi T. Clinicopathological and embryological considerations of single ectopic ureters opening into Gartner's duct cyst: a unique subtype of single vaginal ectopia. J Urol 1987;137:969.
69. Dwyer PL, Rosamilia A. Congenital urogenital anomalies that are associated with the persistence of Gartner's duct: a review. Am J Obstet Gynecol 2006; 195:354.
70. Sheih CP, Li YW, Liao YJ, et al. Diagnosing the combination of renal dysgenesis, Gartner's duct cyst and ipsilateral Müllerian duct obstruction. J Urol 1998; 159:217.
71. Albers P, Foster RS, Bihrle R, et al. Ectopic ureters and ureteroceles in adults. Urology 1995;45:870.
72. Touijer AK, Dalbagni G. Role of voided urine cytology in diagnosing primary urethral carcinoma. Urology 2004;63:33.
73. Aleksic I, Rais-Bahrami S, Daugherty M, et al. Primary urethral carcinoma: a Surveillance, Epidemiology, and End Results data analysis identifying predictors of cancer-specific survival. Urol Ann 2018;10:170.
74. Swartz MA, Porter MP, Lin DW, et al. Incidence of primary urethral carcinoma in the United States. Urology 2006;68:1164.
75. Visser O, Adolfsson J, Rossi S, et al. Incidence and survival of rare urogenital cancers in Europe. Eur J Cancer 2012;48:456.
76. Libby B, Chao D, Schneider BF. Non-surgical treatment of primary female urethral cancer. Rare Tumors 2010;2:158.
77. Wiener JS, Walther PJ. A high association of oncogenic human papillomaviruses with carcinomas of the female urethra: polymerase chain reaction-based analysis of multiple histological types. J Urol 1994;151:49.
78. Altman D, Rogers RG, Yin L, et al. Cancer risk after midurethral sling surgery using polypropylene mesh. Obstet Gynecol 2018;131:469.
79. Gakis G, Efstathiou JA, Daneshmand S, et al. Oncological outcomes of patients with concomitant bladder and urethral carcinoma. Urologia Internationalis 2016; 97:134.
80. Network, N. C. C.: bladder cancer. 6. 2020. Available at: https://www.nccn.org/professionals/physician_gls/pdf/bladder.pdf.
81. Gakis G, Bruins HM, Cathomas R, et al. European Association of Urology guidelines on primary urethral carcinoma-2020 update. Eur Urol Oncol 2020;3:424.
82. Gourtsoyianni S, Hudolin T, Sala E, et al. MRI at the completion of chemoradiotherapy can accurately evaluate the extent of disease in women with advanced urethral carcinoma undergoing anterior pelvic exenteration. Clin Radiol 2011;66: 1072.
83. Brierley JD, Gospodarowicz MK, Wittekind C. Urethra. Available at: https://onlinelibrary.wiley.com/doi/10.1002/9780471420194.tnmc45.pub3.   Accessed February 26, 2017.

84. Compérat E, Varinot J. Immunochemical and molecular assessment of urothelial neoplasms and aspects of the 2016 World Health Organization classification. Histopathology 2016;69:717.
85. Derksen JW, Visser O, de la Rivière GB, et al. Primary urethral carcinoma in females: an epidemiologic study on demographical factors, histological types, tumour stage and survival. World J Urol 2013;31:147.
86. Champ CE, Hegarty SE, Shen X, et al. Prognostic factors and outcomes after definitive treatment of female urethral cancer: a population-based analysis. Urology 2012;80:374.
87. DiMarco DS, DiMarco CS, Zincke H, et al. Surgical treatment for local control of female urethral carcinoma. Urol Oncol Semin Orig Invest 2004;22:404.
88. DiMarco DS, DiMarco CS, Zincke H, et al. Outcome of surgical treatment for primary malignant melanoma of the female urethra. J Urol 2004;171:765.
89. Garden AS, Zagars GK, Delclos L. Primary carcinoma of the female urethra. Results of radiation therapy. Cancer 1993;71:3102.
90. Milosevic MF, Warde PR, Banerjee D, et al. Urethral carcinoma in women: results of treatment with primary radiotherapy. Radiother Oncol 2000;56:29.
91. Sharma DN, Gandhi AK, Bhatla N, et al. High-dose-rate interstitial brachytherapy for female peri-urethral cancer. J Contemp Brachytherapy 2016;8:41.
92. Dalbagni G, Donat SM, Eschwège P, et al. Results of high dose rate brachytherapy, anterior pelvic exenteration and external beam radiotherapy for carcinoma of the female urethra. J Urol 2001;166:1759.
93. Hara I, Hikosaka S, Eto H, et al. Successful treatment for squamous cell carcinoma of the female urethra with combined radio- and chemotherapy. Int J Urol 2004;11:678.
94. Gakis G, Morgan TM, Daneshmand S, et al. Impact of perioperative chemotherapy on survival in patients with advanced primary urethral cancer: results of the international collaboration on primary urethral carcinoma. Ann Oncol 2015;26:1754.
95. Cahn DB, Handorf E, Ristau BT, et al. Contemporary practice patterns and survival outcomes for locally advanced urethral malignancies: A National Cancer Database Analysis. Urol Oncol 2017;35:670.e15.
96. Vapnek JM, Turzan CW. Primary malignant lymphoma of the female urethra: report of a case and review of the literature. J Urol 1992;147:701.
97. Sisler K, Knutson A, McLennan M. Primary small cell neuroendocrine tumor within a urethral diverticulum. Obstet Gynecol 2019;133:308.
98. D''Arrigo L, Costa A, Fraggetta F, et al. Carcinosarcoma of the female urethra. Urol Int 2016;96:370.
99. Cai T, Li Y, Jiang Q, et al. Paraganglioma of the vagina: a case report and review of the literature. OncoTargets Ther 2014;7:965.
100. Papeš D, Altarac S. Melanoma of the female urethra. Med Oncol 2013;30:329.

Ultrasonographic Imaging of the Pelvic Floor

Trang X. Pham, MD, Lieschen H. Quiroz, MD*

KEYWORDS

- Pelvic floor ultrasonography • 3D ultrasonography • Levator ani • Anal sphincter
- Pelvic mesh

KEY POINTS

- Knowledge of pelvic floor anatomy is essential in understanding the clinical application of pelvic floor ultrasonography.
- Ultrasonography can be performed by transperineal, introital, or endoluminal routes (endovaginal or endoanal).
- Pelvic ultrasonography is an essential adjunct tool in the evaluation of pelvic floor disorders.

 Video content accompanies this article at http://www.obgyn.theclinics.com.

INTRODUCTION

Pelvic floor and voiding disorders are prevalent in the aging population.[1–3] The evaluation of pelvic floor disorders sometimes requires a multifaceted approach for comprehensive assessment. In addition to a clinical examination, imaging modalities such as ultrasonography can be an invaluable adjunct in providing real-time assessment of anatomic and functional status of the pelvic floor. Ultrasonography is the most widely used imaging technology in obstetrics and gynecology. Advantages to this modality include the lack of ionizing radiation, low cost, and wide availability, with minimum patient discomfort. This article serves as a review of ultrasonographic techniques and their utility in the evaluation of pelvic floor and voiding disorders.

Female Pelvic Medicine and Reconstructive Surgery, Department of Obstetrics and Gynecology, University of Oklahoma Health Sciences, 800 Stanton L. Young Boulevard, Suite 2400, Oklahoma City, OK 73104, USA
* Corresponding author.
E-mail address: Lieschen-quiroz@ouhsc.edu

Obstet Gynecol Clin N Am 48 (2021) 617–637
https://doi.org/10.1016/j.ogc.2021.05.014
0889-8545/21/© 2021 Elsevier Inc. All rights reserved.

obgyn.theclinics.com

PELVIC FLOOR ANATOMY

Female pelvic floor anatomy consists of a network of support structures anchored by the bony pelvis to maintain pelvic visceral organ support. These support structures involve an interplay of innervated muscles, ligaments, and connective tissue that accommodates for childbirth and facilitates urinary and defecatory function. Central to pelvic floor support is the levator ani complex that is prone to injury during vaginal childbirth. The levator ani complex is innervated by the levator ani nerve, which originates from S3-S5. Damage to the levator ani muscles is associated with an increased risk of pelvic organ prolapse.[4] Vaginal childbirth increases the risk of levator ani injury compared with other delivery modes.[5] Magnetic resonance imaging (MRI) anatomic studies led to detailed descriptions of the levator ani complex composed of muscle subdivisions, based on their origin and insertion (**Fig. 1**).[6] The latest development in imaging of the pelvic floor has emerged from the three-dimensional (3D) capabilities of ultrasonography. Based on the literature on endoluminal 3D ultrasonography, the levator ani is described as having 3 subdivisions: the puborectalis, pubococcygeus (also referred to as pubovisceral muscle), and the iliococcygeus (**Fig. 2**).[7] The puborectalis muscle originates from the inferior pubic ramus and passes posteriorly to form a sling around the vagina and rectum. This muscle forms the anorectal angle and while contracted, promotes the closure of the urogenital hiatus. The pubococcygeus muscle originates on the posterior inferior pubic rami and inserts on the midline-visceral organs and the anococcygeal raphe. The iliococcygeus muscle originates from the arcus tendineus levator ani and travels medially to insert into the anococcygeal raphe in the midline. Intact pelvic floor musculature allows for closure of the urogenital hiatus during a contraction by compressing the vagina, urethra, and rectum against the pubic bone.[7–9] The anatomy of the anorectum is also important to understand, especially in

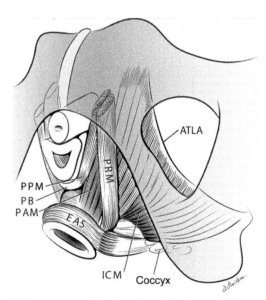

Fig. 1. Musculoskeletal anatomy of the female pelvic floor. ATLA, arcus tendineus levator ani; EAS, external anal sphincter; ICM, iliococcygeus muscle; PAM, puboanalis muscle; PB, perineal body; PPM, puboperinealis muscle; PRM, puborectalis muscle. (Copyright © DeLancey 2003.)

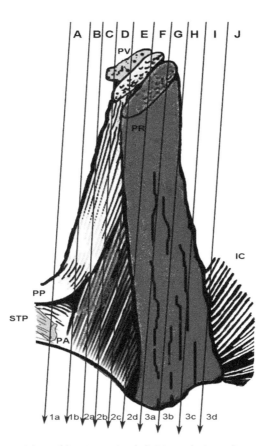

Fig. 2. The relative position of levator ani subdivisions during ultrasonographic imaging. Levels 1 to 3 are identified below the figure. The *A–J* markings on top of the figure correspond to the ultrasonograohic images shown in **Fig. 4**. IC, iliococcygeus; PA, puboanalis; PP, puboperinealis; STP, superficial transverse perinea. Illustration: John Yanson. (*From* Appearance of the levator ani muscle subdivisions in endovaginal three-dimensional ultrasonography. Shobeiri SA, Leclaire E, Nihira MA, Quiroz LH, O'Donoghue D. Obstet Gynecol. 2009 Jul;114(1):66-72. https://doi.org/10.1097/AOG.0b013e3181aa2c89. PMID: 19546760) with permission [Wolters Kluwer].)

the setting of anal incontinence and obstetric anal sphincter lacerations. The internal anal sphincter (IAS) is the continuation of the longitudinal circular smooth muscle of the rectum and maintains up to 80% of the anal resting tone under autonomic control. The puborectalis muscle, as mentioned previously, forms a sling around the posterior aspect of the rectum, more specifically around the proximal aspect of the IAS. Surrounding the distal anal canal is the external anal sphincter (EAS), which abuts the puborectalis muscle and overlaps with the distal aspect of the IAS.[10] Understanding pelvic floor anatomy is essential to the performance and interpretation of pelvic floor ultrasonography.

ULTRASONOGRAPHIC INDICATIONS AND TECHNIQUES

Indications for pelvic floor ultrasonography evaluation include urinary incontinence, voiding dysfunction, recurrent urinary tract infections, persistent dysuria, levator ani assessment after childbirth, obstetric perineal injury, anal incontinence, as well as evaluation of vaginal cysts or masses and visualization of synthetic implants (**Box 1**).[11] The American Institute of Ultrasound in Medicine (AIUM) and the International Urogynecologic Association (IUGA) suggest practice guidelines and parameters to standardize the performance of urogynecologic ultrasonographic examinations. The standardization of these techniques helps disseminate quality data and offers insight into the pathophysiology of pelvic floor disorders. Ultrasonography requires no special preparation on the part of the patient. In general, the patient is instructed to have a comfortable, but moderate amount of urine in the bladder. Positioning is preferably in the low lithotomy position, or occasionally in the lateral recumbent position.[11]

Transperineal Ultrasonography

An abdominal transducer, 4-dimensional volume, mechanical, or matrix transducer, is placed on the perineum. The transducer can be oriented longitudinally on the perineum after separating the labia to evaluate the bladder neck, urethra, prolapse, and levator ani complex (**Fig. 3**A). An alternate view of the two-dimensional (2D) imaging with transperineal transducer is depicted in **Fig. 3**B. Assessment of the anal canal and sphincters can be accomplished with the transducer oriented posteriorly and in a transverse manner. In addition, introital pelvic floor ultrasonography can be performed with an endovaginal microconvex transducer that is positioned at the vaginal introitus or perineum. The pelvic floor structures (levator ani muscle anatomy and periurethral area) can be assessed with the transducer directed cranially. Alternatively,

---

Box 1
Indications for pelvic floor ultrasonography

- Urinary incontinence
- Recurrent urinary tract infections
- Persistent dysuria
- Symptoms of voiding dysfunction
- Symptoms of pelvic organ prolapse
- Obstructed defecation
- Anal incontinence
- Vaginal discharge or bleeding after pelvic floor surgery
- Pelvic or vaginal pain after pelvic floor surgery
- Dyspareunia
- A vaginal cyst or mass
- Synthetic implants (slings, meshes, and bulking agents)
- Levator ani muscle assessment after childbirth
- Obstetric perineal injury
- Obstetric anal sphincter injury
- A perineal cyst or mass

AIUM/IUGA practice parameter for the performance of Urogynecological ultrasound examinations: Developed in collaboration with the ACR, the AUGS, the AUA, and the SRU. Int Urogynecol J. 2019.

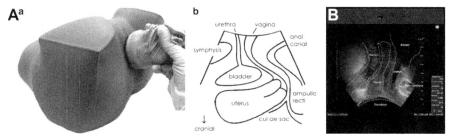

Fig. 3. (*A*) Transducer placement (*left*) and field of vision (*right*) for translabial/perineal ul-trasonography, midsagittal plane. (*B*) Alternate sagittal view with a transperineal trans-ducer. (*From* [*A*] Dietz HP. The role of 2D and 3D dynamic ultrasound in pelvic organ prolapse. Journal of Minimally Invasive Gynecology 2010; 17: 282–294, PMID 20171938 with permission [Elsevier]. Original Fig. 1.)

when the transducer is oriented posteriorly, the anal sphincter structures can be visualized.[11]

Basic transperineal evaluation of the pelvic floor requires the use of a 2D system capable of B-mode (brightness mode) and cineloop function with a 3.5- to 5-MHz curved array transducer.[12] (B-mode shows the signal amplitude as the brightness of a point, providing images of a cross-sectional slice.) To measure residual urine and detrusor wall thickness on the bladder dome, the labia are parted and the abdominal transducer is placed on the perineum (**Fig. 4**). The position should be optimal to obtain a midsagittal view that includes the inferoposterior symphyseal margin and urethra anteriorly and the anal canal posteriorly. Residual urine is determined by measurement

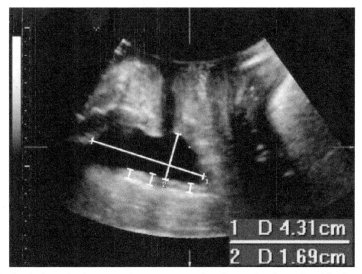

Fig. 4. Sagittal view single-screen image at rest for determination of residual urine (lines perpendicular to each other) and the detrusor wall thickness (3 short vertical measure-ments). (*From* AIUM/IUGA practice parameter for the performance of Urogynecological ul-trasound examinations: Developed in collaboration with the ACR, the AUGS, the AUA, and the SRU. Int Urogynecol J. 2019 Sep;30(9):1389-1400. https://doi.org/10.1007/s00192-019-03954-5. PMID: 31111173 [Original Fig. 2] With permission.)

of the bladder length and the perpendicular anteroposterior diameter.[11] Next, a dynamic assessment of the pelvic floor can be effectively accomplished with split screen images at rest and with Valsalva to capture bladder neck descent, urethral rotation, and the retrovesical angle. Furthermore, real-time evaluation of pelvic floor descent (including bladder, uterus, and rectal ampulla/pouch of Douglas) can be performed in the supine or standing position. A descent of the pelvic organs is measured against the inferior symphyseal margin while the patient maintains maximal Valsalva for at least 6 seconds.[11] Four-dimensional imaging of the pelvic floor can be used to assess the hiatal area and ballooning as well as levator ani integrity.[12] A split screen image may be useful to demonstrate pelvic floor structures at rest and the extent of prolapse with maximum Valsalva. The image encompassing the levator hiatus should include the dimensions between the posterior symphysis pubis and anterior anorectal angle.[11] Levator ani integrity can be demonstrated while the patient contracts the pelvic floor and the plane of minimal hiatal dimensions is identified (**Fig. 5**).[13] A tomographic ultrasonographic image of the puborectalis component is assessed with 2.5-mm interslice intervals. A diagnosis of levator ani avulsion requires at least 3 slices showing abnormal insertion of the puborectalis muscle on the pubic ramus (**Fig. 6**). Anal sphincter integrity can be assessed with the transducer oriented transversely and directed posteriorly with a distance of 1 cm between the skin and the EAS. **Fig. 7** shows the placement of transducer to allow for transperineal ultrasonography of the anal sphincter complex.[14] Tomographic ultrasonographic imaging may also be used to assess the sphincter complex, ideally with pelvic floor contraction, using acquired volumes at 60° and 70°, to optimize the resolution. Three-dimensional acquisition provides volume data sets that can be arbitrarily sliced in all 3 orthogonal planes (A, B, or C planes, which are axial, sagittal, and coronal planes, respectively). An orthogonal view is, by definition, a radiographic view obtained 90° to the original view. **Fig. 8** shows the tomographic assessment of the anal sphincter complex. The interslice intervals should be adjusted to ensure that the captured cranial slice does not include

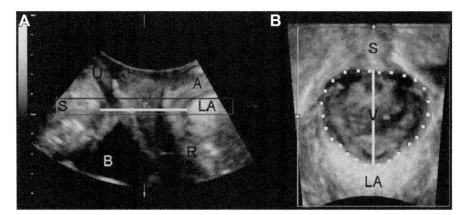

Fig. 5. Split screen four-dimensional acquisition for organ descent and hiatal ballooning. The region of interest (*box* in *A*) is set between the symphysis (S) on the left and the levator ani (LA) on the right. A, anal canal; B, bladder; R, rectal ampulla; U, urethra; V, vagina. The dotted contour in (*B*) is the hiatus in the plane of minimal dimensions; the solid line in (*A*) and (*B*) is the minimal hiatal diameter in the midsagittal (anteroposterior) plane. (*From* AIUM/IUGA practice parameter for the performance of Urogynecological ultrasound examinations: Developed in collaboration with the ACR, the AUGS, the AUA, and the SRU. Int Urogynecol J. 2019 Sep;30(9):1389-1400. https://doi.org/10.1007/s00192-019-03954-5. PMID: 31111173.)

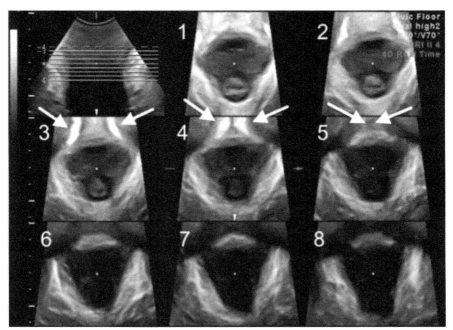

Fig. 6. Translabial/perianeal ultrasonography for the evaluation of levator ani integrity. Tomographic ultrasonographic imaging in the C (axial) plane for assessment of levator integrity. Slice 1 is the caudal slice; slice 8 is the most cranial slice. The arrows indicate the symphysis pubis. (*From* AIUM/IUGA practice parameter for the performance of Urogynecological ultrasound examinations: Developed in collaboration with the ACR, the AUGS, the AUA, and the SRU. Int Urogynecol J. 2019 Sep;30(9):1389-1400. https://doi.org/10.1007/s00192-019-03954-5. PMID: 31111173.)

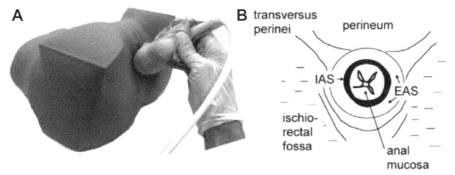

Fig. 7. Pane A shows placement of the transducer, Pane B shows a schematic of the represented structures. Placement of the transducer to allow for transperineal ultrasonography of the anal sphincter complex. (*From* Exoanal Imaging of the Anal Sphincters. Dietz HP. J Ultrasound Med. 2018 Jan;37(1):263-280. https://doi.org/10.1002/jum.14246. Epub 2017 May 22. PMID: 28543281).

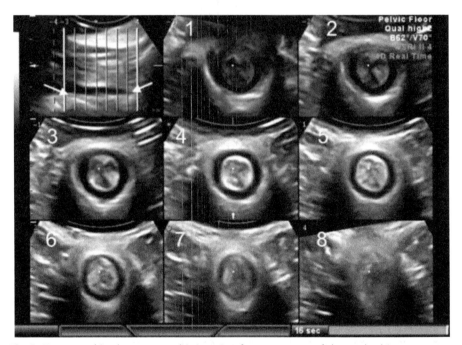

Fig. 8. Tomographic ultrasonographic imaging for assessment of the anal sphincter: asymptomatic. nullipara. The top left image in the midsagittal plane shows lacement of the 8 transverse slices, which encompass the entire EAS from slices 2 to 7, with the possible exception of the most superficial part of the subcutaneous EAS. A "residual defect" of the sphincter is diagnosed if 4 of 6 panels from 2 to 7 show a defect of greater than 30° circumference. (*From* Dietz HP. Exoanal imaging of the anal sphincters. J Ultrasound Med 2018; 37:263–280, Wiley.)

the EAS ventrally and the dorsal slice does not include the IAS. Introital pelvic floor ultrasonographic imaging with an endovaginal transducer can be used to obtain similar images.[11]

Endovaginal Ultrasonography

We recommend to always perform a multicompartmental approach. First, a 2D and dynamic assessment of the pelvic floor is done with a transperineal curved array transducer. To follow, the endoluminal transducer in placed in the vagina until the vesicourethral junction is visualized. A linear or radial array 360° 3D transducer is inserted into the vagina for evaluation of the bladder neck, urethra, levator ani muscles, anal canal, and anal sphincter complex. **Fig. 9** shows a normal example of a sagittal view with an endovaginal transducer.

Owing to the close proximity of the tissues, endoluminal ultrasonography allows for high-definition images of detailed anatomy in the pelvic floor. The anterior and posterior compartments of the pelvic floor can be evaluated for mesh implants or vaginal wall masses. One should be careful that the evaluation of pelvic organ descent may be hindered by the presence of the intracavitary transducer. Hence, dynamic assessment is preferred for confirmation of the presence of prolapse or pelvic organ descent. Pelvic floor dyssynergia can be diagnosed by measuring the distance from the transducer to the levator plate at rest and with pelvic floor contraction. Although there is no set criteria, pelvic floor dyssynergia is described as a nonrelaxing or paradoxic

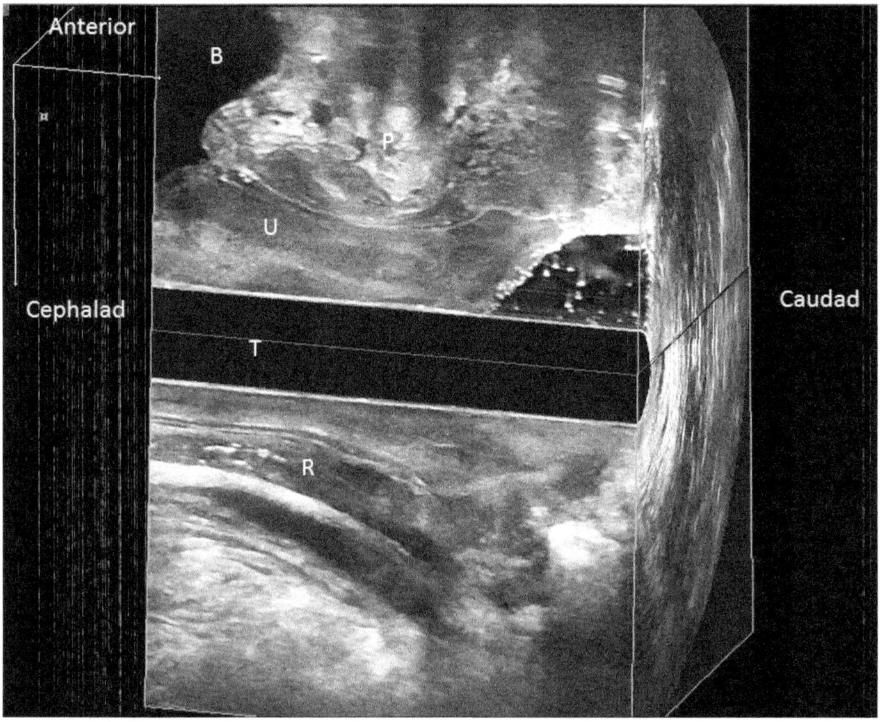

Fig. 9. Sagittal view with an endoluminal transducer. B, bladder; P, pubic symphysis; R, rectum; T, transducer; U, urethra. Yellow delineates the urethral lumen.

contraction of the pelvic floor of the puborectalis and is measured as a decrease in the distance between transducer and the levator plate. Three-dimensional imaging with the endovaginal technique can obtain images including the vesicourethral junction to the perineal body and evaluate levator ani integrity, vaginal masses, and the presence of mesh and other foreign bodies.[11]

Endoanal Ultrasonography

An endoanal transducer with linear or radial array 360° 3D transducer is inserted in the anal canal for evaluation of the anal sphincter complex. Evaluation can be performed with the patient in supine position or left lateral position. In lithotomy, the transducer is inserted at a 45° angle until the levator plate is visualized posteriorly. Imaging of the anal sphincter complex is discussed in a later section of this review article.

CLINICAL UTILITY

A multitude of indications for ultrasonographic evaluation of the pelvic floor exists, as previously discussed. Different ultrasonographic modalities can be used to examine the pelvic floor compartments including the anorectal structures, each offering its own set of advantages and disadvantages depending on the anatomic structure of interest.

Anterior Compartment

The assessment of the anterior compartment of the pelvic floor is accomplished with either transperineal or endovaginal ultrasonography. The transperineal approach may be favored over endovaginal, particularly in instances in which the target anatomy can be distorted by the placement of an endovaginal transducer. Examples include assessment of bladder neck descent, urethral hypermobility, evaluation of cystocele, and anterior vaginal wall masses, such as urethral diverticula.[12]

Bladder and Urethra

Cystocele or bladder wall descent is evaluated with transperineal ultrasonography. Maximal descent of the bladder upon Valsalva is measured as a vertical distance against a horizontal line drawn through the inferior symphyseal margin and has been correlated with clinical symptoms of prolapse.[15-17] The position of the bladder neck can be determined relative to the inferoposterior margin of the symphysis pubis at rest and with Valsalva[18] (Video 1). Transperineal ultrasonography may have some utility in the assessment of urinary incontinence via evaluation of the bladder and urethra. Urethral mobility with bladder neck descent measured with Valsalva from the resting phase has been shown to be significant in patients that demonstrate stress urinary incontinence on urodynamics study.[19] No definition of "normal" for bladder neck descent exists, although a distance greater than 30 mm is proposed as this is less than the 95th percentile of findings in young nulligravid continent women.[20] Urethral length can be assessed with transperineal or endovaginal ultrasonography. In one study, an elongated urethral length assessed by transperineal ultrasonography was associated with stress incontinence regardless of the urodynamic functional urethral length, suggesting greater tissue insufficiency in incontinent women.[21] These findings suggest that ultrasonography may be a less-invasive surrogate in the evaluation of stress urinary incontinence than urodynamics. In addition, occult stress urinary incontinence has been correlated with urethral mobility measured by the change in vesicourethral angle and bladder neck funneling with Valsalva by 3D transperineal ultrasonography.[22]

Several studies have suggested that bladder or detrusor wall thickness may be associated with detrusor overactivity and thus may have some utility in the diagnosis and monitoring of therapy.[23,24] The ultrasonographic measurements and techniques for measuring bladder wall hypertrophy have not yet been standardized. An endovaginal approach compared with transperineal or suprapubic approach to ultrasonographic evaluation of bladder wall hypertrophy seems to have less interobserver and intraobserver variability.[25] Other studies have not demonstrated a strong correlation between bladder wall thickness and detrusor overactivity. Urodynamics remains superior to ultrasonography in the evaluation of women with overactive bladder.[25,26] Therefore, further investigation may be warranted regarding the utility of bladder wall thickness measurement as a surrogate for detrusor overactivity.

Levator Ani Integrity

As previously discussed, the paired levator ani muscles and network of connective tissue attached to rigid landmarks of the bony pelvis provide support for the pelvic organs. Pelvic floor trauma, especially in the setting of obstetric injury, can lead to a multitude of pelvic floor disorders. Levator ani defects have an established association with pelvic organ prolapse, urinary and/or fecal incontinence, and sexual dysfunction.[27-30] The borders of the levator ani hiatus are composed of the symphysis pubis anteriorly and the puborectalis portion of the levator ani postero-laterally (**Fig. 10**). The levator ani muscle and the levator hiatus are currently assessed with axial views on 3D ultrasonography. The levator hiatus, as the largest potential herniating point in the pelvic floor, plays an important role in its association with pelvic organ prolapse.

Three-dimensional transperineal and endovaginal ultrasonography are widely used modalities to evaluate levator ani defects. Levator trauma is measured in several ways,

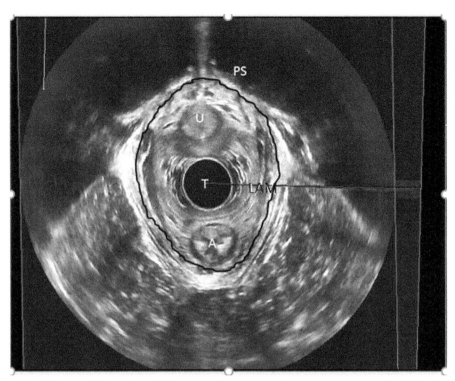

Fig. 10. Axial view with 3D endovaginal ultrasonography. P, pubic symphysis; R, rectum; T, transducer; U, urethra. The levator ani hiatus is delineated in black.

either as the presence or absence of levator avulsion or as a "pelvic floor deficiency."[12] The term "levator ani deficiency" implies a measurable gradient versus the term "avulsion," which may imply an all-or-none phenomenon.[31,32] A levator ani deficiency scoring system using 3D endovaginal ultrasonography has been validated, with a higher score corresponding to worsening defects[32,33] (**Fig. 11**). Increased levator ani deficiency (worse score) is shown to be associated with clinically significant prolapse.[31] Example of severe levator ani deficiency, compared with a normal levator ani complex, as visualized by 3D endovaginal ultrasonography is shown in **Fig. 12**A, B. In addition, the actual *timing* between the inciting event (ie, levator trauma) and the clinical presentation of symptomatic prolapse may play a role. Rostaminia and colleagues[34] demonstrated in a cross-sectional study that increasing age is a major risk factor for pelvic organ prolapse in women diagnosed with significant levator ani defects and that symptomatic women with severe defects were on average 18 years older than their younger counterparts. Other factors such as increasing levator hiatus and levator ballooning have been found to have a strong association with pelvic organ prolapse and were inversely related to pelvic muscle strength.[4]

The levator urethral gap is another measurement used in the literature to describe levator ani avulsion with transperineal ultrasomography.[35] A study by Kozma and colleagues[36] found that the levator-urethral gap measured by 3D transperineal ultrasonography was significantly larger in women with prolapse in all 3 compartments compared with single compartment. Potential differences in levator trauma definitions may contribute to inconsistencies in the association between levator trauma and symptomatic pelvic floor disorders.

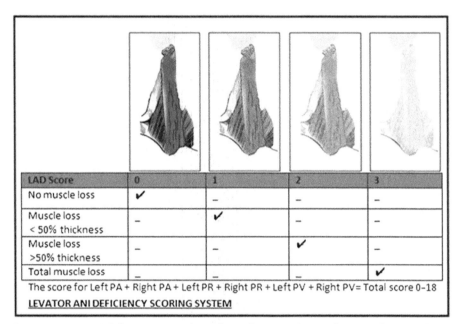

LAD Score	0	1	2	3
No muscle loss	✔	–	–	–
Muscle loss < 50% thickness	–	✔	–	–
Muscle loss >50% thickness	–	–	✔	–
Total muscle loss	–	–	–	✔

The score for Left PA + Right PA + Left PR + Right PR + Left PV + Right PV= Total score 0–18

LEVATOR ANI DEFICIENCY SCORING SYSTEM

Fig. 11. Levator ani deficiency score. PA, puboanalis; PR, puborectalis; PV, pubovisceral muscle. (*From* Santiago, A.C., O'Leary, D.E., Quiroz, L.H. et al. Is there a correlation between levator ani and urethral sphincter complex status on 3D ultrasonography?. Int Urogynecol J 26, 699–705 (2015). https://doi.org/10.1007/s00192-014-2577-5.)

Anterior Vaginal Wall Mass

The differential diagnosis of anterior vaginal wall masses can include urethral diverticulum, urethral leiomyoma, ureteroceles, Mullerian duct remnants, Gartner duct cysts, and Skene gland cysts. A clinical examination may be insufficient to discern the cause of vaginal wall masses. Long and colleagues[37] present a case of a suburethral

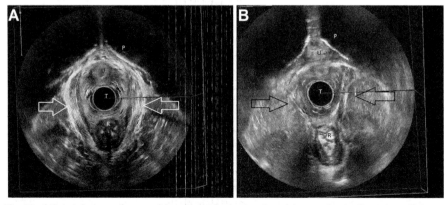

Fig. 12. (*A*) Axial view of normal levator ani muscles. P, pubic symphysis; R, rectum; T, transducer; U, urethra. The white arrows point toward the normal levator ani musculature. (*B*) Axial view of several levator defects. P, pubic symphysis; R, rectum; T, transducer; U, urethra. The black arrows point toward where levator ani musculature would have been found.

Mullerian cyst noted on transperineal ultrasonography that was mistaken as a cystocele on physical examination. Another difficult diagnosis is that of a urethral diverticulum. Patients with this condition are often subject to delayed diagnosis given the array of presenting symptoms, including lower urinary tract symptoms, voiding dysfunction, dysuria, and dyspareunia, that may be attributed to other causes. In addition to a urethroscopy, imaging either by magnetic resonance or ultrasonography is necessary to assess the location, size, and characteristics of the mass (septation, calcifications, wall thickening, solid components, etc.) that may influence the management plan. **Fig. 13**A, B show sagittal and multiplanar views of a complex urethral diverticulum. Translabial ultrasonography has been found to be a suitable alternative to MRI for characterization of urethral diverticulum.[38] The findings of a cystic structure on translabial ultrasonography, noted to be crossing the urethral rhabdosphincter has a high positive predictive value for diagnosis of a urethral diverticulum on urethroscopy.[38] Leiomyoma is an uncommon cause of anterior vaginal wall mass; however, when present, it may cause symptoms such as voiding dysfunction and dyspareunia. On transperineal ultrasonography, these leiomyomas appear as well-defined homogeneous and hypoechoic solid lesions in the anterior vaginal wall. Proximity of leiomyomas to the urethra on ultrasonography can help delineate urethral leiomyomas from anterior vaginal wall leiomyoma.[39] Thus pelvic floor ultrasonography is a useful adjunct to a clinical examination in identifying anterior vaginal wall pathologies.

Central Compartment

Sonographic assessment of the central compartment is primarily limited to the transperineal approach given the potential anatomic distortion with an endovaginal approach. As with the anterior compartment, levator ani avulsions have also been associated with clinical and sonographic prolapse in the central compartment.[40] In the central compartment, ultrasonography may bridge the gap when clinical findings are incongruent with symptoms. In order for apical or central descent to be recognized on physical examination, the uterus or vaginal vault is required to prolapse an additional distance, compared with the anterior or posterior compartment prolapse. Even if uterine and vaginal vault prolapse are clinically obvious, transperineal

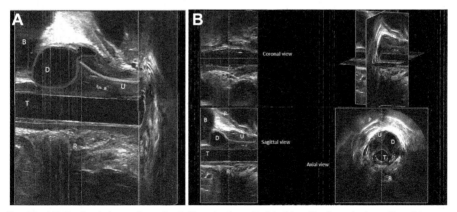

Fig. 13. (*A*) Sagittal view of urethral diverticulum. B, bladder; D, diverticulum; P, pubic symphysis; R, rectum; T, transducer; U, urethra. Yellow delineates the urethral lumen, the diverticulum is highlighted in red. (*B*) Multiplanar view with 3D endoluminal ultrasonography. B, bladder; D, diverticulum; P, pubic symphysis; R, rectum; T, transducer; U, urethra. The diverticulum is highlighted in red.

ultrasonography may demonstrate descent of an acutely anteverted uterus that may compress the anorectum and lead to symptoms of obstructed defecation. Conversely, a retroverted uterus with an anteriorized cervix may be associated with voiding dysfunction.[12] Ultrasonography may also be useful in assessing central enteroceles[41]; this is especially useful in the evaluation of prolapse symptoms in posthysterectomy prolapse, wherein evaluation of vaginal vault descent and any associated anterior and posterior herniations can be visualized with ultrasonography.

Posterior Compartment

Ultrasonography is a useful alternative to MRI in the evaluation of the posterior compartment. Anal sphincter integrity and posterior vaginal wall prolapse are commonly assessed and can be primarily evaluated with transperineal and endoanal ultrasonography.

Anal Sphincter

Endoanal ultrasonography is considered the gold standing of imaging modalities to detect obstetric anal sphincter injuries (OASI). OASI are associated with fecal and anal incontinence. A digital rectal examination is inaccurate in determining EAS defects less than 90°.[42] Imaging assessment is useful in establishing a care plan for symptomatic patients. Evaluation of the anal canal is divided into 3 levels in the axial plane on endoanal ultrasonography. The upper level of assessment includes the mixed echogenic appearance of the puborectalis muscle surrounding the complete ring of hypoechoic IAS. The IAS and surrounding hyperechoic EAS should be visible in the midlevel (**Fig. 14**). Finally, the lower level of assessment should only involve the distal

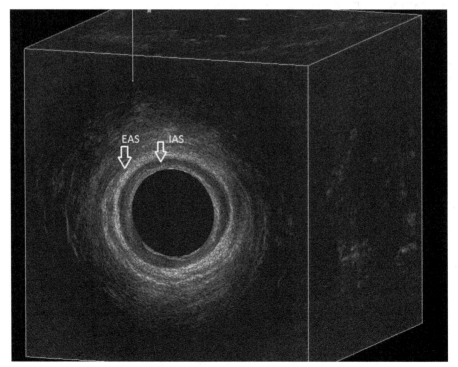

Fig. 14. Three-dimensional endoanal ultrasonography showing normal hypoechogenic internal anal sphincter (IAS) and hyperechogenic external anal sphincter (EAS).

EAS.[10] **Fig. 15** shows an example of an intact internal sphincter and a defect noted in the EAS. Alternatively, introital or transperineal ultrasonography have a high negative predictive value in detecting OASI.[43] Strong agreement exists between endoanal and transperineal ultrasonography in the assessment of the anal sphincter complex for OASI.[44] Therefore, in experienced hands, transperineal or introital ultrasonography may be suitable alternatives to screen for sphincter integrity if endoanal ultrasonography is not immediately available.

Posterior Vaginal Wall Prolapse

Integrated pelvic floor ultrasonographic involving endovaginal, transperineal, and endoanal ultrasonography has been found to have comparable accuracy to defecation proctography in the detection of posterior vaginal wall defects, including rectocele, enterocele, intussusception.[41,45,46] Hainsworth and colleagues[41] found that total pelvic floor ultrasonography had a positive predictive value of 73% in diagnosing rectoceles compared with proctography. In this same study, rectoceles identified on multiple ultrasonographic modalities were more likely to require surgery than those identified by single ultrasonographic modality. The authors recommend the use of total pelvic floor ultrasonography as a first-line investigation of pelvic floor defecatory dysfunction. Moreover, enteroceles found on ultrasonography were noted to be functionally significant on proctography.[45] Three-dimensional endoanal ultrasonography can also identify anal fistulas and perianal infectious diseases.[47]

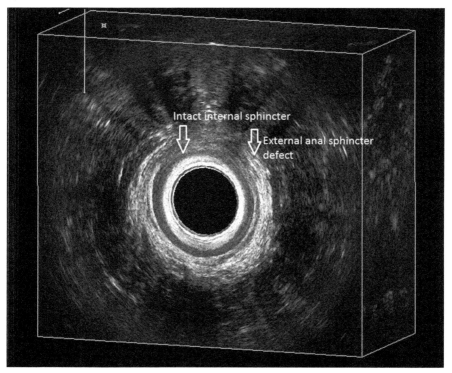

Fig. 15. Three-dimensional endoanal ultrasonography showing a defect in the external anal sphincter (EAS) and an intact internal anal sphincter (IAS).

Implanted Vaginal Material

With the introduction of implanted products for repair of prolapse and stress inconti-nence, ultrasonography is useful to evaluate complications following implant place-ment such as pain, voiding dysfunction, and lower urinary tract symptoms. The highly echogenic appearance of synthetic implants such as polypropylene mesh per-mits its visualization on ultrasonography. **Fig. 16** is an example of a transperineal ul-trasonography documenting the remnants of a mesh sling in a patient with a history of "sling removal" and persistent voiding dysfunction symptoms. The ultrasono-graphic image shows the presence of most of the sling with a 1-cm gap in the midline.

Dynamic assessment of the urethra can also be provided with ultrasonography (Video 2). Three-dimensional transperineal or endovaginal ultrasonography allows for characterization of mesh appearance, position, and dimensions and may be useful in patients with recurrent prolapse after mesh augmentation.[48–50] Ultrasonography de-lineates the position and configuration (ie, folded appearance) of the mesh that, in conjunction with a clinical examination, identifies the area of interest for intervention.[51]

Fig. 17 shows an example of "sling mapping," which includes specifying the length of the urethra and the location of the sling relative to the bladder neck. This figure also includes the incidental finding of anterior vaginal mesh and a posterior vaginal mass. In addition to pelvic mesh for prolapse, the course and type of midurethral sling (eg, transobturator, retropubic, single-incision sling) can be identified with static and dynamic transperineal and endovaginal ultrasonography.[52] Findings on ultrasonogra-phy can be correlated with pain, voiding dysfunction, or recurrent incontinence. Mesh

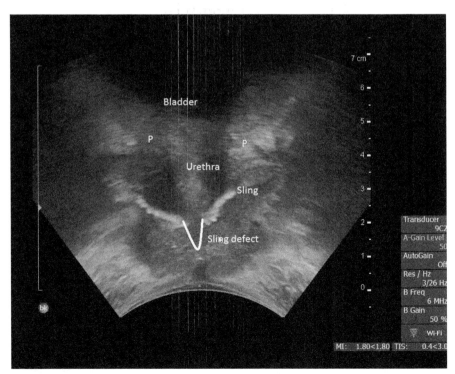

Fig. 16. Transperineal ultrasonography, coronal view showing a missing gap or defect in the sling.

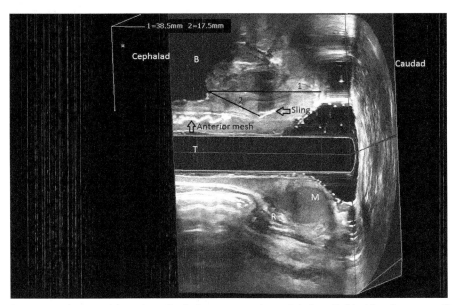

Fig. 17. Axial view with endovaginal ultrasonography, axial view. B, bladder; R, rectum; T, transducer. Black arrows point to a midurethral sling and anterior mesh. Measurement #1 is the length of the urethra (38.5 mm), and measurement #2 is the distance of the sling distal to the bladder neck (17.5 mm). M, incidental finding of a posterior vaginal mass not connected to her rectum.

erosion in the lower urinary tract can also be visible on ultrasonography, especially in the presence of calcifications.[53] Furthermore, ultrasonographic imaging can confirm the presence or absence of other implanted materials such as urethral bulking agents, which is useful in the surgical planning and counseling.[54]

SUMMARY

As ultrasound technology continues to evolve, different modalities, particularly transperineal ultrasonography, have become more versatile in the assessment of pelvic floor anatomy and pathologic condition. These pathologies include pelvic organ prolapse, urinary and anal incontinence, and vaginal implants as discussed in this review. Therefore pelvic floor ultrasonography, in conjunction with a clinical assessment, can provide a comprehensive approach in the evaluation and management of patients in a urogynecologic setting.

CRITICAL CARE POINTS

- Pelvic floor ultrasonography is an important adjunct to physical examination in cases of complex pelvic floor disorders.
- Pelvic floor ultrasonography is widely available, cost effective, and provides essential imaging information, while minimizing patient risk and discomfort.
- Pelvic floor ultrasonography should always be considered in the evaluation and surgical planning of vaginal mesh complications.

DISCLOSURE

T.X. Pham: None. L.H. Quiroz: Grant/Research Support: Cook Cellebrate; Renovia. Consultant BK Medical. Royalties: UpToDate.

SUPPLEMENTARY DATA

Supplementary data to this article can be found online at https://doi.org/10.1016/j.ogc.2021.05.014.

REFERENCES

1. Nygaard I, Barber MD, Burgio KL, et al. Pelvic Floor Disorders Network. Prevalence of symptomatic pelvic floor disorders in US women. JAMA 2008;300(11): 1311–6.
2. Alshiek J, Jalalizadeh M, Wei Q, et al. Ultrasonographic age-related changes of the pelvic floor muscles in nulliparous women and their association with pelvic floor symptoms: A pilot study. Neurourol Urodyn 2019;38(5):1305–12.
3. Geller EJ, Babb E, Nackley AG, et al. Incidence and Risk Factors for Pelvic Pain After Mesh Implant Surgery for the Treatment of Pelvic Floor Disorders. J Minim Invasive Gynecol 2017;24(1):67–73.
4. Handa VL, Roem J, Blomquist JL, et al. Pelvic organ prolapse as a function of levator ani avulsion, hiatus size, and strength. Am J Obstet Gynecol 2019;221(1): 41.e1–7.
5. de Araujo CC, Coelho SA, Stahlschmidt P, et al. Does vaginal delivery cause more damage to the pelvic floor than cesarean section as determined by 3D ultrasound evaluation? A systematic review. Int Urogynecol J 2018;29(5):639–45.
6. Kearney R, Sawhney R, DeLancey JO. Levator ani muscle anatomy evaluated by origin-insertion pairs. Obstet Gynecol 2004 Jul;104(1):168–73.
7. Shobeiri SA, Rostaminia G, White D, et al. The determinants of minimal levator hiatus and their relationship to the puborectalis muscle and the levator plate. BJOG 2013;120(2):205–11. Erratum in: BJOG. 2013 Apr;120(5):655. PMID: 23157458.
8. Shobeiri SA, Leclaire E, Nihira MA, et al. Appearance of the levator ani muscle subdivisions in endovaginal three-dimensional ultrasonography. Obstet Gynecol 2009 Jul;114(1):66–72.
9. Shobeiri SA, Chesson RR, Gasser RF. The internal innervation and morphology of the human female levator ani muscle. Am J Obstet Gynecol 2008;199(6): 686.e1–6.
10. Sultan AH, Monga A, Lee J, et al. An International Urogynecological Association (IUGA)/International Continence Society (ICS) joint report on the terminology for female anorectal dysfunction. Int Urogynecol J 2017 Jan;28(1):5–31.
11. AIUM/IUGA practice parameter for the performance of Urogynecological ultrasound examinations : Developed in collaboration with the ACR, the AUGS, the AUA, and the SRU. Int Urogynecol J 2019;30(9):1389–400.
12. Dietz HP. Ultrasound in the assessment of pelvic organ prolapse. Best Pract Res Clin Obstet Gynaecol 2019;54:12–30.
13. Dietz HP, Shek C, Clarke B. Biometry of the pubovisceral muscle and levator hiatus by three-dimensional pelvic floor ultrasound. Ultrasound Obstet Gynecol 2005 Jun;25(6):580–5.
14. Dietz HP. Exoanal Imaging of the Anal Sphincters. J Ultrasound Med 2018;37(1): 263–80.

15. Dietz HP, Haylen BT, Vancaillie TG. Female pelvic organ prolapse and voiding function. Int Urogynecol J Pelvic Floor Dysfunct 2002;13(5):284–8.
16. Dietz HP, Kamisan Atan I, Salita A. Association between ICS POP-Q coordinates and translabial ultrasound findings: implications for definition of 'normal pelvic organ support. Ultrasound Obstet Gynecol 2016;47(3):363–8.
17. Volløyhaug I, Rojas RG, Mørkved S, et al. Comparison of transperineal ultrasound with POP-Q for assessing symptoms of prolapse. Int Urogynecol J 2019;30(4): 595–602.
18. Dietz HP. Pelvic floor ultrasound: a review. Am J Obstet Gynecol 2010;202(4): 321–34.
19. Minardi D, Piloni V, Amadi A, et al. Correlation between urodynamics and perineal ultrasound in female patients with urinary incontinence. Neurourol Urodyn 2007; 26(2):176–82, discussion 183-4.
20. Dietz HP, Eldridge A, Grace M, et al. Pelvic organ descent in young nulligravid women. Am J Obstet Gynecol 2004;191(1):95–9.
21. Najjari L, Janetzki N, Kennes L, et al. Comparison of Perineal Sonographically Measured and Functional Urodynamic Urethral Length in Female Urinary Incontinence. Biomed Res Int 2016;2016:4953091.
22. Yin Y, Xia Z, Feng X, et al. Three-Dimensional Transperineal Ultrasonography for Diagnosis of Female Occult Stress Urinary Incontinence. Med Sci Monit 2019;25: 8078–83.
23. Abou-Gamrah A, Fawzy M, Sammour H, et al. Ultrasound assessment of bladder wall thickness as a screening test for detrusor instability. Arch Gynecol Obstet 2014;289(5):1023–8.
24. Oelke M, Khullar V, Wijkstra H. Review on ultrasound measurement of bladder or detrusor wall thickness in women: techniques, diagnostic utility, and use in clinical trials. World J Urol 2013;31(5):1093–104.
25. Latthe P, Middleton L, Rachaneni S, et al, BUS Collaborative Group. Ultrasound bladder wall thickness and detrusor overactivity: a multicentre test accuracy study. BJOG 2017;124(9):1422–9.
26. Rachaneni S, McCooty S, Middleton LJ, et al. Bladder Ultrasound Study (BUS) Collaborative Group. Bladder ultrasonography for diagnosing detrusor overactivity: test accuracy study and economic evaluation. Health Technol Assess 2016;20(7):1–150.
27. Weinstein MM, Pretorius DH, Jung SA, et al. Transperineal three-dimensional ultrasound imaging for detection of anatomic defects in the anal sphincter complex muscles. Clin Gastroenterol Hepatol 2009;7(2):205–11.
28. DeLancey JO, Morgan DM, Fenner DE, et al. Comparison of levator ani muscle defects and function in women with and without pelvic organ prolapse. Obstet Gynecol 2007;109(2 Pt 1):295–302.
29. DeLancey JO, Kearney R, Chou Q, et al. The appearance of levator ani muscle abnormalities in magnetic resonance images after vaginal delivery. Obstet Gynecol 2003;101(1):46–53.
30. DeLancey JO, Trowbridge ER, Miller JM, et al. Stress urinary incontinence: relative importance of urethral support and urethral closure pressure. J Urol 2008; 179(6):2286–90, discussion 2290.
31. Rostaminia G, White D, Hegde A, et al. Levator ani deficiency and pelvic organ prolapse severity. Obstet Gynecol 2013;121(5):1017–24.
32. Santiago AC, O'Leary DE, Quiroz LH, et al. Is there a correlation between levator ani and urethral sphincter complex status on 3D ultrasonography? Int Urogynecol J 2015;26(5):699–705.

33. Oversand SH, Staff AC, Sandvik L, et al. Levator ani defects and the severity of symptoms in women with anterior compartment pelvic organ prolapse. Int Urogynecol J 2018;29(1):63–9.
34. Rostaminia G, Peck JD, Quiroz LH, et al. Characteristics associated with pelvic organ prolapse in women with significant levator ani muscle deficiency. Int Urogynecol J 2016;27(2):261–7.
35. Dietz HP, Abbu A, Shek KL. The levator-urethra gap measurement: a more objective means of determining levator avulsion? Ultrasound Obstet Gynecol 2008; 32(7):941–5.
36. Kozma B, Larson K, Scott L, et al. Association between pelvic organ prolapse types and levator-urethra gap as measured by 3D transperineal ultrasound. J Ultrasound Med 2018;37(12):2849–54.
37. Long CY, Wang CL, Hsu CS. Anterior vaginal cyst mimicking a cystocele assessed by transperineal ultrasound. Eur J Obstet Gynecol Reprod Biol 2012; 165(1):128–9.
38. Gillor M, Dietz HP. Translabial ultrasound imaging of urethral diverticula. Ultrasound Obstet Gynecol 2019;54(4):552–6.
39. Cicilet S, Joseph T, Furruqh F, et al. Urethral leiomyoma: a rare case of voiding difficulty. BMJ Case Rep 2016;2016, bcr2016216728.
40. Atan IK, Lin S, Dietz HP, et al, ProLong Study Group. Levator Avulsion Is Associated With Pelvic Organ Prolapse 23 Years After the First Childbirth. J Ultrasound Med 2018;37(12):2829–39.
41. Hainsworth AJ, Solanki D, Hamad A, et al. Integrated total pelvic floor ultrasound in pelvic floor defaecatory dysfunction. Colorectal Dis 2017;19(1):O54–65.
42. Dobben AC, Terra MP, Deutekom M, et al. Anal inspection and digital rectal examination compared to anorectal physiology tests and endoanal ultrasonography in evaluating fecal incontinence. Int J Colorectal Dis 2007;22(7):783–90.
43. Taithongchai A, Sultan AH, Wieczorek PA, et al. Clinical application of 2D and 3D pelvic floor ultrasound of mid-urethral slings and vaginal wall mesh. Int Urogynecol J 2019;30(9):1401–11.
44. Stuart A, Ignell C, Örnö AK. Comparison of transperineal and endoanal ultrasound in detecting residual obstetric anal sphincter injury. Acta Obstet Gynecol Scand 2019;98(12):1624–31.
45. Hainsworth AJ, Solanki D, Morris SJ, et al. Is there Any Association Between Symptoms and Findings on Imaging in Pelvic Floor Defaecatory Dysfunction? A Prospective Study. Colorectal Dis 2021;23(1):237–45.
46. Chamié LP, Ribeiro DMFR, Caiado AHM, et al. Translabial US and Dynamic MR Imaging of the Pelvic Floor: Normal Anatomy and Dysfunction. Radiographics 2018;38(1):287–308.
47. Iacobellis F, Reginelli A, Berritto D, et al. Pelvic floor dysfunctions: how to image patients? Jpn J Radiol 2020;38(1):47–63.
48. Javadian P, Quiroz LH, Shobeiri SA. In Vivo Ultrasound Characteristics of Vaginal Mesh Kit Complications. Female Pelvic Med Reconstr Surg 2017;23(2):162–7.
49. Yune JJ, Quiroz L, Nihira MA, et al. The Location and Distribution of Transurethral Bulking Agent: 3-Dimensional Ultrasound Study. Female Pelvic Med Reconstr Surg 2016;22(2):98–102.
50. Hegde A, Smith AL, Aguilar VC, et al. Three-dimensional endovaginal ultrasound examination following injection of Macroplastique for stress urinary incontinence: outcomes based on location and periurethral distribution of the bulking agent. Int Urogynecol J 2013;24(7):1151–9.

51. Eisenberg VH, Steinberg M, Weiner Z, et al. Three-dimensional transperineal ultrasound for imaging mesh implants following sacrocolpopexy. Ultrasound Obstet Gynecol 2014;43(4):459–65.
52. Rodrigues CA, Bianchi-Ferraro AMHM, Zucchi EVM, et al. Pelvic Floor 3D Ultrasound of Women with a TVT, TVT-O, or TVT-S for Stress Urinary Incontinence at the Three-year Follow-up. Rev Bras Ginecol Obstet 2017;39(9):471–9. English.
53. Chan L, Tse V. Pelvic floor ultrasound in the diagnosis of sling complications. World J Urol 2018;36(5):753–9.
54. Taithongchai A, van Gruting IMA, Volløyhaug I, et al. Comparing the diagnostic accuracy of 3 ultrasound modalities for diagnosing obstetric anal sphincter injuries. Am J Obstet Gynecol 2019;221(2):134.e1–9.

Sexual Function After Pelvic Reconstructive Surgery

Danielle D. Antosh, MD*, Nadia N. Megahed, MD

KEYWORDS

- Dyspareunia • Pelvic organ prolapse • Reconstructive surgery • Sexual activity
- Sexual function

KEY POINTS

- Overall sexual function scores either improve or remain unchanged after all types of pelvic organ prolapse surgery.
- Dyspareunia prevalence appears to be lower after all types of pelvic reconstructive surgery than its prevalence preoperatively.
- De novo dyspareunia after prolapse repair is low, ranging from 0% to 9%, except posterior repair (limited data).
- Persistent dyspareunia in women is higher after transvaginal mesh repair than after native tissue repair.

INTRODUCTION

Sexual dysfunction is common among women presenting to urogynecologists with pelvic floor complaints. According to a prospective study of women presenting to a female pelvic medicine and reconstructive surgery (FPMRS) practice, approximately 64% were classified as having sexual dysfunction.[1] In addition to sexual concerns being common in this patient population, patients undergoing pelvic reconstructive surgery for pelvic organ prolapse (POP) view improvement in sexual function after surgery as a very important goal.[2] According to a qualitative study by Dunivan and colleagues, women reported worsening sexual function as a severe adverse event after surgery, feeling it was similar in severity to ICU admission.[2] Because of patient importance, surgeons must discuss this in the informed consent prior to surgery.

Pelvic floor surgery alters vaginal anatomy, which has varying effects on female sexual function. An open discussion with patients is important and should address their current sexual function and activity and their goals for future sexual function. The purpose of this article is to review published data to help guide surgeons on patient counseling regarding sexual function and dyspareunia after pelvic reconstructive surgery

Department of Obstetrics and Gynecology, Houston Methodist Hospital, 6550 Fannin Street, Suite 2221, Houston, TX 77030, USA
* Corresponding author.
E-mail address: ddantosh@houstonmethodist.org

Obstet Gynecol Clin N Am 48 (2021) 639–651
https://doi.org/10.1016/j.ogc.2021.05.015
0889-8545/21/© 2021 Elsevier Inc. All rights reserved.

obgyn.theclinics.com

for POP. The article will also review how various types and routes of prolapse surgery, such as vaginal native tissue (NT) repair, transvaginal mesh (TVM), biological grafts, and sacrocolpopexy (SCP) affect sexual function and activity.

SEXUAL ACTIVITY BEFORE AND AFTER SURGERY

Sexual activity is an important component of sexual function to assess in one's practice. Approximately 46% of women presenting to FPMRS practices are sexually active.[1] A patient may be sexually inactive for many reasons, some of which may be related to their pelvic floor disorder. Others may be inactive for reasons entirely unrelated to their medical problems, such as lack of a partner. Providers should assess sexual activity and function routinely in all patients undergoing pelvic floor surgery, as this will lead to a discussion about the patient's sexual function goals. If a patient is not sexually active, the provider should inquire about the reason and determine whether the patient intends or desires to be sexually active after the surgery. Some common reasons for sexual inactivity reported in the literature are lack of a partner, partner-related problems (such as erectile dysfunction), prolapse or incontinence-related complaints, and pain.

Most studies that report on sexual activity do not define what is meant by "activity." Similarly, many studies do not specify whether this means sexually active with a partner, with penetrative intercourse, or sexually active with oneself. According to the International Urogynecological Association/International Continence Society's "Joint Report on the Terminology for the Assessment of Sexual Health of Women with Pelvic Floor Dysfunction," sexual activity status should be self-defined and not limited to women who engage in sexual intercourse.[3]

Sexual activity varies preoperatively and postoperatively after pelvic reconstructive surgery depending on the surgery type. Based on a systematic review of POP trials and sexual function, the range of sexual activity preoperatively was 38% to 54%, and postoperatively it ranged from 25% to 57%.[4] Unfortunately, in the vast majority of studies in this review, only overall rates were reported without individual-level data. One cannot assume the women who were sexually active preoperatively are the same as those who were sexually active postoperatively. Furthermore, few studies reported on reasons for sexual inactivity. Reported reasons for sexual inactivity include lack of partner, partner-related problems, personal preference, prolapse complaints, and pain.[5–11] According to this systematic review, sexual activity rates were higher after vaginal mixed NT repair, posterior repair, and biological grafts, while sexual activity rates were lower after anterior repair, sacrospinous ligament suspensions, TVM, and SCP.[4] The lower prevalence of sexual activity after many POP surgeries could not be deciphered from the results of the systematic review because most trials do not report reasons for inactivity. However, pain as the primary reason for sexual inactivity was reported in 16 studies at approximately 8%.[4]

CHANGES IN OVERALL SEXUAL FUNCTION AFTER PELVIC ORGAN PROLAPSE SURGERY

Four systematic reviews reported on sexual function and dyspareunia after pelvic reconstructive surgery for POP.[4,12–14] All concluded that overall sexual function, as assessed by validated sexual function questionnaires, remained unchanged or improved postoperatively. A recently published systematic review of prospective POP trials included 74 manuscripts representing 67 original POP comparative studies looking at sexual function outcomes before and after surgery.[4] Approximately 58% of published manuscripts reported using validated sexual questionnaires. Changes in overall sexual function were assessed with validated sexual function questionnaires. For the meta-analysis on changes in sexual function in this review, the Pelvic Organ Prolapse/Urinary Incontinence Sexual Questionnaire Short Form (PISQ-12) was used because it was the questionnaire most frequently reported in trials.[4] Mixed NT repair is defined as surgery with a combination of any of the following: anterior or posterior repair, uterosacral suspensions, and sacrospinous ligament suspensions.

Based on a prior systematic review, changes in sexual function according to surgery are shown in **Table 1**.[4] Importantly, no surgery type, including TVM, had a significant worsening effect on sexual function. Of all surgery types, TVM had the smallest mean positive change in sexual function. Improvement in sexual function after POP surgery may be attributed largely to a resolution of bulge symptoms and incontinence during sex. While prolapse-related complaints may improve, pain may not, leaving preoperative and postoperative sexual function scores similar overall.

DYSPAREUNIA AFTER PELVIC FLOOR SURGERY

Dyspareunia, or pain with intercourse, is one of the most common sexual function outcomes reported in POP surgical trials. Pelvic reconstructive surgery alters and restores vaginal anatomy, but it can also lead to scarring, shortening, or narrowing of the vagina, which can lead to dyspareunia. However, dyspareunia is also commonly reported by patients prior to POP surgery as well. In a systematic review, baseline dyspareunia was reported in approximately 22% to 36% of patients prior to prolapse surgery.[4] In order to report total postoperative dyspareunia, preoperative dyspareunia must be accounted for. It is also important to understand the rates of persistent dyspareunia, defined as postoperative sexual pain in women who had pain prior to surgery, as well as the rates of de novo or new-onset dyspareunia in women who did not have pain prior to surgery. The International Urogynecological Association (IUGA) and the International Continence Society published a joint report on assessing sexual health in women with pelvic floor dysfunction and recommended a minimum of reporting preoperative and postoperative sexual activity, pain/dyspareunia, and overall sexual function based on a validated sexual function questionnaire.[3]

Based on a recent systematic review of 67 studies on sexual function in POP surgery, the rates of preoperative total dyspareunia, postoperative total dyspareunia,

Table 1 Sexual function changes after prolapse surgery			
	Sexual Function Change After Surgery	Mean Change in PISQ-12	95% CI, P Value
Mixed Native Tissue Repair	IMPROVED	4.8	95% CI 2.9–6.7, P<.001
Anterior Repair	IMPROVED	3.2	95% CI 0.4–6.1, P = .025
Uterosacral Ligament Suspension	IMPROVED	2.9	95% CI 1.2–4.7, P<.001
Sacrospinous Ligament Suspensions	IMPROVED	2.9	95% CI 0.1–5.8, P = .043
Sacrocolpopexy	IMPROVED	5.3	95% CI 1.5–9.2, P = .007
Posterior Repair	UNCHANGED	5.8	95% CI -1.5 to 13.1, P = .12
Transvaginal Mesh	UNCHANGED	0.9	95% CI -1.6 to 3.4, P = .48
Biological Grafts	UNCHANGED	12	95% CI -3.6 to 27.6, P = .13

persistent dyspareunia, and de novo dyspareunia are listed in **Table 1**.[4] Data for persistent dyspareunia were extracted from individual studies. While not all studies in the review reported on both preoperative and postoperative dyspareunia, in those who did, the prevalence of postoperative dyspareunia was lower than the prevalence of preoperative dyspareunia in all surgery types. There are low-quality data on persistent dyspareunia. As for de novo dyspareunia, the prevalence is low and ranged from 0% to 9% after POP surgery except for posterior repair, where rates were not reported in randomized trials.[15–18] Only 1 prospective nonrandomized study reported on this outcome in posterior repair, which found 33% de novo dyspareunia.[19] However, this cohort included levatorplasties in an undisclosed proportion of posterior repair, which is a known risk factor for dyspareunia. Therefore, the systematic review had limited evidence on de novo dyspareunia for traditional posterior repair involving standard midline plication of the posterior compartment. Based on other studies not included in the systematic review, de novo dyspareunia after traditional posterior repair can range from 4% to 19%.[20] This randomized trial also looked at the applicability of postoperative vaginal dilator use 4 weeks after posterior repair and its effect on de novo dyspareunia. De novo dyspareunia rates in women who used vaginal dilators versus those who did not postoperatively showed no difference (**Table 2**).

COMPARING SEXUAL FUNCTION AFTER VARIOUS TYPES OF PROLAPSE SURGERY

A secondary analysis of a systematic review on sexual function after POP surgery was performed comparing various types/routes of prolapse surgery with other prolapse repair regarding sexual function, dyspareunia, and sexual activity.[4] The studies included were randomized controlled trials and prospective nonrandomized comparative trials. Four comparisons were sufficient for meta-analysis: TVM versus mixed NT repair (24 studies); NT repair versus sacrocolpopexy (SCP) (5 studies); TVM versus SCP (3 studies); and NT repair versus vaginal biological grafts (7 studies).

In the most robust comparison of TVM and NT repair, change in sexual activity (preoperatively or postoperatively) and sexual function scores (assessed by PISQ-12) did not vary between groups. Total overall dyspareunia prevalence was similar postoperatively between groups. However, persistent dyspareunia (in those who had baseline dyspareunia) was higher in women after TVM (48% vs 31%, 4 studies, n = 988). De novo dyspareunia was similar between TVM and NT repair groups.

In comparing NT repair with SCP, no differences were observed between groups in sexual activity (preoperatively and postoperatively), total dyspareunia (preoperatively or postoperatively), de novo dyspareunia, or changes in PISQ-12 sexual function scores after surgery.

In trials comparing TVM and SCP, there was no difference in sexual activity (preoperatively or postoperatively), de novo dyspareunia, or persistent dyspareunia. However, based on 1 study, total postoperative dyspareunia was higher in patients after TVM than after SCP (29% vs 15%).[24] Changes in PISQ-12 sexual function scores were similar between groups.

In comparing NT repair with vaginal biological grafts, no differences were observed in sexual activity (preoperatively and postoperatively) or total dyspareunia (preoperatively or postoperatively). Changes in PISQ-12 sexual function scores were similar between groups.

There are few differences in sexual function and activity between these surgery types. Choice of surgery type should be based on patient factors and goals, as well as efficacy, and not necessarily on sexual function.

Table 2
Dyspareunia in women before and after prolapse surgery based on a systematic review[a]

	Preoperative Total Dyspareunia	Postoperative Total Dyspareunia	Persistent Dyspareunia	De Novo Dyspareunia
Mixed Native Tissue Repair 18 papers, 15 studies (13 RCTs, 2 nRCS) N = 1803	24% 9 studies N = 898	13% 12 studies N = 870	71% 1 study[21] N = 7	9% 5 studies N = 234
Anterior Repair 16 papers, 12 studies (10 RCTs, 2 nRCS) N = 744	28% 3 studies N = 99	14% 5 studies N = 117	10% 2 studies[7,22] N = 31	5% 7 studies N = 223
Posterior Repair 9 papers/studies (4 RCTs, 5 nRCS) N = 4304	36% 5 studies N = 136	32% 6 studies N = 178	12% 1 study[19] N = 922	33% 1 study[a] N = 1206
Uterosacral Ligament Suspensions 4 papers/studies (2 RCTs, 2 nRCS) N = 278	26% 1 study N = 110	10% 1 study N = 110	24% 1 study[23] N = 78	9% 2 studies N = 78
Sacrospinous Ligament Suspensions 11 papers, 10 studies (7 RCTs, 3 nRCS) N = 553	29% 1 study N = 31	9% 5 studies N = 194	57% 1 study[5] N = 7	8% 2 studies N = 37
Transvaginal Synthetic Mesh 37 papers, 33 studies (26 RCTs, 7 nRCS) N = 2725	22% 13 studies N = 658	15% 21 studies N = 988	28% 4 studies[7,19,21,22] N = 60	9% 14 studies N = 433
Vaginal Biological Grafts 10 papers, 9 studies (8 RCTs, 1 nRCS) N = 782	28% 7 studies N = 506	11% 9 studies N = 557	NR	0% 1 study N = 28
Sacrocolpopexy 18 papers, 16 studies (9 RCTs and 7 nRCS) N = 1147	31% 5 studies N = 192	18% 9 studies N = 295	44% 1 study[5] N = 9	6% 3 studies N = 118

Abbreviations: NR, not reported; nRCS, nonrandomized comparative study; RCT, randomized controlled trial.
[a] This study was a prospective nonrandomized comparative trial, but posterior repair groups included levatorplasties.

DOMAINS OF SEXUAL FUNCTION

Various domains of female sexual function include desire, arousal, lubrication, satisfaction/enjoyment, orgasm, partner-related domains, and pain. Most POP surgical trials assess overall sexual function using validated questionnaires, but few report on individual items on the questionnaires that may reflect changes in these various domains. Based on the recent systematic review, orgasm, sexual desire, sexual arousal, and sexual satisfaction were individually reported in too few studies to meta-analyze.[4] Another study reports domains most affected in women with POP are arousal, orgasm, and dyspareunia.[25] One prospective trial of 70 women evaluated sexual function in women after NT repair, found that desire, arousal, lubrication, satisfaction, and pain improved significantly postoperatively, while orgasm showed no change.[26] This study also looked at partner-related domains and found that in male partners, sexual interest, drive, and overall satisfaction improved, while erection, ejaculation, and orgasm remained unchanged. Another prospective trial of vaginal NT repair showed that women had improved desire, arousal, lubrication, satisfaction, and orgasm, while dyspareunia had increased at a 3-month follow-up.[27] A secondary analysis of an RCT evaluating postoperative sexual function after NT repair and SCP using the Golombok Rust Inventory of Sexual Satisfaction (GRISS) questionnaire found that anorgasmia, satisfaction, and partner avoidance had improved 3 months after surgery.[28] Most reported studies have small sample sizes, and therefore, the effect of POP surgery on these other sexual function domains is largely unknown. Future larger, multi-center research trials are needed in this area.

HOW TO MEASURE SEXUAL FUNCTION IN PELVIC RECONSTRUCTIVE SURGERY

Overall sexual function should be assessed in FPMRS practice and POP surgical trials using validated sexual function questionnaires. **Table 3** lists several validated, commonly used sexual function questionnaires. The Female Sexual Function Index (FSFI) and GRISS are non-condition-specific validated questionnaires widely used in the literature to study female sexual function. The FSFI, although non-condition-specific, addresses 6 domains of sexual function including, desire, arousal, lubrication, orgasm, satisfaction, and pain.[29] The Pelvic Organ Prolapse/ Urinary Incontinence Sexual Questionnaire (PISQ) was the first validated sexual function questionnaire condition-specific to women with POP and urinary incontinence.[30] In addition to assessing sexual function domains listed above, it assesses for coital incontinence and partner avoidance due to vaginal bulge symptoms. A short form of the questionnaire, the PISQ-12, was later developed and is the most common questionnaire utilized in POP surgical trials currently.[4,31] The Pelvic Organ Prolapse/Urinary Incontinence Sexual Questionnaire, IUGA-Revised is also condition-specific but differs from the PISQ and PISQ-12, as sexually inactive women can also fill out the questionnaire, and it is more generalizable to all women presenting to urogynecology clinics. The Body Image in Pelvic Organ Prolapse questionnaire addresses body image within the setting of POP. Even though this questionnaire does not address the majority of domains, it could be useful as an adjunct because recent studies have attributed the improvement in sexual function after surgical correction of POP to improvements in body image.[32,33] The optimal questionnaire for practice and surgical trials depends on the research question and the study population while balancing the length of questionnaires and burden for patients.

Table 3
Validated questionnaires for female sexual function

Questionnaire Name	Year of Validation	Number of Questions/ Items	Scoring	Population	Limitations	Strengths	Condition-Specific to Pelvic Organ Prolapse or Incontinence
Body Image in Pelvic Organ Prolapse[34]	2014	21	Likert scale Higher scores indicating worse body image	Sexually active and non-sexually active women	• Validated in predominantly white population	Only validated condition-specific genital body image questionnaire	Yes
Female Sexual Function Index[29]	2000	19	Likert scale Calculate domain-specific scores and multiplying sum by the domain factor; sum these for a total score Higher scores indicate better sexual function	Sexually active women in the last 4 wk	Complex scoring system	Specific domain scoring	No

(continued on next page)

Table 3
(continued)

Questionnaire Name	Year of Validation	Number of Questions/ Items	Scoring	Population	Limitations	Strengths	Condition-Specific to Pelvic Organ Prolapse or Incontinence
The Golombok Rust Inventory of Sexual Satisfaction[35]	1985	28	Pseudo-stanine scale Score of 5 or above on individual question indicates dysfunction Higher scores indicate worse sexual function	Heterosexual couples Sexually active	• Designed for use with therapists and counseling • Assessment given to couples in a heterosexual relationship	• Comprehensive • Addresses specific male factors of sexual dysfunction as well as female factors • Used to monitor changes that occur with intervention within heterosexual couples	No
International Consultation on Incontinence Questionnaire—Female Sexual Matters Associated with Lower Urinary Tract Symptoms Module[36]	2004	4	Likert scale Scores are additionally weighted to assess perceived impact of symptoms Higher scores indicate worse sexual function	Sexually active women in the last 4 wk	• Not comprehensive • Validated in women with surgery for SUI	• short length	Yes

	Year	Items	Scale/Scoring	Population	Disadvantages	Advantages	Validated
International Consultation on Incontinence Questionnaire—Vaginal Symptoms Module[37]	2006	14	Likert scale. Scores are additionally weighted to assess perceived impact of symptoms. Subset of vaginal symptoms, sexual matters, and quality of life scores. Higher scores indicate worse sexual function	Sexually active women (in last 4 wk)	• lengthy	• Comprehensive • Addresses multiple symptoms related to pelvic dysfunction and prolapse	Yes
Pelvic Organ Prolapse/Urinary Incontinence Sexual Questionnaire (PISQ)[30]	2001	31	Likert scale. Higher scores indicate better sexual function	Heterosexual Sexually active women	• Length of questionnaire	• First condition-specific questionnaire • Comprehensive	Yes
Short form PISQ[31]	2003	12	Likert scale. Higher scores indicate better sexual function	Heterosexual sexually active women	• Only validated in heterosexual activity • Not validated in women w/anal incontinence	• Concise, easy use in clinical practice	Yes

(continued on next page)

Table 3
(continued)

Questionnaire Name	Year of Validation	Number of Questions/Items	Scoring	Population	Limitations	Strengths	Condition-Specific to Pelvic Organ Prolapse or Incontinence
PISQ, IUGA-Revised[38]	2013	33	Likert scale Cut-off score for impaired sexual function	Sexually active and non-sexually active women	• Length of questionnaire	• Addresses anal incontinence • Includes non-sexually active women • Uses gender-neutral items • Created with international team	Yes
Sexual Function Questionnaire[39]	2002	31	Likert scale Score ranges that indicate higher likelihood of sexual dysfunction Higher scores indicate worse sexual function	Sexually active last 4 wk	Length of questionnaire	Designed around 7 domains Specific domain scoring	No
Sexual Quality of Life—Female[40]	2005	18	Likert scale Higher scores indicating better sexual function	Sexually active women	Does not address pelvic dysfunction or symptoms	Assesses dysfunction and its relation to quality of life Addresses sexual function outside of partner-specific practices (ex: masturbation)	No

SUMMARY

Overall sexual function remains unchanged or improved after all types of POP surgery. High rates of baseline dyspareunia are reported in patients with prolapse before surgery. While the prevalence of total dyspareunia is lower after surgery than preoperatively, there is a small but substantial risk of developing de novo dyspareunia after surgery. The rate of de novo dyspareunia after posterior repair can be as high as 19%, whereas de novo dyspareunia after POP surgery in other compartments with and without mesh ranges from 0% to 9%. It is important to counsel patients on changes in sexual function after surgery, as this is an important goal for most women.

CLINICS CARE POINTS

- Surgeons should counsel patients on changes in sexual function and dyspareunia, as improvement in sexual function is an important goal for most women undergoing reconstructive surgery.
- There are few differences in sexual function and activity between POP surgery types. The choice of surgery type should be based on patient factors and goals as well as efficacy and not necessarily on sexual function.

DISCLOSURE

The authors have no financial disclosures.

REFERENCES

1. Pauls RN, Segal JL, Silva WA, et al. Sexual function in patients presenting to a urogynecology practice. Int Urogynecol J Pelvic Floor Dysfunct 2006;17(6): 576–80.
2. Dunivan GC, Sussman AL, Jelovsek JE, et al. Gaining the patient perspective on pelvic floor disorders' surgical adverse events. Am J Obstet Gynecol 2019; 220(2):185.e10.
3. Rogers RG, Pauls RN, Thakar R, et al. An international Urogynecological association (IUGA)/international continence society (ICS) joint report on the terminology for the assessment of sexual health of women with pelvic floor dysfunction. Int Urogynecol J 2018;29(5):647–66.
4. Antosh DD, Kim-Fine S, Meriwether KV, et al. Changes in sexual activity and function after pelvic organ prolapse surgery: a systematic review. Obstet Gynecol 2020;136(5):922–31.
5. Maher CF, Qatawneh AM, Dwyer PL, et al. Abdominal sacral colpopexy or vaginal sacrospinous colpopexy for vaginal vault prolapse: a prospective randomized study. Am J Obstet Gynecol 2004;190(1):20–6.
6. Lo TSW, Wang AC. Abdominal colposacropexy and sacrospinous ligament suspension for severe uterovaginal prolapse: A comparison. J Gynecol Surg 2009; 14:59–64.
7. de Tayrac R, Cornille A, Eglin G, et al. Comparison between trans-obturator transvaginal mesh and traditional anterior colporrhaphy in the treatment of anterior vaginal wall prolapse: results of a French RCT. Int Urogynecol J 2013;24(10): 1651–61.

8. Nieminen K, Hiltunen R, Heiskanen E, et al. Symptom resolution and sexual function after anterior vaginal wall repair with or without polypropylene mesh. Int Urogynecol J Pelvic Floor Dysfunct 2008;19(12):1611–6.

9. Geoffrion R, Hyakutake MT, Koenig NA, et al. Bilateral sacrospinous vault fixation with tailored synthetic mesh arms: clinical outcomes at one year. J Obstet Gynaecol Can 2015;37(2):129–37.

10. Glazener C, Breeman S, Elders A, et al. Clinical effectiveness and cost-effectiveness of surgical options for the management of anterior and/or posterior vaginal wall prolapse: two randomised controlled trials within a comprehensive cohort study - results from the PROSPECT Study. Health Technol Assess 2016; 20(95):1–452.

11. Lukacz ES, Warren LK, Richter HE, et al. Quality of Life and Sexual Function 2 Years After Vaginal Surgery for Prolapse. Obstet Gynecol 2016;127(6):1071–9.

12. Dietz V, Maher C. Pelvic organ prolapse and sexual function. Int Urogynecol J 2013;24(11):1853–7.

13. Jha S, Gray T. A systematic review and meta-analysis of the impact of native tissue repair for pelvic organ prolapse on sexual function. Int Urogynecol J 2015; 26(3):321–7.

14. Liao SC, Huang WC, Su TH, et al. Changes in Female Sexual Function After Vaginal Mesh Repair Versus Native Tissue Repair for Pelvic Organ Prolapse: A Meta-Analysis of Randomized Controlled Trials. J Sex Med 2019;16(5):633–9.

15. Sung VW, Rardin CR, Raker CA, et al. Porcine subintestinal submucosal graft augmentation for rectocele repair: a randomized controlled trial. Obstet Gynecol 2012;119(1):125–33.

16. Paraiso MF, Barber MD, Muir TW, et al. Rectocele repair: a randomized trial of three surgical techniques including graft augmentation. Am J Obstet Gynecol 2006;195(6):1762–71.

17. Nieminen K, Hiltunen KM, Laitinen J, et al. Transanal or vaginal approach to rectocele repair: a prospective, randomized pilot study. Dis Colon Rectum 2004; 47(10):1636–42.

18. Farid M, Madbouly KM, Hussein A, et al. Randomized controlled trial between perineal and anal repairs of rectocele in obstructed defecation. World J Surg 2010;34(4):822–9.

19. Madsen LD, Nüssler E, Kesmodel US, et al. Native-tissue repair of isolated primary rectocele compared with nonabsorbable mesh: patient-reported outcomes. Int Urogynecol J 2017;28(1):49–57.

20. Antosh DD, Gutman RE, Park AJ, et al. Vaginal dilators for prevention of dyspareunia after prolapse surgery: a randomized controlled trial. Obstet Gynecol 2013; 121(6):1273–80.

21. Gutman RE, Nosti PA, Sokol AI, et al. Three-year outcomes of vaginal mesh for prolapse: a randomized controlled trial. Obstet Gynecol 2013;122(4):770–7.

22. Vollebregt A, Fischer K, Gietelink D, et al. Primary surgical repair of anterior vaginal prolapse: a randomised trial comparing anatomical and functional outcome between anterior colporrhaphy and trocar-guided transobturator anterior mesh. BJOG 2011;118(12):1518–27.

23. Ucar MG, İlhan TT, Şanlıkan F, et al. Sexual functioning before and after vaginal hysterectomy to treat pelvic organ prolapse and the effects of vaginal cuff closure techniques: a prospective randomised study. Eur J Obstet Gynecol Reprod Biol 2016;206:1–5.

24. Lucot JP, Fauconnier A. Reply to Maurizio Bologna, Amerigo Vitagliano, and Mauro Cervigni's Letter to the Editor re: Jean-Philippe Lucot, Michel Cosson,

Georges Bader, et al. Safety of Vaginal Mesh Surgery Versus Laparoscopic Mesh Sacropexy for Cystocele Repair: Results of the Prosthetic Pelvic Floor Repair Randomized Controlled Trial. Eur Urol 2018;74:167-76: Is There Enough Evidence To Prove Higher Safety of Laparoscopic Sacropexy in Comparison to Vaginal Surgery for Cystocele Mesh Repair? Eur Urol 2018;74(3):e73–176.

25. Handa VL, Cundiff G, Chang HH, et al. Female sexual function and pelvic floor disorders. Obstet Gynecol 2008;111(5):1045–52.

26. Kuhn A, Brunnmayr G, Stadlmayr W, et al. Male and female sexual function after surgical repair of female organ prolapse. J Sex Med 2009;6(5):1324–34.

27. Azar M, Noohi S, Radfar S, et al. Sexual function in women after surgery for pelvic organ prolapse. Int Urogynecol J Pelvic Floor Dysfunct 2008;19(1):53–7.

28. Geynisman-Tan J, Kenton K, Komar A, et al. Recovering sexual satisfaction after prolapse surgery: a secondary analysis of surgical recovery. Int Urogynecol J 2018;29(11):1675–80.

29. Rosen R, Brown C, Heiman J, et al. The Female Sexual Function Index (FSFI): a multidimensional self-report instrument for the assessment of female sexual function. J Sex Marital Ther 2000;26(2):191–208.

30. Rogers RG, Kammerer-Doak D, Villarreal A, et al. A new instrument to measure sexual function in women with urinary incontinence or pelvic organ prolapse. Am J Obstet Gynecol 2001;184(4):552–8.

31. Rogers RG, Coates KW, Kammerer-Doak D, et al. A short form of the Pelvic Organ Prolapse/Urinary Incontinence Sexual Questionnaire (PISQ-12). Int Urogynecol J Pelvic Floor Dysfunct 2003;14(3):164–8 [discussion: 168].

32. Lowder JL, Ghetti C, Nikolajski C, et al. Body image perceptions in women with pelvic organ prolapse: a qualitative study. Am J Obstet Gynecol 2011;204(5): 441–5.

33. Lowenstein L, Gamble T, Sanses TV, et al. Changes in sexual function after treatment for prolapse are related to the improvement in body image perception. J Sex Med 2010;7(2 Pt 2):1023–8.

34. Lowder JL, Ghetti C, Oliphant SS, et al. Body image in the Pelvic Organ Prolapse Questionnaire: development and validation. Am J Obstet Gynecol 2014;211(2): 174–9.

35. Rust J, Golombok S. The Golombok-Rust Inventory of Sexual Satisfaction (GRISS). Br J Clin Psychol 1985;24(Pt 1):63–4.

36. Brookes ST, Donovan JL, Wright M, et al. A scored form of the Bristol Female Lower Urinary Tract Symptoms questionnaire: data from a randomized controlled trial of surgery for women with stress incontinence. Am J Obstet Gynecol 2004; 191(1):73–82.

37. Price N, Jackson SR, Avery K, et al. Development and psychometric evaluation of the ICIQ Vaginal Symptoms Questionnaire: the ICIQ-VS. BJOG 2006;113(6): 700–12.

38. Rogers RG, Espuna Pons ME. The Pelvic Organ Prolapse Incontinence Sexual Questionnaire, IUGA-revised (PISQ-IR). Int Urogynecol J 2013;24(7):1063–4.

39. Quirk FH, Heiman JR, Rosen RC, et al. Development of a sexual function questionnaire for clinical trials of female sexual dysfunction. J Womens Health Gend Based Med 2002;11(3):277–89.

40. Symonds T, Boolell M, Quirk F. Development of a questionnaire on sexual quality of life in women. J Sex Marital Ther 2005;31(5):385–97.

Defecatory Dysfunction

Erin C. Crosby, MD*, Katherine E. Husk, MD

KEYWORDS

- Abnormal defecation • Chronic constipation • Defecatory dysfunction
- Obstructed defecation

KEY POINTS

- Comprehension of the normal physiologic process of defecation is critical to understanding disorders of defecation.
- Defecatory dysfunction broadly encompasses all disordered defecation aside from fecal incontinence.
- Evaluation should include a focused history and physical examination, with strong consideration of adjunctive testing or imaging.
- Management options range from conservative, such as dietary changes, lifestyle modifications, medications, pelvic floor physical therapy, to surgical management.

BACKGROUND

Normal defecation occurs as a result of a coordinated process involving the rectum, anus, anal sphincter complex and pelvic floor muscles. When gas, liquid, or solid stool moves into the rectum, it stimulates pressure receptors in the colon, rectum, and puborectalis muscle, which then stimulates the rectoanal inhibitory reflex (RAIR). Stated simply, RAIR is when the internal anal sphincter relaxes and cells in the anal canal sample the rectal contents. Information about the rectal contents is communicated to the brain, which determines whether defecation should occur. If defecation is not appropriate, the external anal sphincter and levator ani muscle contract and the rectum relaxes, allowing rectal contents to continue to be stored. If it is decided that defecation is to occur, the puborectalis muscle relaxes, which straightens the anorectal angle. The pelvic floor descends slightly, and the external anal sphincter relaxes. The anal contents are then evacuated. When defecation is complete, the anal sphincter complex contracts and the pelvic floor rises.[1]

The term chronic constipation, as defined most recently by the Rome IV diagnostic criteria (**Box 1**),[2–6] encompasses a broad range of symptoms including straining with defecation, decreased frequency of bowel movements, hard stool consistency, a

Department of Obstetrics and Gynecology, Division of Urogynecology and Pelvic Reconstructive Surgery, Albany Medical College, 391 Myrtle Avenue, Suite 200, Albany, NY 12208, USA
* Corresponding author.
E-mail address: crosbye@amc.edu

Obstet Gynecol Clin N Am 48 (2021) 653–663
https://doi.org/10.1016/j.ogc.2021.05.016
0889-8545/21/© 2021 Elsevier Inc. All rights reserved.

Box 1
Rome IV criteria for constipation disorders[4-7]

Diagnostic Criteria for Functional Constipation
  Symptom onset at least 6 months prior, with criteria fulfilled during the last 3 months
  1. Must include $\geq$ 2 of the following:
    a Straining during greater than 25% of defecation episodes
    b Lumpy or hard stools (Bristol Stool Scale type 1–2) > 25% of defecations
    c Sensation of incomplete emptying greater than 25% defecations
    d Sensation of anorectal obstruction or blockage greater than 25% of defecations
    e Manual maneuvers needed for greater than 25% of defecations
    f. Less than 3 bowel movements per week
  2. Loose stools rarely present without use of laxatives
  3. Insufficient criteria to meet irritable bowel syndrome diagnosis

Diagnostic Criteria for Constipation-Predominant Irritable Bowel Syndrome
  1. Recurrent abdominal pain, at least 1 day/week (on average) in the last 3 months, associated with $\geq$ 2 of the following:
    a Related to defecation
    b Associated with a change in frequency of bowel movements
    c Associated with a change in the appearance/consistency of stool
  2. Greater than 25% of bowel movements with Bristol Stool Scale type 1–2 and less than 25% bowel movements with Bristol Stool Scale type 6–7

---

feeling of anorectal blockage, a feeling of incomplete emptying with defecation, and needing to splint or perform digital maneuvers to defecate.[7-9] Defecatory dysfunction has a similarly broad definition, including essentially any defecatory disorder aside from fecal incontinence.[10] Chronic versus acute constipation is characterized by at least 6 months of symptoms,[7] and can be primary, including idiopathic and functional, or secondary.[9] One of the major updates to the Rome IV criteria is that the authors advocate for decreased usage of the term "functional" to describe certain disorders secondary to concerns that this may over-simplify complex and multifactorial conditions.[4]

Constipation disorders can be characterized through symptoms and testing, including colonic transit studies and assessments of rectal evacuation.[9] The American Gastroenterological Association criteria focus heavily on testing to define three groups: normal transit constipation, slow transit constipation, and other defecatory disorders including pelvic floor dysfunction.[9] In this setting, colonic transit studies are used to distinguish between normal and slow colonic transit, whereas rectal evacuation studies identify defecatory disorders. Others advocate a focus on symptoms, behaviors,[10] and the Rome criteria to classify patients,[9] although the most recent Rome criteria (Rome IV criteria) do incorporate test results.[2,3] Using this model, certain diagnoses would be characterized by symptoms alone, such as functional constipation and constipation-predominant irritable bowel syndrome (IBS).[9] Defecatory disorders include constipation symptoms with abnormal evacuation,[9] and obstructed defecation can result from both anatomic (eg, rectocele, enterocele, colonic masses, rectal prolapse, internal rectal intussusception) or functional (eg, pelvic floor dyssynergia, nonrelaxing puborectalis syndrome) abnormalities.[7,11]

Anatomic abnormalities include changes to the vaginal or rectal structure that result in mechanical obstruction. Posterior compartment prolapse, including rectocele, enterocele, rectal intussusception, and rectal prolapse can cause obstructed defecation. Women with these types of prolapse often have symptoms of straining, incomplete emptying, and needing to splint or manually evacuate.[12] Many women with posterior compartment prolapse do not have defecatory dysfunction, and the defecatory symptom that best correlates with prolapse is needing to splint or manually evacuate.[13]

EVALUATION
History and physical

Initial evaluation should begin with a thorough review of symptoms, past medical history, past surgical history, family history of colorectal cancers or other disorders, dietary practices, medication use, prior trial of any bowel regimen, and review of any recent screening, such as colonoscopy.[7,10] Questions about all potential aspects of defecation should be included, with particular focus on the clinical components covered in the Rome IV criteria. This includes stool consistency, needing to strain, needing to splint or perform digital maneuvers to defecate, abdominal or anorectal pain, frequency of bowel movements, and if sensation of incomplete evacuation or obstruction is present, consideration whether or not patients meet Rome IV criteria for IBS.[2–4,7] IBS and functional constipation diagnoses may have significant overlap and should be thought of on a continuum.[4] Use of the Bristol Stool Scale to reliably assess stool consistency and consideration of a bowel diary to characterize the frequency of defecation can be helpful.[9] A 7-day bowel diary should capture the number of bowel movements, stool consistency, presence and degree of straining, presence of pain and/or bloating, and any utilization of digital maneuvers for defecation.[14] Certain features may suggest a particular diagnosis. For example, splinting or performing digital maneuvers to defecate suggest obstructed defecation, while hard stool consistency and bloating suggest slow transit constipation or other motility issues.[10] The presentation of defecatory dysfunction related to prolapse varies significantly, and may include straining, splinting, or performing other manual manipulation during defecation, sensation of incomplete evacuation, and/or feeling of anorectal blockage. Of these, the need to splint is the only symptom that consistently correlates with posterior wall prolapse.[7,13] A validated Constipation Severity Instrument distinguishes individuals based on symptoms and captures aspects related to obstructive defecation, colonic inertia or slow transit, and pain.[15] Symptoms do not consistently predict specific diagnoses, and therefore other methods of evaluation should be considered.[9] Certain concerning features should prompt more immediate referral to gastroenterology or potentially colorectal surgery. These include melena, hematochezia or rectal bleeding, significant family history of colon cancer, unintentional weight loss, anemia, a positive fecal occult blood test, or acute change in bowel habits, such as with stool caliber or frequency of bowel movements, particularly in older individuals aged 50 years or older.[7,9,10]

   The physical examination should include evaluation for pelvic organ prolapse with the Pelvic Organ Prolapse Quantification (POP-Q) assessment with a focus on the posterior vaginal wall, confirmation of normal sacral reflexes, and evaluation of pelvic floor muscle tone, strength, and coordination. Rectal examination should assess for anal sphincter tone, squeeze pressure, and Valsalva pressure, presence of a rectocele assessed as weakness in the rectovaginal wall, masses, fissures, hemorrhoids, and assessment of the pelvic floor musculature, particularly the puborectalis during squeeze and Valsalva.[7,10,14] During the squeeze portion, the puborectalis should elevate and there should be increased tone of the external anal sphincter.[9] The patient should then be instructed to attempt Valsalva during the digital rectal examination, and in a normal individual, both the puborectalis and the external anal sphincter should relax, with associated descent of the perineum by 2 to 4 cm.[9,16,17] Inherent limitations with the physical examination exist, and that many of these disorders lack reliable pelvic examination indicators. In addition, the degree of association between examination findings and bowel symptoms is uncertain.[7] Digital rectal examination findings may be predictive of rectal balloon expulsion test results; however, this appears to be significantly associated with examiner expertise as sensitivity and specificity decrease significantly when the examiner is less skilled.[9] Although it is not always necessary to include imaging or other testing as part of the evaluation, these tests can be a helpful adjunct, particularly if the individual's symptoms do not align with the physical examination[7] or when the presentation is otherwise unclear.

Colonoscopy

Colonoscopy is important in those patients who are not up to date on appropriate screening and/or if bowel symptoms arose only after the most recent colonoscopy. In addition, if concerning features potentially suggestive of colorectal cancer present or if constipation is unable to be sufficiently managed with conservative or medical management, colonoscopy may be appropriate.[9]

Colonic Transit Studies

This testing modality is used to assess colonic transit time and is completed using several different techniques. Patients should be instructed to discontinue laxative-type components of a bowel regimen including suppositories, enemas, and laxatives for at least 5 days before the testing, as use of these medications can impact results.[7] When using radio-opaque markers, the patient will ingest a capsule that contains 24 radio-opaque markers, with x-ray performed on the abdomen 120 hours later on day 5 after ingestion.[14] The transit study is considered abnormal if greater than 5 radio-opaque markers remain in the colon at the time of radiograph evaluation (**Fig. 1**).[14,18] An alternate technique involves ingestion of a capsule containing 24

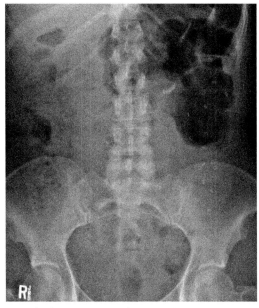

Fig. 1. Colonic transit study demonstrating slow-transit constipation.

radio-opaque markers on days 1, 2, and 3, then assessing for the remaining markers on days 4 and 7.[9] When using this technique, retaining greater than 68 markers on either day is considered abnormal.[9] The location of any remaining radio-opaque markers may suggest an etiology for the constipation. For example, markers distributed throughout the colon likely represent slow-transit constipation, whereas markers concentrated in the rectosigmoid suggest outlet obstruction.[7] Transit time can also be assessed through the use of wireless motility capsules (WMC). For this test, the patient ingests a capsule that wirelessly transmits information about pH, temperature, and pressure recordings, without requiring exposure to radiation.[14] Use of wireless capsules allows for assessment of both regional and whole-gut transit time, with validated normal values of less than 59 hours for colonic transit and less than 73 hours for whole-gut transit time.[14] Evaluation of these two transit study techniques appears to demonstrate good agreement between the findings on a radio-opaque marker study and WMC study for a given individual.[19] Colonic manometry is an experimental method used to assess resting and dynamic changes in colonic motility, particularly after ingesting a meal, in select patients at certain hospital centers.[18,19] One major limitation of transit studies is that approximately two-thirds of individuals with dyssynergia will also have slow-transit constipation[20] and this testing often cannot reliably distinguish between those with isolated dyssynergic defecation versus slow-transit constipation. In these cases, anorectal manometry may be a helpful adjunct.[14]

Anorectal Manometry

Anorectal manometry is a physiologic test that involves the use of pressure-sensitive catheters, introduced with a small inflated balloon in the rectum, that allow for measurement of rectal sensation, rectal compliance, relaxation of the internal anal sphincter, and assessment of attempted balloon expulsion.[7] Individuals complete a bowel preparation with an enema to empty the bowels before completing the study.[7] During the testing, the individual is asked to squeeze, push, and relax, and each point anal sphincter pressure measurements are captured.[7] Finally, during the rectal balloon expulsion test portion, a balloon is inserted into the rectum and then inflated with water (usually 50 mL), and the ability to evacuate this balloon, and the time to accomplish evacuation, is assessed.[7] During Valsalva associated with normal evacuation, the intrarectal pressure should increase, while there is a concomitant decrease in external anal sphincter pressure,[14] resulting in a rectoanal gradient that is negative in healthy controls.[9] Normal time to evacuation should be less than 1 minute, with some slight variation in the range of normal values depending on the measurement technique used.[7,9,21,22] Although the rectal balloon expulsion test does have high sensitivity and specificity for diagnosing defecatory dysfunction, results can be impacted in the setting of significant prolapse[9,23] or in settings where the test environment does not reflect normal practices.[9] The anal sphincter may fail to relax on anorectal manometry in some normal controls,[24] perhaps due to discomfort or embarrassment during testing.

Defecography

Defecography provides information about anatomic changes during attempted defecation, such as evaluating for the presence of rectocele, rectal prolapse, intussusception, or other dynamic changes including dyssynergia, descent of the perineum, and change in the anorectal angle during defecation.[9,14] During the study, anorectal junction and anorectal angle assessment is performed during rest, evacuation, and recovery, often using the pubococcygeal line (a line drawn from the inferior pubic symphysis to the last coccygeal joint),[25] the midpubic line (the longitudinal axis of the pubic symphysis roughly correlating to the level of the hymenal remnant), or the ischial tuberosities as reference points (**Fig. 2**).[7] Defecography can be completed with videofluoroscopy after instillation of a barium enema or with magnetic resonance (MR) defecography, which does not involve radiation.[14] Before defecography, the rectum should be emptied.[7] If performing fluoroscopic defecography, oral ingestion of dilute barium is started 30 to 45 minutes before the study to allow opacification of the small bowel.[7] Just ahead of starting the study, rectal contrast, which is mixed with paste to more closely resemble stool consistency, is inserted, and if vaginal opacification is needed, contrast can be intermixed with ultrasound gel and inserted vaginally.[7,26] Similarly, with MRI

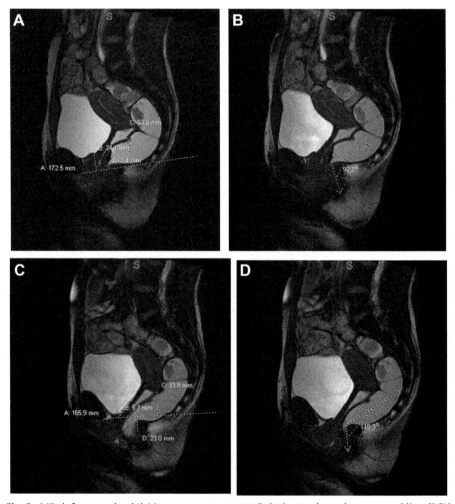

Fig. 2. MR defecography. (*A*) Measurements at rest. Relative to the pubococcygeal line (PCL) indicated by A. B = Distance from bladder base to PCL. C = Distance from cervix to PCL. D = Distance from anorectal junction to PCL. (*B*) Anorectal angle with Kegel (squeeze). (*C*) Measurements with maximum strain. Relative to the PCL indicated by A. B = Distance from bladder base to PCL. C = Distance from cervix to PCL. D = Distance from anorectal junction to PCL. (*D*) Anorectal angle with maximum strain.

defecography, viscous contrast material should be inserted into the rectum for visu-alization.[7] After emptying the rectum, it is possible to assess for rectal prolapse, rectocele, and enterocele, with the latter two evaluated by recognized grading sys-tems.[7,27] In addition to structural findings, features suggestive of pelvic floor dyssy-nergia include delayed evacuation (>30 seconds), narrowing of the anal canal during straining as a result of a nonrelaxed puborectalis, and inadequate widening of the anorectal angle.[7,28] Significant interobserver variability for fluoroscopic defe-cography exists.[14] MR defecography findings are often more readily reproduced,[29] and have improved ability to assess anatomy and function concomitantly,[30] and providing a more detailed assessment of the pelvic floor.[14] Use of MR permits simultaneous assessment of the pelvic bony landmarks and musculature, which is critical for the evaluation of dynamic motion of the pelvic floor.[9] MR defecography is significantly more costly.[14] In addition, defecography may not adequately identify defecatory disorders, as it is well-recognized that approximately two-thirds of normal individuals will have abnormal findings on defecography.[31] Defecography can identify a rectocele during defecation in many normal, asymptomatic women.[7,32] Furthermore, defecography findings do not consistently correlate with physical examination findings or prolapse symptoms.[7,33–36] Because of this, defe-cography is often used in combination with other defecatory evaluations rather than as the sole testing modality.[14]

THERAPEUTIC OPTIONS
Conservative management options

First-line treatment for defecatory disorders includes dietary and behavioral modifica-tion and oral medications. Patients with chronic constipation should be counseled on the benefits of soluble fiber and exercise. Evidence that increased hydration is benefi-cial in the treatment of constipation is lacking.[37] Fiber intake should be between 25 and 35 g per day in total, and soluble fibers such as psyllium and ispaghula husk tend to be better tolerated than insoluble fibers like bran.[38] Fiber intake should be titrated up slowly with patients increasing by 3 to 4 g daily to avoid side-effects like bloating and abdom-inal discomfort.[39] Exercise is recommended and a recent meta-analysis showed an improvement in constipation symptoms with walking and other physical movement.[40] Toileting behaviors should be addressed. Colonic motility is increased after meals and patients should be encouraged to attempt defecation at that time. The use of a step stool is helpful to elevate the knees slightly higher than the hips, and deep breathing and mindfulness can also help relax the pelvic floor muscles.[41]

Oral laxatives can be used as they are inexpensive and readily available. Osmotic laxatives are preferred to stimulant ones, and polyethylene glycol has been found to be superior to lactulose. Osmotic laxatives can cause bloating, gas, and abdominal discomfort. Stimulant laxatives such as bisacodyl and senna can be used if osmotic laxatives are not effective, but have a higher risk of causing abdominal pain and cramping. Both osmotic and stimulant laxatives can cause loose stools. If standard laxatives are not effective, prosecretory agents can be used, such as linaclotide, ple-canatide, and lubiprostone. Another option is prucalopride, which is a serotonin 5HT4 agonist that increases motility. It is well-tolerated and common side-effects resolve af-ter the first week of therapy.[39]

Biofeedback Therapy

Biofeedback is a process that gives auditory, visual, or verbal feedback to rehabilitate pelvic floor function.[42] It improves pelvic floor muscle coordination, strengthens the pelvic floor, and restores rectal sensation.[41] Although studies have not shown clear evidence of benefit in idiopathic constipation, biofeedback has shown benefit in several studies on defecatory dysfunction. Anorectal manometry, surface electromyography, and rectal balloons should be used as needed during biofeedback. Biofeedback has been shown to reduce dyssynergia and laxative use in patients with defecatory dysfunction, as well as improve satisfaction with bowel habits.[42] Biofeedback should be encouraged if it is affordable and geographically accessible to the patient, especially before a surgical intervention is considered.

Surgical Management

Surgical management of posterior compartment prolapse is most commonly performed through either the transvaginal route or through the transanal approach. Transvaginal repair can be done with a traditional posterior colporrhaphy or a site-specific defect repair. Posterior colporrhaphy is performed by incising the posterior vaginal wall in the midline and approximating the rectovaginal fascia with absorbable suture. Site-specific defect repair is performed by incising the posterior vaginal wall in the midline, identifying the specific areas of defect in the rectovaginal fascia and correcting them. A concomitant perineorrhaphy can be performed with either technique. Several studies have compared the two techniques, and posterior colporrhaphy showed greater improvements in bulge symptoms and anatomic outcomes compared with a site-specific repair and so is preferred. Relief of defecatory symptoms has not been adequately assessed in comparative studies between the two techniques.[43]

Transanal repair is performed by making an incision in the anterior rectal mucosa, creating and then trimming a rectal mucosal flap, closing the rectal mucosa, and performing a plication of the rectovaginal septum. Comparative studies between transanal repair and native tissue posterior colporrhaphy show greater improvements in constipation, incomplete evacuation and straining with posterior colporrhaphy, as well as a greater improvement in posterior vaginal wall anatomy.[44,45] Therefore, transvaginal posterior colporrhaphy is preferred. Other procedures are described for defecatory dysfunction, but they lack sufficient evidence to support their recommendation. Laparoscopic sacrocolpoperineopexy is not recommended for patients with defecatory dysfunction as several studies have shown that defecatory symptoms do not improve with the correction of posterior vaginal wall anatomy.[46–48] The stapled transanal rectal resection procedure has not been compared with other techniques and comparative statements cannot be made. Insufficient evidence supports the use of biologic grafts in the posterior compartment to improve obstructed defecation symptoms.[48] Botulinum toxin A has been used to treat dyssynergic defecation; however, a recent systematic review showed varied success with this treatment.[49]

CLINICS CARE POINTS

- A careful history and physical examination often reveal the cause of defecatory dysfunction, but imaging and other testing modalities should be used when the cause is not clear.
- Conservative therapy such as a bowel regimen, healthy toileting habits, and physical therapy should be maximized before consideration of surgical therapy.
- Transvaginal native-tissue posterior colporrhaphy is the preferred surgical treatment of posterior compartment prolapse.

DISCLOSURE

The authors have nothing to disclose.

REFERENCES

1. Wani RA, Thakur N. Physiology of Defecation. In: Chowdri NA, Parray FQ, editors. Benign anorectal disorders: a Guide to diagnosis and management. India: Springer; 2016.
2. Rao SS, Bharucha AE, Chiarioni G, et al. Functional Anorectal Disorders. Gastroenterology 2016;150(6). 1430–1442.e4.
3. Mearin F, Lacy BE, Chang L, et al. Bowel Disorders. Gastroenterology 2016; 150(6). 1393–1407.e5.
4. Simren M, Palsson OS, Whitehead WE. Update on Rome IV Criteria for Colorectal Disorders: Implications for Clinical Practice. Curr Gastroenterol Rep 2017; 19(4):15.
5. Ikee R, Yano K, Tsuru T. Constipation in chronic kidney disease: it is time to reconsider. Ren Replace Ther 2019;5(51):1–10.
6. Drossman DA, Hasler WL. Rome IV-Functional GI Disorders: Disorders of Gut-Brain Interaction. Gastroenterology 2016;150(6):1257–61.
7. Ridgeway BM, Weinstein MM, Tunitsky-Bitton E. American Urogynecologic Society Best-Practice Statement on Evaluation of Obstructed Defecation. Female Pelvic Med Reconstr Surg 2018;24(6):383–91.
8. Longstreth GF, Thompson WG, Chey WD, et al. Functional bowel disorders. Gastroenterology 2006;130(5):1480–91.
9. Bharucha AE, Wald A. Chronic Constipation. Mayo Clin Proc 2019;94(11): 2340–57.
10. Brown H, Grimes C. Current Trends in Management of Defecatory Dysfunction, Posterior Compartment Prolapse, and Fecal Incontinence. Curr Obstet Gynecol Rep 2016;5(2):165–71.
11. Times ML, Reickert CA. Functional anorectal disorders. Clin Colon Rectal Surg 2005;18(2):109–15.
12. Grimes CL, Lukacz ES. Posterior vaginal compartment prolapse and defecatory dysfunction: are they related? Int Urogynecol J 2012;23(5):537–51.
13. Erekson EA, Kassis NC, Washington BB, et al. The Association Between Stage II or Greater Posterior Prolapse and Bothersome Obstructive Bowel Symptoms. Female Pelvic Med Reconstr Surg 2010;16(1):59–64.
14. Rao SS, Rattanakovit K, Patcharatrakul T. Diagnosis and management of chronic constipation in adults. Nat Rev Gastroenterol Hepatol 2016;13(5):295–305.
15. Varma MG, Wang JY, Berian JR, et al. The constipation severity instrument: a validated measure. Dis Colon Rectum 2008;51(2):162–72.
16. Orkin BA, Sinykin SB, Lloyd PC. The digital rectal examination scoring system (DRESS). Dis Colon Rectum 2010;53(12):1656–60.
17. Tantiphlachiva K, Rao P, Attaluri A, et al. Digital rectal examination is a useful tool for identifying patients with dyssynergia. Clin Gastroenterol Hepatol 2010;8(11): 955–60.
18. Remes-Troche JM, Rao SS. Diagnostic testing in patients with chronic constipation. Curr Gastroenterol Rep 2006;8(5):416–24.
19. Camilleri M, Thorne NK, Ringel Y, et al. Wireless pH-motility capsule for colonic transit: prospective comparison with radiopaque markers in chronic constipation. Neurogastroenterol Motil 2010;22(8):874–82.e233.

20. Rao SS, Tuteja AK, Vellema T, et al. Dyssynergic defecation: demographics, symptoms, stool patterns, and quality of life. J Clin Gastroenterol 2004;38(8): 680–5.
21. Rao SS, Hatfield R, Soffer E, et al. Manometric tests of anorectal function in healthy adults. Am J Gastroenterol 1999;94(3):773–83.
22. Noelting J, Ratuapli SK, Bharucha AE, et al. Normal values for high-resolution anorectal manometry in healthy women: effects of age and significance of rectoanal gradient. Am J Gastroenterol 2012;107(10):1530–6.
23. Prichard DO, Lee T, Parthasarathy G, et al. High-resolution Anorectal Manometry for Identifying Defecatory Disorders and Rectal Structural Abnormalities in Women. Clin Gastroenterol Hepatol 2017;15(3):412–20.
24. Minguez M, Herreros B, Sanchiz V, et al. Predictive value of the balloon expulsion test for excluding the diagnosis of pelvic floor dyssynergia in constipation. Gastroenterology 2004;126(1):57–62.
25. Kelvin FM, Maglinte DD, Hale DS, et al. Female pelvic organ prolapse: a comparison of triphasic dynamic MR imaging and triphasic fluoroscopic cystocolpoproctography. AJR Am J Roentgenol 2000;174(1):81–8.
26. Maglinte DD, Bartram C. Dynamic imaging of posterior compartment pelvic floor dysfunction by evacuation proctography: techniques, indications, results and limitations. Eur J Radiol 2007;61(3):454–61.
27. Wiersma TG, Mulder CJ, Reeders JW. Dynamic rectal examination: its significant clinical value. Endoscopy 1997;29(6):462–71.
28. Thompson JR, Chen AH, Pettit PD, et al. Incidence of occult rectal prolapse in patients with clinical rectoceles and defecatory dysfunction. Am J Obstet Gynecol 2002;187(6):1494–9, discussion 1499–1500.
29. Reiner CS, Tutuian R, Solopova AE, et al. MR defecography in patients with dyssynergic defecation: spectrum of imaging findings and diagnostic value. Br J Radiol 2011;84(998):136–44.
30. Dvorkin LS, Hetzer F, Scott SM, et al. Open-magnet MR defaecography compared with evacuation proctography in the diagnosis and management of patients with rectal intussusception. Colorectal Dis 2004;6(1):45–53.
31. Freimanis MG, Wald A, Caruana B, et al. Evacuation proctography in normal volunteers. Invest Radiol 1991;26(6):581–5.
32. Shorvon PJ, McHugh S, Diamant NE, et al. Defecography in normal volunteers: results and implications. Gut 1989;30(12):1737–49.
33. Weber AM, Walters MD, Ballard LA, et al. Posterior vaginal prolapse and bowel function. Am J Obstet Gynecol 1998;179(6 Pt 1):1446–9, discussion 1449–1450.
34. Carter D, Gabel MB. Rectocele–does the size matter? Int J Colorectal Dis 2012; 27(7):975–80.
35. Altman D, Lopez A, Kierkegaard J, et al. Assessment of posterior vaginal wall prolapse: comparison of physical findings to cystodefecoperitoneography. Int Urogynecol J Pelvic Floor Dysfunct 2005;16(2):96–103, discussion 103.
36. Jelovsek JE, Barber MD, Paraiso MF, et al. Functional bowel and anorectal disorders in patients with pelvic organ prolapse and incontinence. Am J Obstet Gynecol 2005;193(6):2105–11.
37. Muller-Lissner SA, Kamm MA, Scarpignato C, et al. Myths and misconceptions about chronic constipation. Am J Gastroenterol 2005;100(1):232–42.
38. Ford AC, Moayyedi P, Lacy BE, et al. American College of Gastroenterology monograph on the management of irritable bowel syndrome and chronic idiopathic constipation. Am J Gastroenterol 2014;109(Suppl 1):S2–26, quiz S27.

39. Aziz I, Whitehead WE, Palsson OS, et al. An approach to the diagnosis and management of Rome IV functional disorders of chronic constipation. Expert Rev Gastroenterol Hepatol 2020;14(1):39–46.
40. Gao R, Tao Y, Zhou C, et al. Exercise therapy in patients with constipation: a systematic review and meta-analysis of randomized controlled trials. Scand J Gastroenterol 2019;54(2):169–77.
41. Pratt T, Mishra K. Evaluation and management of defecatory dysfunction in women. Curr Opin Obstet Gynecol 2018;30(6):451–7.
42. Narayanan SP, Bharucha AE. A Practical Guide to Biofeedback Therapy for Pelvic Floor Disorders. Curr Gastroenterol Rep 2019;21(5):21.
43. Grimes CL, Schimpf MO, Wieslander CK, et al. Surgical interventions for posterior compartment prolapse and obstructed defecation symptoms: a systematic review with clinical practice recommendations. Int Urogynecol J 2019;30(9): 1433–54.
44. Nieminen K, Hiltunen KM, Laitinen J, et al. Transanal or vaginal approach to rectocele repair: a prospective, randomized pilot study. Dis Colon Rectum 2004; 47(10):1636–42.
45. Farid M, Madbouly KM, Hussein A, et al. Randomized controlled trial between perineal and anal repairs of rectocele in obstructed defecation. World J Surg 2010;34(4):822–9.
46. Ramanah R, Ballester M, Chereau E, et al. Anorectal symptoms before and after laparoscopic sacrocolpoperineopexy for pelvic organ prolapse. Int Urogynecol J 2012;23(6):779–83.
47. Fox SD, Stanton SL. Vault prolapse and rectocele: assessment of repair using sacrocolpopexy with mesh interposition. BJOG 2000;107(11):1371–5.
48. Mowat A, Maher D, Baessler K, et al. Surgery for women with posterior compartment prolapse. Cochrane Database Syst Rev 2018;3:CD012975.
49. Chaichanavichkij P, Vollebregt PF, Scott SM, et al. Botulinum toxin type A for the treatment of dyssynergic defaecation in adults: a systematic review. Colorectal Dis 2020;49(22):1832–41.

Urinary Incontinence in Older Women

A Syndrome-Based Approach to Addressing Late Life Heterogeneity

Candace Parker-Autry, MD[a],*, George A. Kuchel, MD[b]

KEYWORDS

- Frailty • Geriatric syndrome • Urinary incontinence • Elderly

KEY POINTS

- Urinary incontinence is not a normal part of aging.
- Among many older women, urinary incontinence can be considered to present as a geriatric syndrome; intimately associated with physical function impairments, mobility disability, and cognitive decline.
- Urinary incontinence is a key determinant of health, thus assessment and treatment based on symptom bother may promote unhealthy aging.

INTRODUCTION

Healthy aging allowing for high level of function, independence, and quality of life should be the priority of all health care providers who care for women regardless of their specialty. Aging is an inevitable aspect of life, yet how each individual ages and its impact on that person's health and function is highly variable, potentially affecting every aspect of a women's life. Health care has been successful at increasing the lifespan of older Americans; thus, the older population is growing exponentially. Integrating healthy aging practices into the field of female pelvic medicine and reconstructive surgery is imperative as adults older than 65 years will make up more than 20% of the entire US population by 2034,[1] and the majority will be women evidenced by the life expectancy of US women being 81 years compared with 76 years in men.[2]

Many older women fulfill matriarchal duties of caregiving for their spouses, financially supporting their adult children, or taking over to parent grandchildren. Informal caregiving is physically and emotionally demanding and may result in ignoring health

[a] Department of Urology, Wake Forest School of Medicine, 1 Medical Center Boulevard, Winston-Salem, NC 27103, USA; [b] UConn Center on Aging, University of Connecticut, 263 Farmington Avenue, Farmington, CT 06030, USA
* Corresponding author.
E-mail address: cparkera@wakehealth.edu

Obstet Gynecol Clin N Am 48 (2021) 665–675
https://doi.org/10.1016/j.ogc.2021.05.017
0889-8545/21/© 2021 Elsevier Inc. All rights reserved.
obgyn.theclinics.com

problems when symptoms arise and delayed presentation for health care.[3] In fact, more than 50% of older women live with disabilities such as poor physical performance, difficulty with function or executing tasks, dementia, or other cognitive impairments. For these reasons, we must prioritize aging healthily. Prioritizing their health will promote the health of their families and thus our overall society.[3]

As we consider how to best address healthy aging in women, urinary incontinence (UI) is a top priority; identified to be a 'giant of aging' better known as a geriatric syndrome because of its high prevalence, multifactorial etiology, and high impact on the lives of older adults. Older women often present with *more severe UI symptoms* that have a *greater negative impact on their lives*. In addition, their *UI symptoms* may be *less responsive to standard treatments*.[4] The refractory nature of UI in this population may be partly attributed to both its complexity and interindividual heterogeneity as a multifactorial geriatric syndrome whose etiology is poorly understood and whose characteristics remain to be fully defined clinically. The *'Geriatric Incontinence Syndrome' (GIS)* was coined to name this *under-recognized clinical phenotype of UI* as distinct from the 'condition' of UI seen in younger or functionally intact women. The goal of this article is to review the supporting evidence of UI being a geriatric syndrome and to explore the potential impact of treatment efficacy on complex GIS.

URINARY INCONTINENCE IS ASSOCIATED WITH UNHEALTHY AGING

Unfortunately, in our current model of health care, issues pertaining to healthy aging and function often do not receive sufficient emphasis. More than 50% of women who live beyond 70 years do so with physical disabilities, difficulty with independent execution of daily tasks, and dementia or other cognitive impairments. After the age of 65 years, more than 50% of all women will develop some measure of UI through their geriatric years.[5] Symptoms in this population are often more severe, more bothersome, and more often refractory to standard treatments.[6] The general outlook on incontinence currently is "laissez-faire"; only prompting investigation and treatment when its impact becomes visible and sufficiently worrisome and/or bothersome. In clinical practice, we emphasize 'bother' as an essential element for treatment. This approach ignores the reality that the involuntary loss of urine that defines UI is a key determinant of health, independence, and quality of life with aging.[5,7] It may also promote normalizing UI among older women with resultant underreporting and underdiagnosis, likely contributing to the observation that only 3% of providers may be actively screening for UI symptoms during wellness visits.[8]

There is growing evidence indicating that UI is both a consequence of and a risk factor for broader disability and loss of independence. With aging, contributors to UI are multifactorial, more often reflecting poor health and a dysfunction of multiple different systems. This is the crux of its designation as a geriatric syndrome in older adults.[9] The term "geriatric syndrome" is used to capture those clinical conditions in older persons that fail to fit into typical discrete disease categories. Although heterogeneous, geriatric syndromes are multifactorial involving multiple organ systems with a substantial impact on quality of life and disability. They are highly prevalent in older adults and often lead to frailty. They pose significant challenges in the diagnosis and management of conditions because the chief complaint does not always represent the disconnect between the site of the underlying physiologic insult and the resulting clinical symptom. For example, when an infection involving the urinary tract precipitates delirium, the cognitive and behavioral changes reflect the diagnosis of delirium and determines many functional outcomes.

Therefore, geriatric syndromes can be viewed as *multifactorial conditions* that have *share risk factors* of aging, increasing the risk of frailty, and its downstream conse-quences of loss of independence, institutionalization, and death. Geriatric syndromes cross organ systems and discipline-based boundaries and thus challenge traditional perspectives on diagnosis and management. Although UI has been termed a *geriatric syndrome* by many, it remains a *poorly characterized clinical phenotype of UI currently not well distinguished from UI the condition related to pelvic floor dysfunction (PFD)*. Specifically, the concomitant presence of incontinence, functional impairment, mobility disability, or cognitive decline may define geriatric syndrome of incontinence that is intimately associated with loss of independence, institutionalization, and frailty.[10] Despite this knowledge, there has been a disparate amount of knowledge gained on geriatric incontinence as compared with the other well-characterized geri-atric syndromes of falls and dementia (**Fig. 1**).

To promote greater understanding and appreciation of UI as a geriatric syndrome, leading to improved care and outcomes, we must identify the varied multidimensional contributors to UI in late life. The development of UI among older women may indicate a loss of functional reserve historically isolated to the pelvic floor, but many factors outside of the pelvic floor are important. We must comprehensively consider the pro-cess of aging and the cumulative impact of predisposing, inciting, and intervening fac-tors that occur with life to understand why and when UI among geriatric women (age >70 years) may be a geriatric syndromic instead of a pelvic floor condition.

URINARY INCONTINENCE EVOLVES OVER THE LIFESPAN

Throughout a woman's lifecycle from the embryonic through adulthood stages, the lower urinary tract and pelvic floor undergo anatomic and functional changes. These changes in conjunction with life events such as pregnancy, menopause, metabolic changes in body composition, and aging may contribute to pelvic floor dysfunction and the development of UI, the most prevalent pelvic floor disorder in women.

John DeLancey and colleagues created a 3-phase lifespan model as a conceptual framework of how predisposing, inciting, and intervening factors of life may result in pelvic floor disorders (PFDs)[11] (**Fig. 2**).[11] According to this concept, after pelvic floor maturation in early adulthood, there is a set functional reserve capacity and symptom threshold below which symptoms of PFDs such as UI begin. The functional capacity and the symptom thresholds vary individually based on "independent, interactive, and cumulative" effects of biological and lifestyle factors during childhood, adolescence, and adult life.[11]

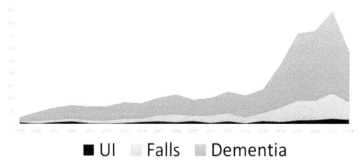

■ UI ░ Falls ▓ Dementia

Fig. 1. Twenty-year review of publications on geriatric incontinence (black) in comparison to other geriatric syndromes of falls (gray) and dementia (blue).

Lifespan Analysis of Pelvic Floor Function

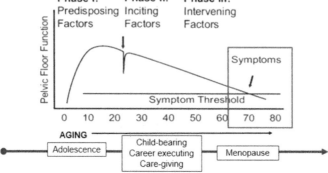

Fig. 2. Graphical display of the phases of a women's life and the role of natural and inciting events that may influence the development of PFDs. Modified conceptual framework of lifespan analysis if pelvic floor function. *Phase 1* represents life phases from an embryo through adolescence and represents predisposing factors such as genetics and environment. *Phase 2* extends from young adulthood through menopause. It is during this phase that inciting factors such as pregnancy, childbirth, pelvic surgery or radiation, chronic increases in intra-abdominal pressure/strain (constipation, obesity, heavy lifting), and estrogen deficiency may cumulatively decrease pelvic floor function towards the symptom threshold of irreversible pelvic floor dysfunction. *Phase 3* begins after the menopausal transition and represent age-related intervening factors such as physical function impairments, cognitive decline, mobility disability, and chronic medical conditions. It is important to understand that these factors should be considered "independently, interactively, and cumulatively". This phase considers the cumulative impact of phase 1 predisposing factors, phase 2 inciting factors, and age-related conditions on pelvic floor function. For many women, the symptom threshold is crossed and irreversible pelvic floor dysfunctions present. (*From* Delancey, J.O., et al., Graphic integration of causal factors of pelvic floor disorders: an integrated life span model. Am J Obstet Gynecol, 2008. 199(6): p. 610 e1-5; with permission.)

Phase 1 represents the life-phases from an embryo through adolescents and represents predisposing factors such as genetics and environment that may predispose women to develop PFDs later in life.

The factor with the most identifiable potential impact is genetic predisposition. Isali and colleagues performed a systematic review of gene expression in stress UI (SUI) and reported on 4 studies that examined 18,411 genes. Of those, 11 genes were identified as being overexpressed in women with SUI and 2 genes were underexpressed. Many of the genes identified had co-expressive interactions involved in intermediate filament, cytoskeleton, and extracellular matrix organization.[12]

Phase 2 is the longest and most prone life-phase, during which *inciting factors* may cumulatively decrease the threshold to develop PFDs. Pregnancy and childbirth are the most common inciting factor in this phase. It is plausible that the concomitant impact of phase 1 predisposing factors and the severity of birth trauma may lower the pelvic floor functional reserve capacity toward the symptom threshold and thus determine the level of pelvic floor recovery. **Fig. 3** demonstrates different scenarios (lines A, B, and C) that may affect the onset of UI during pregnancy or after delivery with emphasis on a few key points. First, genetic predisposition for poor pelvic floor function may affect the resilience of the pelvic floor after the inciting event of pregnancy/childbirth and thus the onset of PFD symptoms. Scenario 'A' may represent

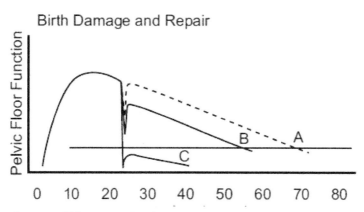

Fig. 3. Application of lifespan model phase 2. Multiple scenarios of birth injury and repair are demonstrated, line (*A*) represents a single delivery with birth damage resulting in brief decline in pelvic floor function from normal reserve with spontaneous recovery almost to baseline; (*B*) represents birth injury with recovery to a lower pelvic floor reserve and function; (*C*) represents birth injury that results in loss of pelvic floor function below the symptom threshold with the onset of permanent pelvic floor dysfunction. (*From* Delancey, J.O., et al., Graphic integration of causal factors of pelvic floor disorders: an integrated life span model. Am J Obstet Gynecol, 2008. 199(6): p. 610 e1-5; with permission.)

most women, whereas they have baseline normal pelvic floor function and capacity, undergo birth damage with resultant decrease in pelvic floor function that is rapidly returned near their baseline and this does not affect their projected point at crossing the symptom threshold. However, in scenario 'B,' there is less resilience of the pelvic floor and the birth injury results in a more permanent loss of pelvic floor function with a more rapid progression toward crossing the symptom threshold. Scenario 'C' represents 20% to 30% of women who have normal baseline pelvic floor function, but likely with poor physiologic reserve due to predisposing or inciting factors. In this scenario, the birth injury results in a decrease in pelvic floor function below the symptom threshold level and PFDs become more permanent. Baseline factors that may increase the risk of this scenario and outcome are vaginal delivery, birthweight greater than 4180 g, and head circumference greater than 35 cm. B, BMI $\geq$25 kg/m^2, and age $\geq$29 years had increased risk of incident UI at 6 months.[13]

As women move beyond their childbearing years into the premenopausal years, there are changes in life priorities with rearing children and/or career progression. The presence of UI symptoms may be a distraction and source of depleted confidence in the workplace. The frequent toileting breaks, use of pads, and daytime purposeful dehydration may negatively influence work performance in incontinent middle-aged women.[14,15] In addition, SUI is predominant[16,17] and 30% of women have symptoms that prevent participation in high-impact exercises.[18] This may result in greater incidence of obesity in this population. Furthermore, as women approach menopause, there is often increased total body adiposity thereby resulting in increased body mass index (BMI) and abdominal fat. Aune and colleagues performed a systematic review of 14 population-based cohort studies (both retrospective and prospective) and generated a dose-response risk associated with adiposity measures. Adiposity increased the risk of UI by 20% per 5-unit increase in BMI, 18% per 10 cm increase in waist circumference, and 34% per 10 kg increase in weight gain over time. Mixed UI (presence of urgency and stress UI) increased by 52% per 5 unit increase in BMI.[17]

Phase 3 accounts for aging, the multifactorial process involving complex interactions among biological, environmental, and molecular mechanisms. With aging, there is often an accelerated rate of dysfunction because of DNA damage, alterations in gene and noncoding RNA expression, genotoxicity, oxidative stress, and the incidence of shorter telomeres.[19] These are often concepts that we fail to consider when managing women over the age of 70 years who have developed UI. During this life-phase, there is a potential accelerated deterioration of pelvic floor function, the rate of which may be dictated by the cumulative impact of predisposing and inciting factors. It is plausible that during this phase of life, conditions such as chronic constipation, abdominal obesity, changes in neuromuscular health from chronic conditions such as type 2 diabetes mellitus, may accelerate pelvic floor dysfunction, thereby contributing to the onset of incontinence with aging. Conclusively, it is therefore more likely that UI develops in this phase of life because of the cumulative impact of biological changes coupled with genetic factors, and accelerated by other intervening factors of unhealthy aging.

URINARY INCONTINENCE: AN UNDERSTUDIED AND POORLY CHARACTERIZED GERIATRIC SYNDROME

Aging and the contribution of varied chronic conditions and frailty may be the most important intervening factor that diminishes the impact of mid-life inciting factors. The incidence of having at least 1 pelvic floor disorder increases with age, from 10% in women ages 20 to 39 years, to 37% among women ages 60 to 79 years, and up to 50% among women older than 80 years.[20] Most of these women will have UI, the most common of all pelvic floor disorders.[21] Although it is well accepted that parity is a known risk factor for UI among premenopausal women, after menopause this association dissipates.[21] Among nulliparous women, the incidence of bothersome UI symptoms was 32% in women ages 55 to 64 years.[21]

It is unclear why the incidence of UI increases with aging. However, physiologically, age-related changes in the lower urinary tract of women have been observed.[10] Detrusor muscle strength declines with aging[22]; likely due to the structural changes resulting in fibrosis and cell differentiation associated with estrogen deficiency.[23] The urethra undergoes specific changes in intrinsic sphincter and extrinsic muscle function. With aging, there is an estrogen deficiency associated with loss of urethral vascular density and blood flow.[24,25] With this loss, there is decreased urethral coaptation evidenced by the decreasing urethral closure pressure by 15 cm H_2O per decade of aging; thus, increasing the risk of urethral incontinence with aging.[26] Urethral length also shortens as a result of decreases in circular smooth muscle and longitudinal skeletal muscle mass associated with global skeletal muscle dysfunction or sarcopenia that increases with aging.[27] These age-related changes may be improved with intravaginal estrogen that may improve urethral closure pressure by improving submucosal vascular density, thus improving urethral coaptation.[28]

The clinical phenotype of the geriatric incontinence syndrome is complex because of a proposed cumulative impact of multiple intervening factors discussed earlier. We applied the concept the cumulative deficit model to conceptualize the development of the clinical phenotype of the GIS (Fig. 4). Considering this model, it is plausible that targeted interventions for this GIS should consider all these risk factors to treat geriatric incontinence. Below, we review the evidence to support each aspect in this framework.

Pelvic Floor Dysfunction Contributes to the Development of Geriatric Incontinence Syndrome

Changes to the aging pelvic floor can be the result of neuromuscular changes. In a study by Aukee and colleagues measured pelvic floor function in 31 women with

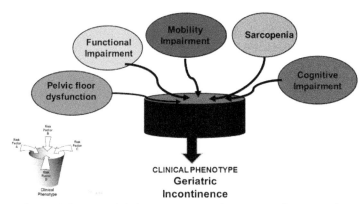

Fig. 4. Cumulative deficit model defining important factors contributing to the presence of the geriatric incontinence syndrome phenotype of UI.

SUI and 35 controls with vaginal surface EMG during 3 rapid contractions in both the sitting and standing positions. They found significantly lower amplitudes of contraction in both positions among patients with SUI compared with those who did not have SUI (17 microV sitting and 12 microV standing for SUI versus 19.5 microV sitting and 18.2 microV standing in the control patients, P = .006). Electromyography signal is age-dependent and associated with neuronal and muscle loss. In a study of female cadavers (average age of 47 years ranging from 15 to 78 years), sagittal specimens were obtained and stained from 13 cadaveric urethras. Results showed that nerve density decreased with advancing age (P = .004) and the decreased nerve density within the striated sphincter correlated with a decrease in muscle cells (P = .02) (14). As urethral strength is an important factor in the continence mechanism, understanding potential causes of compromised urethral function is necessary for future research.

The decrease in ovarian estrogen production during the menopausal transition results in a significant decline in systemic estrogen. The genitourinary syndrome of menopause is a persistent consequence of menopause that results in anatomic and physiologic changes in the urethra, bladder, and vagina. Unlike the vasomotor symptoms that may be transient, the postmenopausal period may in turn result in worsening of urethral function over time, contributing to the development of geriatric incontinence syndrome. The female urethra and vagina share embryologic origin, with estrogen-sensitive stratified squamous epithelium within the mucosa. With the loss of systemic estrogen, decreased urethral closure (coaptation) contributes to symptoms of urinary urgency, urge incontinence, or stress UI. Intravaginal replacement of estrogen via cream or ring can decrease UI episodes by 65% to 75%[29]; by way of improving urethral vascular flow,[30] and urethral coaptation with decreased urinary urgency symptoms.[28,31]

Physical Function Impairments are Common Among Older Women with Urinary Incontinence

Up to 62% of older incontinent women will have disability and difficulty with completing activities of daily living and a 3-fold high risk of losing their independence.[32] We examined a large cohort of healthy women older than 70 years, without baseline physical function impairments or UI. As these women aged over 4 years, those who developed UI symptoms were more likely to experience a concomitant decline in physical performance specifically with functional decline in standing balance. There was also a greater increase in concomitant development of clinically significant skeletal muscle weakness and declining skeletal muscle mass that may indicate the onset of sarcopenia.[33] Women with UI at baseline also demonstrated a more significant decline in physical performance compared with their continent peers. These data suggest that as women develop UI after the age of 70 years, they have weakened skeletal muscle function leading to physical function impairments and poor balance. These findings may explain the tightly observed associations between mobility impairment, falls, and UI symptoms.

Sarcopenia is an Understudied but Biologically Plausible Contributor to the Geriatric Incontinence Syndrome

Sarcopenia is a progressive and generalized skeletal muscle disorder that may result in loss of muscle mass, strength, and function. Although it has been previously associated with other geriatric syndromes to include falls and physical disability, we were the first to describe its association with UI.[34] Erdogan and colleagues examined a cross-section of women older than 60 years with UI and evaluated the prevalence of sarcopenia determined by bioimpedance analysis. They observed that 49% of their cohort had UI symptoms and that sarcopenia was independently associated with UI symptoms after adjusting for BMI and muscle mass.[35]

Mobility Impairment is Associated with Urinary Incontinence in Older Women

Mobility impairment has also been an important factor that may be present because of common changes in skeletal muscle health with aging. Mobility impairment featuring lower extremity weakness has a 2-fold higher prevalence among women with UI symptoms and with a history of falling.[32,36] Omae and colleagues observed a significant association with gait speed and a higher likelihood of having urinary urgency and urge incontinence in a cross-sectional analysis. Fritel also examined a large cohort of women older than 75 years to explore the association between functional limitations related to mobility and UI. They observed significant associations between balance and gait impairments among those with urgency UI symptoms.

Cognitive Impairment is Understudied but Presents Concomitantly Among Older Incontinence Women

There is also a 1.4 higher risk of cognitive impairment among older women with UI.[37] The underlying mechanisms that connect UI and cognitive impairment have not been fully elucidated, but may be a consequence of cerebral dysfunction leading to loss of the brain's inhibitory influence over the micturition reflex. There is a paucity of data reporting on the associations of UI and cognitive decline among older adults outside of dementia in institutionalized adults. Among institutionalized adults, UI is a marker of unhealthy aging and is associated with dementia in up to 90% of adults.[38] The combination of dementia and UI creates a significant challenge for caregivers at home and nurses in institutions. Unfortunately, the paucity of data on the relationship between these two conditions significantly limits effective treatments.

FUTURE DIRECTIONS

The geriatric incontinence syndrome represents a refractory UI phenotype, whose etiology is multifactorial and extends beyond the pelvic floor-based etiology of the condition of UI. When present concomitantly with functional or cognitive impairments, mobility disability, or clinically significant weakness, UI transforms from a condition into a geriatric syndrome. It is likely that the geriatric incontinence syndrome is the predominant type of UI that we treat in our clinical practice of older women. Thus, it is imperative that we recognize this reality to prioritize learning more about how these disabilities may affect the care of older women with UI.

UI in older women is heterogeneous. Although common, the development of UI symptoms is not a normal part of aging. Despite evidence of the aforementioned physiologic changes, more than 50% of older women remain continent. In addition, it is not assumed that every older woman with UI will have the geriatric incontinence syndrome. However, for some women, the UI that develops with aging represents a complex syndrome resulting from the cumulative impact of predisposing and inciting events in addition to changes unique to unhealthy aging. Risk factors for developing UI after the age of 65 years include high BMI, functional impairment, impaired mobility, and cognitive impairment or dementia.[9] These risk factors are interdependent and may overlap with other physiologic changes, resulting in a different clinical phenotype of UI, unique to aging women, previosly defined as a geriatric syndrome. It is clinically imperative that we better define and distinguish the geriatric incontinence syndrome from the condition of UI because of potential negative future consequences associated with the onset of frailty. In fact, it is plausible that this geriatric incontinence syndrome may be an early marker of frailty as it may relate to the severity of risk factors for other geriatric syndromes such as falls.[39]

Current nonsurgical and surgical treatment approaches were developed in younger cohorts but are applied to women of all ages. The average age of women included in the major studies of the effectiveness of standard treatments for incontinence was 55 to 65 years. Therefore, we know very little about how to treat UI specifically for women older than 70 years. Furthermore, we have only explored the surface of how UI in older women may be influenced by known age-related changes in the pelvic floor, urethra, global skeletal muscle, cognition, and overall physical function. These changes may reflect the proposed refractory nature of the geriatric incontinence syndrome phenotype. Robust comparative studies are urgently needed to understand how the presence of this geriatric incontinence syndrome may affect our current approach to treating older incontinence women.

DISCLOSURE

None.

REFERENCES

1. Vespa, J., The U.S. Joins Other Countries With Large Aging Populations 2018.
2. 2017 National Population Projections Tables. 2017 [cited 2020 January 22,]; U.S. Census Bureau data].
3. Capistrant BD. Caregiving for Older Adults and the Caregivers' Health: an Epidemiologic Review. Curr Epidemiol Rep 2016;3(1):72–80.
4. Erekson EA, Cong X, Townsend MK, et al. Ten-Year Prevalence and Incidence of Urinary Incontinence in Older Women: A Longitudinal Analysis of the Health and Retirement Study. J Am Geriatr Soc 2016;64(6):1274–80.
5. Nitti VW. The prevalence of urinary incontinence. Rev Urol 2001;3(Suppl 1): S2–S6.
6. Veronese N, Au fnm, Soysal P, et al. Association between urinary incontinence and frailty: a systematic review and meta-analysis. Eur Geriatr Med 2018;9(5): 571–8.

7. Shaw C, Rajabali S, Tannenbaum C, et al. Is the belief that urinary incontinence is normal for ageing related to older Canadian women's experience of urinary incontinence? Int Urogynecol J 2019;30(12):2157–60.
8. Duralde ER, Walter LC, Van Den Eeden SK, et al. Bridging the gap: determinants of undiagnosed or untreated urinary incontinence in women. Am J Obstet Gynecol 2016;214(2):266.e1-9.
9. Inouye SK, Studenski S, Tinetti ME, et al. Geriatric syndromes: clinical, research, and policy implications of a core geriatric concept. J Am Geriatr Soc 2007;55(5):780–91.
10. DuBeau CE, Kuchel GA, Johnson T, et al. Incontinence in the frail elderly: report from the 4th International Consultation on Incontinence. Neurourol Urodyn 2010;29(1):165–78.
11. Delancey JO, Kane Low L, Miller JM, et al. Graphic integration of causal factors of pelvic floor disorders: an integrated life span model. Am J Obstet Gynecol 2008;199(6):610–5.e1-5.
12. Isali I, Mahran A, Khalifa AO, et al. Gene expression in stress urinary incontinence: a systematic review. Int Urogynecol J 2020;31(1):1–14.
13. Wesnes SL, Hannestad Y, Rortveit G. Delivery parameters, neonatal parameters and incidence of urinary incontinence six months postpartum: a cohort study. Acta Obstet Gynecol Scand 2017;96(10):1214–22.
14. Fultz N, Girts T, Kinchen K, et al. Prevalence, management and impact of urinary incontinence in the workplace. Occup Med (Lond) 2005;55(7):552–7.
15. Tang DH, Colayco DC, Khalaf KM, et al. Impact of urinary incontinence on healthcare resource utilization, health-related quality of life and productivity in patients with overactive bladder. BJU Int 2014;113(3):484–91.
16. Nygaard IE, Shaw JM. Physical activity and the pelvic floor. Am J Obstet Gynecol 2016;214(2):164–71.
17. Da Roza T, Brandão S, Mascarenhas T, et al. Volume of training and the ranking level are associated with the leakage of urine in young female trampolinists. Clin J Sport Med 2015;25(3):270–5.
18. Nygaard I, Girts T, Fultz NH, et al. Is urinary incontinence a barrier to exercise in women? Obstet Gynecol 2005;106(2):307–14.
19. Wagner KH, Cameron-Smith D, Wessner B, et al. Biomarkers of aging: from function to molecular biology. Nutrients 2016;8(6):338.
20. Nygaard I, Barber MD, Burgio KL, et al. Prevalence of symptomatic pelvic floor disorders in US women. JAMA 2008;300(11):1311–6.
21. Al-Mukhtar Othman J, Åkervall S, Milsom I, et al. Urinary incontinence in nulliparous women aged 25-64 years: a national survey. Am J Obstet Gynecol 2017;216(2):149.e1-11.
22. Pfisterer MH, Griffiths DJ, Schaefer W, et al. The effect of age on lower urinary tract function: a study in women. J Am Geriatr Soc 2006;54(3):405–12.
23. Taylor JA 3rd, Kuchel GA. Detrusor underactivity: Clinical features and pathogenesis of an underdiagnosed geriatric condition. J Am Geriatr Soc 2006;54(12):1920–32.
24. Yang JM, Yang SH, Huang WC. Functional correlates of Doppler flow study of the female urethral vasculature. Ultrasound Obstet Gynecol 2006;28(1):96–102.
25. Siracusano S, Bertolotto M, Cucchi A, et al. Application of ultrasound contrast agents for the characterization of female urethral vascularization in healthy pre- and postmenopausal volunteers: preliminary report. Eur Urol 2006;50(6):1316–22.

26. Trowbridge ER, Wei JT, Fenner DE, et al. Effects of aging on lower urinary tract and pelvic floor function in nulliparous women. Obstet Gynecol 2007;*109*(3): *715*–20.

27. Clobes A, DeLancey JO, Morgan DM. Urethral circular smooth muscle in young and old women. Am J Obstet Gynecol 2008;*198*(5):*587*.e1-5.

28. Bhatia NN, Bergman A, Karram MM. Effects of estrogen on urethral function in women with urinary incontinence. Am J Obstet Gynecol 1989;*160*(1):*176*–81.

29. Fantl JA, Cardozo L, McClish DK. Estrogen therapy in the management of urinary incontinence in postmenopausal women: a meta-analysis. First report of the Hormones and Urogenital Therapy Committee. Obstet Gynecol 1994;*83*(1):*12*–8.

30. Marsh AP, Miller ME, Saikin AM, et al. Lower extremity strength and power are associated with 400-meter walk time in older adults: The InCHIANTI study. J Gerontol A Biol Sci Med Sci 2006;*61*(11):*1186*–93.

31. Krause MP, Albert SM, Elsangedy HM, et al. Urinary incontinence and waist circumference in older women. Age Ageing 2010;*39*(1):*69*–73.

32. Erekson EA, Ciarleglio MM, Hanissian PD, et al. Functional disability and compromised mobility among older women with urinary incontinence. Female Pelvic Med Reconstr Surg 2015;*21*(3):*170*–5.

33. Parker-Autry C, Houston DK, Rushing J, et al. The decline in physical performance and onset of sarcopenia is associated with the development of urinary incontinence in older community dwelling women. Neurourol Urodyn 2016;*35*: *S251*–2.

34. Parker-Autry C, Houston DK, Rushing J, et al. Characterizing the Functional Decline of Older Women With Incident Urinary Incontinence. Obstet Gynecol 2017;*130*(5):*1025*–32.

35. Erdogan T, Bahat G. Incidence of sarcopenia and dynapenia according to stage in patients with idiopathic Parkinson's disease. Neurol Sci 2019;*40*(3):*625*.

36. Greer JA, Xu R, Propert KJ, et al. Urinary incontinence and disability in community-dwelling women: a cross-sectional study. Neurourol Urodyn 2015; *34*(6):*539*–43.

37. Tinetti ME, Inouye SK, Gill TM, et al. Shared risk factors for falls, incontinence, and functional dependence. Unifying the approach to geriatric syndromes. JAMA 1995;*273*(17):*1348*–53.

38. Rose A, Thimme A, Halfar C, et al. Severity of urinary incontinence of nursing home residents correlates with malnutrition, dementia and loss of mobility. Urol Int 2013;*91*(2):*165*–9.

39. Holroyd-Leduc JM, Mehta KM, Covinsky KE. Urinary incontinence and its association with death, nursing home admission, and functional decline. J Am Geriatr Soc 2004;*52*(5):*712*–8.

Neuromodulation

Karen Noblett, MD, MBA*, Carly Crowder, MD

KEYWORDS

- Sacral neuromodulation • Urinary urgency incontinence • Urinary retention
- Fecal incontinence • InterStim • Axonics

KEY POINTS

- Sacral neuromodulation has evolved into a minimally invasive, outpatient procedure for treatment of refractory voiding dysfunction and fecal incontinence with a positive long-term safety profile.
- Advances in SNM technology have resulted in devices that are longer lived (15 years), rechargeable, and MRI safe.
- Features of the newest SNM devices are described and compared in this article.
- Recently published best practices for implant technique and perioperative care have shown higher conversion rates to IPG placement and higher long-term success.

INTRODUCTION

Sacral neuromodulation (SNM) involves placing a quadripolar lead adjacent to a sacral nerve root (typically S3) that is connected to a neurostimulator that delivers nonpainful, electrical pulses to the sacral nerves to modulate the reflexes that influence the bladder, bowels, sphincters, and pelvic floor musculature to improve or restore function (**Fig. 1**).[1–3] Currently approved and available devices in the United States include InterStim II and Micro (Medtronic, Minneapolis, MN, USA) and the Axonics SNM system (Axonics Modulation Technologies Inc, Irvine, CA, USA), which are shown in **Fig. 2**. The features of the 2 newest, rechargeable systems are comparable with regard to size, longevity of implant life of 15 years in the body, magnetic resonance imaging (MRI) conditions for both 1.5 and 3 T, and the use of constant current for stimulation delivery. There are four noticeable differences between the Axonics and Medtronic systems, which include (1) the charge interval, which is approximately 1 hour once a month for Axonics and 1 hour every 2 weeks for the Medtronic Micro (under standard settings of 1–2 mA, 210 pulse width, and rate of 14 Hz); (2) the patient remote, which for the Axonics device does not require recharging or battery change and can be held at arm's length to communicate with the neurostimulator, whereas

Department of Obstetrics & Gynecology, University of California, Irvine, 101 The City Drive South, Orange, CA 92686, USA
* Corresponding author. 26 Technology Drive, Irvine, CA 92618.
E-mail address: knoblett@axonics.com

Obstet Gynecol Clin N Am 48 (2021) 677–688
https://doi.org/10.1016/j.ogc.2021.05.018
0889-8545/21/© 2021 Elsevier Inc. All rights reserved.

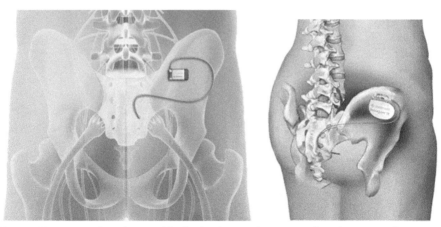

Fig. 1. INS connected to the quadripolar lead at S3. (*Courtesy of* Medtronic, Fridley, MN.)

with the Medtronic system the patient remote comes with 2 components, a Samsung smartphone that is used to change neurostimulator settings and a communicator that needs to be placed over the neurostimulator to allow for communication between the neurostimulator and the Samsung smartphone (both these devices require recharging); (3) the patient programmer for the Medtronic system provides default settings and allows the patient to determine the best program, whereas the Axonics patient programmer uses a proprietary algorithm that takes intraoperative patient information and based on that information suggests the 4 best programs to start with; (4) the Medtronic INS and patient programmer has the capability of providing up to 11 programs for the patient to rotate through, whereas the Axonics system has the capability of providing 2 programs.

SNM is currently approved by the US Food and Drug Administration (FDA) in the United States for urgency incontinence, urinary urgency frequency, nonobstructive urinary retention, and fecal incontinence. The long-term efficacy and safety of the therapy has been well established. Therapeutic response rates ranging from 67% to 82% of patients with urgency incontinence, 57% to 71% with urgency frequency, and 68% to 71% with urinary retention have been reported.[4–8]

SNM is indicated for patients with overactive bladder (OAB) with and without incontinence who fail conservative therapy and/or medical management, including those

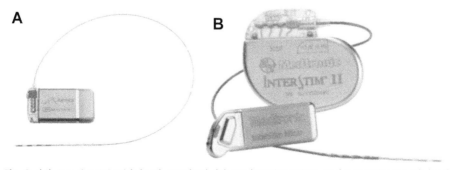

Fig. 2. (*A*) Axonics INS with lead attached. (*B*) Medtronic's Micro and InterStim II with lead attached. (*Courtesy of* Medtronic, Fridley, MN.)

who experience intolerable side effects. SNM is the only viable treatment option other than bladder catheterization for patients with nonobstructive urinary retention (NOUR).[9] Catheterization is uncomfortable and associated with increased risk of bladder infections. SNM has been proved to be an effective alternative to catheterization and has been shown to significantly improve the quality of life for this patient population. Finally, SNM is indicated for fecal incontinence in patients who have failed conservative therapies, even those with anal sphincter defects, and can be ideal in patients who have both urinary and bowel disorders.

The causes of OAB, NOUR, and fecal incontinence are multifactorial and not completely understood. Similarly, the mechanisms through which SNM treats bladder and bowel dysfunction are incompletely delineated. The S3 nerve root is the preferred target for SNM as S3 is the main contributor to pelvic floor innervation.[10] For OAB, SNM most likely functions through both local reflex pathways that influence bladder activity and higher levels in the brain that govern bladder function. Sacral preganglionic outflow to the bladder receives inhibitory input from both somatic and visceral afferents, suggesting that nerves going to the bladder from the sacral nerve roots can be influenced by input from the pudendal nerve before actually affecting the bladder.[11–16] SNM activates these somatic afferents to inhibit detrusor function and improve OAB symptoms. Stimulating the somatic afferent nerves in a sacral spinal root (S3, S4, and/or pudendal) also sends signals to the higher centers in the central nervous system (CNS) that may restore normal communication between the brain and the bladder. Imaging studies indicate that SNM normalizes abnormal brain activity associated with detrusor overactivity.[17] Direct activation of motor neurons innervating the striated urethral sphincter can increase outlet resistance, thus inhibiting bladder reflex activity at the CNS level.[18]

Clinical Care Points

- One of the advantages of SNM is that the patient can undergo a test procedure to determine if the therapy is right for them.
- For surgeons, there is no other existing procedure that offers this advantage. Therapy for SNM is generally completed in 2 phases. In the first phase, a temporary peripheral nerve evaluation (PNE) or tined lead is placed along a sacral nerve root (generally S3) and stimulation with an external pulse generator is conducted for a period of 3 to 14 days.
- Patients who have a 50% or greater improvement in symptoms and are satisfied with the response go on to the second phase wherein a sterile implantable pulse generator (IPG), or implantable neurostimulator (INS), is connected to a tined lead and implanted in the lateral upper buttocks.

Phase 1 Options: Peripheral Nerve Evaluation Versus Tined Lead

Placement of a temporary lead (PNE) is less invasive than placement of a tined lead. A PNE trial can be completed in an office or surgery center and only requires local anesthesia, but monitored anesthesia care is also commonly used. A temporary electrode wire is placed in the S3 foramen with or without fluoroscopic guidance and is generally done bilaterally. A recent randomized clinical trial demonstrated that the outcomes for PNEs performed without fluoroscopy was noninferior to outcomes of those performed with fluoroscopy.[19] The PNE wire is then connected to a temporary, external pulse generator and worn by the patient for 3 to 7 days to evaluate whether the therapy is effective.[20] The PNE is less costly and less invasive to place than a tined lead and does not require a trip to the operating room. However, PNE can be problematic due to lead migration, a shorter trial period, and potentially suboptimal wire placement. If phase 1 results are inconclusive with a PNE lead, another phase 1 trial with a tined lead may be conducted, or the patient may choose to pursue other treatment modalities. If phase 1 results confirm success of the therapy, the PNE lead is replaced with a tined lead in the operating room at the time of the INS implantation.

The second option for phase 1, also called a staged procedure, involves placing a tined lead adjacent to a sacral nerve root under fluoroscopic guidance. Patients are positioned prone in the OR to allow visualization of the S3 nerve responses including great toe dorsiflexion and bellows response. General anesthesia with paralytics and regional anesthesia must be avoided to visualize these responses.[9] The length of the staged lead placement trial is generally 7 to 14 days, and there is no evidence demonstrating benefit of performing a bilateral over a unilateral tined lead trial.[21]

PNE versus a staged trial was evaluated in a prospective trial by Borawski and colleagues.[22] This study showed a significantly increased progression to implant placement with staged procedure versus PNE (88% vs 46%, $P<.02$). Banakhar and Hassouna[23] evaluated the sensitivity, specificity, and predictive values for a staged implant versus PNE. For PNE positive and negative predictive values were 99% and 82.1%, and for staged test they were 90% and 92.9%, respectively.[23,24] This study demonstrated that PNE has a high positive predictive value, which in conjunction with the potential of a simple office-based procedure may be preferable for certain patients. Although the staged procedure may be more costly and requires 2 OR visits, it has the advantage of higher conversion rate to implant and potential for a longer trial period. The decision for PNE versus staged procedure should be individualized for each patient and practice model. Preoperatively, patients should be counseled regarding procedural risks including infection, implant site or leg pain, and potential need for revision or reprogramming.[9]

Placement of Tined Lead and Implantable Pulse Generator or Implantable Neurostimulator

After identification of the bony landmarks, a 3.5- or 5-inch foramen needle is placed such that it is parallel to the medial border of the foramen on the anteroposterior (AP) image and 1 cm above and parallel to the fusion plate on the lateral image (**Fig. 3**). The needle is only advanced to the anterior surface of the sacrum where the stimulation threshold is tested and considered acceptable if 2 mA or less.[9] Once proper response is confirmed, the lead introducer is placed over a directional guide and advanced such that the radiopaque marker is approximately halfway through the bony plate (**Fig. 4**); this can be done under live fluoroscopy or with incremental advancement. Care should be taken not to advance the introducer too deep because this may create a false path for the lead to follow. It is recommended to use the curved stylet when introducing the lead so that it is able to follow the natural path of the nerve. Use of the curved stylet has been shown to have overall less amplitude requirements and is associated with better long-term outcomes when compared with the straight stylet.[25,26] The quadripolar lead, which is self-anchored via deployable tines, is then placed such that ideal motor responses are achieved on all 4 electrodes (**Table 1**). Achieving bellows response before toe flexion at 2 mA or less on all 4 electrodes is considered ideal.[9]

Routine use of intraoperative fluoroscopy is recommended for tined lead positioning to optimize lead placement. Both AP and lateral fluoroscopy views should be used to assess needle and final tined lead wire placement. The ideal lead placement in the AP view is shown with the trajectory of the lead curving out from medial to lateral, and on the lateral view, having a gentle curvature from cephalad to caudad (**Fig. 5**).

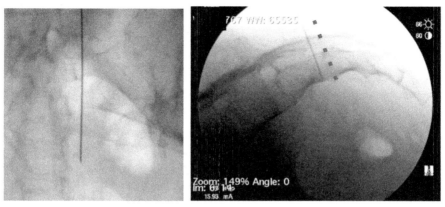

Fig. 3. Ideal needle placement in AP (*left*) and lateral (*right*) views. In the AP view a needle is placed parallel and along the medial border of the foramen. In the lateral view the needle is parallel to the fusion plate of S3 (*red-dotted line*) and is approximately 1 cm above and sitting just at the anterior surface of the sacrum.

Best practices recommend perioperative antibiotics given within 60 minutes of skin incision to be targeted to local skin flora and based on the combination of local hospital antibiogram along with patient's allergies.[9] A large retrospective cohort analysis of sacral nerve stimulation procedures noted a significant reduction in surgical site infections (from 7% to 1.7%) after the implementation of a chlorhexidine wash the night before and the morning of the procedure. In addition, 82% of devices that were explanted as a result of an infection were noted to be colonized with methicillin-resistant *Staphylococcus aureus*, which may influence the selection of prophylactic postoperative antibiotics.[27]

The IPG or INS is typically placed in the lateral upper buttocks in the hollow of the ilium and generally no deeper than 2 cm. Fluoroscopy can assist in appropriate placement of the implantable system to reduce the risk of patient discomfort (**Fig. 6**). Documentation of radiological views of the final tined lead location in both lateral and AP positions, motor and sensory responses achieved, and required stimulus amplitude may aid in trouble-shooting device malfunction in the future.

Surgical techniques for implantation of SNM systems have evolved over time; the International Continence Society has published on best practices for implant

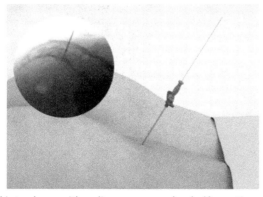

Fig. 4. Passing lead introducer with radio-opaque marker half-way through the sacral plate. (Used with permission of Axonics, Inc.)

Table 1
Sacral nerve sensory and motor responses

	Sensory Response	Motor Response	
		Pelvic Floor	Leg/Foot
S2	Generally none, or may have a sensation in the buttocks	Potential clamp response (anterior to posterior contraction of the perineal structures: a clamplike contraction of the anal sphincter, and in males, a retraction of the penis base)	Rotation of the leg/hip rotation, rotation of the heel, calf contraction
S3*	Pulling in rectum, extending forward to scrotum or labia	Bellows (flattening and deepening of the buttock groove due to lifting and dropping of the pelvic floor)	Flexing great toe, occasional flexing of other toes
S4	Pulling in rectum	Bellows	None

technique.[9] Recent studies in which the new best practices techniques have been adopted have shown higher conversion rates to IPG placement and higher longer-term success rates.[28–30]

EVIDENCE FOR NEUROMODULATION
Bladder

The InSite Trial evaluated the efficacy and safety of Medtronic InterStim SNM with a staged trial for the treatment of urinary urgency incontinence and urinary frequency. A total of 340 subjects were initially included and underwent stimulation testing in this postmarket, multicenter prospective trial. Of these, 272 (80%) had a 50% or greater improvement in symptoms and had an IPG implanted. These responders were followed out to 5 years. The therapeutic success rate was 82% in those available for follow-up and 67% assuming those not available for follow-up were treatment failures. Participants showed improvement in all quality-of-life measurements (ICIQ-OABqol [International Consultation on Incontinence Questionnaire Overactive Bladder] measures), which was sustained over time.[31] The overall safety profile was

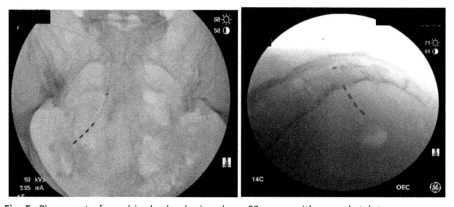

Fig. 5. Placement of quadripolar lead wire along S3 nerve with curved stylet.

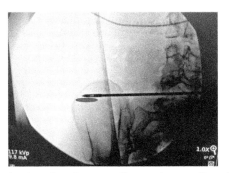 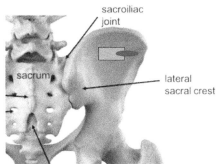

Fig. 6. Using the tunneling tool to confirm the location of the IPG/INS placement. Ideally this is in the hollow of the ilium, approximately 4 cm below the posterior iliac crest.

favorable with only one serious device-related adverse event (AE). Most frequent device-related AEs were undesirable change in stimulation (12%, 32 of 272); implant site pain (7%, 20 of 272); and implant site infection (3%, 9 of 272). Of the 26 events of implant site pain, 13 (50%) required surgical intervention, with only 2 (7.7%) resulting in explant. Ten subjects experienced a surgical site infection, 8 of whom required explantation. The overall surgical intervention rate was 13% with the most common reasons being pain at the surgical site (4%), lack or loss of efficacy (4%), and infection (3%).

The RELAX-OAB study published in 2018 was the first evaluating the new rechargeable SNM system (Axonics r-SNM System). A single-stage implant procedure was completed in 51 patients with OAB. Subjects were followed for 3 months using bladder diaries and quality of life questionnaires.[30] There were 34 patients who responded to an initial test period. At 3-month follow up, 31 of 34 (91%) patients were therapy responders with at least a 50% reduction in urinary voids or incontinence episodes, and these results were maintained out to 1 and 2 years with a continued success rate of 90% in the test responders and a reported satisfaction with therapy by 93% of subjects.[32,33]

The ARTISAN-SNM (Axonics Sacral Neuromodulation System for Urinary Urgency Incontinence Treatment) study was a single-arm, prospective, multicenter, pivotal study evaluating the safety and efficacy of the Axonics System for the treatment of symptoms of urgency urinary incontinence with the primary end point reported at 6-month follow-up study.[28] This study included 129 patients, each implanted with a tined lead and rechargeable SNM system in a nonstaged procedure. Responders were identified as those with at least a 50% improvement from baseline urinary urgency incontinence episodes before treatment initiation at 1 month. At 6-month follow-up, 116 of 129 (90%) were responders with a significant reduction in urinary urgency incontinence episodes from 5.6 to 1.3. The 1- and 2-year results have been published in which 89% and 88% of all implanted participants were responders, respectively.[34,35] These results reflect an as-treated analysis where all subjects were included in the results. When looking at the completers (those available for follow-up) analysis (n = 121) at 2 years, 93% were responders and 82% had a 75% or greater reduction in symptoms. All participants were able to recharge their device at 2 years, and 94% reported that the duration and frequency of recharging was acceptable. There were no serious device-related AEs at 2 years.

Data on the safety and efficacy of the Medtronic Micro are not currently publicly available.

EVIDENCE FOR NEUROMODULATION—BOWEL

SNM has been approved for fecal incontinence since 1994 in Europe and gained FDA approval in the United States in 2011. In 2008, a randomized controlled trial (RCT) using Medtronic InterStim evaluated the efficacy of SNM versus standard medical therapy in patients with severe fecal incontinence. Mean incontinence episodes decreased from 9.5 to 3.1 in the SNM group without any significant improvement in fecal continence in the medical therapy group.[36] Complete continence was achieved in 47.2% of patients. Significant improvement in quality-of-life metrics were observed in the SNM group, whereas the medical therapy group saw no significant improvement in quality-of-life metrics.

In 2010, the safety and efficacy of the InterStim SNM system was evaluated for the indication of fecal incontinence.[37] This prospective, single-arm study enrolled 133 patients to undergo test stimulation. Ninety percent (120 of 133) of subjects ultimately received the SNM implant. At 1-year follow-up, 83% of patients had greater than 50% reduction in incontinence episodes per week compared with baseline. A 5-year follow-up study was completed that showed sustained benefit.[38,39] While the combined device revision, explant, or replacement rate was 35.5%, the morbidity and recurrence rate of alternative therapies and surgical treatment of fecal incontinence is also high.[40]

Initially, SNM was thought not to be applicable to patients with an anatomic sphincter defect, but multiple studies have demonstrated efficacy in patients with sphincter defects up to 180°, and the therapy is currently approved for sphincter defects up to 120°.[37,41–43] SNM effectiveness was prospectively evaluated in patients with and without external anal sphincter defects and found to result in similar effectiveness defined by quality-of-life scores and functional outcomes between groups, further supporting use of SNM in patients with sphincter defects.[44] In 2012, a systematic review of the literature was completed to evaluate the clinical efficacy of SNM for fecal incontinence with the presence of a sphincter defect. Ten studies were included in the review and included 119 patients. The weighted average number of incontinence episodes decreased from 12.1 to 2.3 per week, and the Cleveland Clinic Score decreased from 16.5 to 3.8 after SNM implantation.[45] Efficacy of sphincteroplasty versus SNM in patients with anal sphincter lesions has also been prospectively evaluated with no significant difference in clinical or anorectal manometry parameters posttreatment, thus further supporting SNM as a reasonable approach to fecal incontinence with sphincter lesions.[46–51]

Advances in Therapy: MRI Labeling

Prior versions were not MRI compatible, whereas all 3 currently available SNM devices (Axonics, Medtronic InterStim II, and Medtronic Micro) have 1.5 and 3 T full-body MRI

Table 2					
MRI conditions for the Axonics and Medtronic systems					
1.5 T		Scanner Strength		3 T	
Axonics	Medtronic	Manufacturers		Axonics	Medtronic
2.0	2.0	SAR Limit (W/kg)		1.2	1.4
Not specified	4.0	B1 + rms Limit (µT)		1.7	2.0
30 min	30 min	Allowed Continuous Scan Time		30 min	30 min
5 min	5 min	Wait Time		5 min	5 min

Abbreviation: rms, root mean square.
  Used with permission of Axonics, Inc.

conditional labeling. There are 3 MRI labeling categories: MRI safe (like a Foley catheter), MRI conditionally safe (where conditions need to be met to complete the scan), and MRI unsafe (not approved). A comparison of the Axonics system versus the Medtronic systems conditions is summarized in **Table 2**. As outlined in the chart, both systems are comparable to their MRI conditional labeling.

SUMMARY

SNM provides efficacious treatment of refractory voiding dysfunction and fecal incontinence with a positive long-term safety profile. Although physician and patient uptake of this therapy has been limited historically, recent innovations with longer-lived, rechargeable devices that are MRI safe and provide constant current stimulation may break down some of the traditional barriers to adopting this therapy. Work is ongoing to evaluate the impact of this technology on other pelvic floor disorders, such as bladder pain syndrome, constipation, and neurogenic voiding dysfunction.

DISCLOSURE

K. Noblett: Chief Medical Officer, Axonics Modulation Technologies. C. Crowder: no affiliations or disclosures.

REFERENCES

1. Spinelli M, Sievert KD. Latest technologic and surgical developments in using InterStim Therapy for sacral neuromodulation: impact on treatment success and safety. Eur Urol 2008;54(6):1287–96.
2. Cameron AP, Anger JT, Madison R, et al. Urologic Diseases in America Project. Battery explantation after sacral neuromodulation in the Medicare population. Neurourol Urodyn 2013;32(3):238–41.
3. American Urological Association Guideline: diagnosis and treatment of overactive bladder 9Non-neurogenci) in Adults. 2014. Available at: https://sufuorg.com/docs/guidelines/oab-amendment-061014.aspx.
4. Siegel S, Noblett K, Mangel J, et al. Results of a prospective, randomized, multicenter study evaluating sacral neuromodulation with InterStim therapy compared to standard medical therapy at 6-months in subjects with mild symptoms of overactive bladder. Neurourol Urodyn 2015;34(3):224–30.
5. Brazzelli M, Murray A, Fraser C. Efficacy and safety of sacral nerve stimulation for urinary urge incontinence: a systematic review. J Urol 2006;175:835–41.
6. van Kerrebroeck PE, van Voskuilen AC, Heesakkers JP, et al. Results of sacral neuromodulation therapy for urinary voiding dysfunction: outcomes of a prospective, worldwide clinical study. J Urol 2007;178(5):2029–34.
7. Jonas U, Fowler CJ, Chancellor MB, et al. Efficacy of sacral nerve stimulation for urinary retention: results 18 months after implantation. J Urol 2001;165(1):15–9.
8. High RA, Winkelman W, Panza J, et al. Sacral neuromodulation for symptomatic chronic urinary retention in females: do age and comorbidities make a difference? Int Urogynecol J 2020. https://doi.org/10.1007/s00192-020-04485-0.
9. Goldman HB, Lloyd JC, Noblett KL, et al. International Continence Society best practice statement for use of sacral neuromodulation. Neurourol Urodyn 2018;37(5):1823–48.
10. Benson JT. Sacral nerve stimulation results may be improved by electrodiagnostic techniques. Int Urogynecol J Pelvic Floor Dysfunct 2000;11(6):352–7.

11. DeGroat WC, Saum WR. Synaptic transmission in parasympathetic ganglia in the urinary bladder of the cat. J Physiol 1976;256(1):137–58.

12. De Groat WC. Mechanisms underlying recurrent inhibition in the sacral parasympathetic outflow to the urinary bladder. J Physiol 1976;257:503–13.

13. De Groat WC, Ryall RW. The identification and characteristics of sacral parasympathetic preganglionic neurones. J Physiol 1968;196:563–77.

14. De Groat WC, Ryall RW. Recurrent inhibition in sacral parasympathetic pathways to the bladder. J Physiol 1968;196:579–91.

15. DeGroat WC. Inhibition and excitation of sacral parasympathetic neurons by visceral and cutaneous stimuli in the cat. Brain Res 1971;33:499–503.

16. DeGroat WC. Changes in the organization of the micturition reflex pathway of the cat after transection of the spinal cord. Exp Neurol 1981;71:22.

17. Blok BF, Groen J, Bosch JL, et al. Different brain effects during chronic and acute sacral neuromodulation in urge incontinent patients with implanted neurostimulators. BJU Int 2006;98(6):1238–43.

18. Zhang F, Zhao S, Shen B, et al. Neural pathways involved in sacral neuromodulation of reflex bladder activity in cats. Am J Physiol Ren Physiol 2013;304(6):F710–7.

19. Gupta A, Kinman C, Hobson DTG, et al. The impact of fluoroscopy during percutaneous nerve evaluation on subsequent implantation of a sacral neuromodulator among women with pelvic floor disorders: a randomized, noninferiority trial. Neuromodulation 2020. https://doi.org/10.1111/ner.13164.

20. Hassouna MM, Siegel SW, Anyehoult AA, et al. Sacral neuromodulation in the treatment of urgency-frequency symptoms: a multicenter study on efficacy and safety. J Urol 2000;163:1849–54.

21. Wagner L, Alonso S, Le Normand L, et al. Unilateral versus bilateral sacral neuromodulation test in the treatment of refractory idiopathic overactive bladder: a randomized controlled pilot trial. Neurourol Urodyn 2020;39(8):2230–7.

22. Borawski KM, Foster RT, Webster GD, et al. Predicting implantation with a neuromodulator using two different test stimulation techniques: a prospective randomized study in urge incontinent women. Neurourol Urodyn 2007;26(1):14–8.

23. Banakhar M, Hassouna M. Percutaneous nerve evaluation test versus staged test trials for sacral neuromodulation: sensitivity, specificity, and predictive values of each technique. Int Neurourol J 2016;20(3):250–4.

24. Lightner DJ, Wymer K, Sanchez J, et al. Best practice statement on urologic procedures and antimicrobial prophylaxis. J Urol 2020;203(2):351–6.

25. Jacobs SA, Lane FL, Osann KE, et al. Randomized prospective crossover study of interstim lead wire placement with curved versus straight stylet. Neurourol Urodyn 2014;33(5):488–92.

26. Vaganée D, Kessler TM, Van de Borne S, et al. Sacral neuromodulation using the standardized tined lead implantation technique with a curved vs a straight stylet: 2-year clinical outcomes and sensory responses to lead stimulation. BJU Int 2019;123(5A):E7–13.

27. Brueseke T, Livingston B, Warda H, et al. Risk factors for surgical site infection in patients undergoing sacral nerve modulation therapy. Female Pelvic Med Reconstr Surg 2015;21:198–204.

28. McCrery R, Lane F, Benson K, et al. Treatment of urinary urgency incontinence using a rechargeable SNM system: 6-month results of the ARTISAN-SNM Study. J Urol 2020;203(1):185–92.

29. Adelstein SA, Lee W, Gioia K, et al. Outcomes in a contemporary cohort under-going sacral neuromodulation using optimized lead placement technique. Neuro-urol Urodyn 2019;38(6):1595–601.

30. Blok B, Van Kerrebroeck P, de Wachter S, et al. Three-month clinical results with a rechargeable sacral neuromodulation system for the treatment of overactive bladder. Neurourol Urodyn 2018;37(S2):S9–16.

31. Siegel S, Noblett K, Mangel J, et al. Five-year follow-up results of a prospective, multicenter study of patients with overactive bladder treated with sacral neuromo-dulation. J Urol 2018;199(1):229–36.

32. Blok B, Van Kerrebroeck P, de Wachter S, et al. A prospective, multicenter study of a novel, miniaturized rechargeable sacral neuromodulation system: 12-month results from the RELAX-OAB study. Neurourol Urodyn 2019;38(2):689–95.

33. Blok B, Van Kerrebroeck P, de Wachter S, et al. Two-year safety and efficacy out-comes for the treatment of overactive bladder using a long-lived rechargeable sacral neuromodulation system. Neurourol Urodyn 2020;39(4):1108–14.

34. Benson K, McCrery R, Taylor C, et al. One-year outcomes of the ARTISAN-SNM study with the Axonics System for the treatment of urinary urgency incontinence. Neurourol Urodyn 2020;39(5):1482–8.

35. Pezzella A, McCrery R, Lane F, et al. Two-year outcomes of the ARTISAN-SNM study for the treatment of urinary urgency incontinence using the Axonics rechargeable sacral neuromodulation system. Neurourol Urodyn 2021;40(2):714–21.

36. Tjandra JJ, Chan MK, Yeh CH, et al. Sacral nerve stimulation is more effective than optimal medical therapy for severe fecal incontinence: a randomized, controlled study. Dis Colon Rectum 2008;51:494–502.

37. Wexner SD, Coller JA, Devroede G, et al. Sacral nerve stimulation for fecal incon-tinence: results of a 120-patient prospective multicenter study. Ann Surg 2010;251:441–9.

38. Mellgren A, Wexner SD, Coller JA, et al. Long-term efficacy and safety of sacral nerve stimulation for fecal incontinence. Dis Colon Rectum 2011;54:1065–75.

39. Hull T, Giese C, Wexner SD, et al. Long-term durability of sacral nerve stimulation therapy for chronic fecal incontinence. Dis Colon Rectum 2013;56:234–45.

40. Madoff RD, Parker SC, Varma MG, et al. Faecal incontinence in adults. Lancet 2004;364:621–32.

41. Leroi AM, Parc Y, Lehur PA, et al, Study Group. Efficacy of sacral nerve stimula-tion for fecal incontinence: results of a multicenter double-blind crossover study. Ann Surg 2005;242(5):662–9.

42. Hetzer FH, Hahnloser D, Clavien PA, et al. Quality of life and morbidity after per-manent sacral nerve stimulation for fecal incontinence. Arch Surg 2007;142(1):8–13.

43. Chan MK, Tjandra JJ. Sacral nerve stimulation for fecal incontinence: external anal sphincter defect vs. intact anal sphincter. Dis Colon Rectum 2008;51(7):1015–24 [discussion 1024-5].

44. Boyle DJ, Knowles CH, Lunniss PJ, et al. Efficacy of sacral nerve stimulation for fecal incontinence in patients with anal sphincter defects. Dis Colon Rectum 2009;52(7):1234–9.

45. Ratto C, Litta F, Parello A, et al. Sacral nerve stimulation in faecal incontinence associated with an anal sphincter lesion: a systematic review. Colorectal Dis 2012;14(6):e297–304.

46. Ratto C, Litta F, Parello A, et al. Sacral nerve stimulation is a valid approach in fecal incontinence due to sphincter lesions when compared to sphincter repair. Dis Colon Rectum 2010;53(3):264–72.

47. Lempka SF, Johnson MD, Miocinovic S, et al. Current-controlled deep brain stimulation reduces in vivo voltage fluctuations observed during voltage-controlled stimulation. Clin Neurophysiol 2010;121(12):2128–33.

48. Zander HJ, Graham RD, Anaya CJ, et al. Anatomical and technical factors affecting the neural response to epidural spinal cord stimulation. J Neural Eng 2020;17(3):036019.

49. Merrill DR, Bikson M, Jefferys JG. Electrical stimulation of excitable tissue: design of efficacious and safe protocols. J Neurosci Methods 2005;141(2):171–98.

50. Merrill DR, Tresco PA. Impedance characterization of microarray recording electrodes in vitro. IEEE Trans Biomed Eng 2005;52(11):1960–5.

51. Gill G, Gustafson K. Effects of Tissue impedance on neural activation using "constant-current" versus "constant-voltage" neuromodulation – benchtop study. Poster Presentation. SUFU Miami, FL, February 28 - March 2, 2019.

Moving?

Make sure your subscription moves with you!

To notify us of your new address, find your **Clinics Account Number** (located on your mailing label above your name), and contact customer service at:

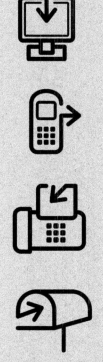

Email: journalscustomerservice-usa@elsevier.com

800-654-2452 (subscribers in the U.S. & Canada)
314-447-8871 (subscribers outside of the U.S. & Canada)

Fax number: 314-447-8029

Elsevier Health Sciences Division
Subscription Customer Service
3251 Riverport Lane
Maryland Heights, MO 63043

*To ensure uninterrupted delivery of your subscription,
please notify us at least 4 weeks in advance of move.

ELSEVIER